Recent Advances in

Histopathology 26

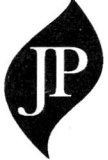

Recent Advances in

Histopathology 26

Fred T Bosman MD PhD
Emeritus Professor of Pathology
Institute of Pathology
University of Lausanne Medical Center
Lausanne, Switzerland

Ivan Damjanov MD PhD
Emeritus Professor
Department of Pathology and Laboratory Medicine
The University of Kansas School of Medicine
Kansas City, Kansas, USA

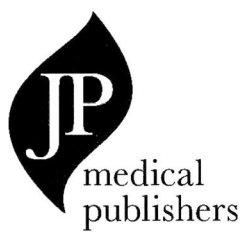

JP
medical
publishers

London • New Delhi

© 2024 Jaypee Brothers Medical Publishers

Published by Jaypee Brothers Medical Publishers,
4838/24 Ansari Road, New Delhi, India

Tel: +91 (011) 43574357   Fax: +91 (011)43574390

Email: info@jpmedpub.com, jaypee@jaypeebrothers.com
Web: www.jpmedpub.com, www.jaypeebrothers.com

JPM is the imprint of Jaypee Brothers Medical Publishers.

The rights of Fred T Bosman and Ivan Damjanov to be identified as the editors of this work have been asserted by them in accordance with the Copyright, Designs and Patents Act 1988.

All brand names and product names used in this book are trade names, service marks, trademarks or registered trademarks of their respective owners. The publisher is not associated with any product or vendor mentioned in this book.

Medical knowledge and practice change constantly. This book is designed to provide accurate, authoritative information about the subject matter in question. However readers are advised to check the most current information available on procedures included and check information from the manufacturer of each product to be administered, to verify the recommended dose, formula, method and duration of administration, adverse effects and contraindications. It is the responsibility of the practitioner to take all appropriate safety precautions. Neither the publisher nor the authors assume any liability for any injury and/or damage to persons or property arising from or related to use of material in this book.

This book is sold on the understanding that the publisher is not engaged in providing professional medical services. If such advice or services are required, the services of a competent medical professional should be sought.

ISBN: 978-1-78779-178-7

British Library Cataloguing in Publication Data
A catalogue record for this book is available from the British Library

Library of Congress Cataloging in Publication Data
A catalog record for this book is available from the Library of Congress

Publishing Manager: Nikita Chauhan

Editorial Assistant: Keshav Kumar

Cover Design: Seema Dogra

Printed in India at Sterling Graphics Pvt. Ltd.

Preface

Two years ago, Mr Jitendar P Vij, the publisher and owner of Jaypee Brothers Medical Publishers (P) Ltd. of New Delhi and London, asked us to help him restart the publication of the venerated British Annual Recent Advances in Histopathology (RAH) which has ceased appearing in print with its volume 24 in 2016. We accepted that challenge, formed an International Editorial Board, developed a publishing plan, solicited articles from all over the world and thus published the first volume of this "new but old series". It was numbered as volume 25 to emphasise the continuity with its predecessors.

We were encouraged by the positive response of our colleagues to volume 25 published in 2022 and decided to continue along the guidelines used while assembling the contributions to the inaugural issue of the new series. Some of the features planned for volume 25 could not materialise, for a number of reasons, but we hope that this issue of RAH will feature many of those and make the series even more attractive. This is yet another reason we are continuing our editorial efforts on RAH.

Some of these novelties will include an interactive website to enable us to correspond online with our readers. Furthermore, we are planning to solicit from our readers their comments and their own contributions, e.g. short case reports from their own pathology practice, or microphotographs from their own histopathology material. We will also publish online material for continuing medical education, such as multiple-choice questions followed by short answers, and additional pictorial material aimed at pathologists either in training or in hospital and university practice. We will be also soliciting ideas for group discussions and possible research projects.

In the volume 26 of RAH, we are presenting a collection of chapters exemplifying the rapid evolution of our discipline. One might think that after 150 years of evolution of histopathology, morphology might no longer provide new impulses to developing 21st century pathology. Not so! Diagnostic modalities change, new therapies induce new iatrogenic conditions, and this is followed attentively by the histopathology community, resulting in a continuous flow of new morphological observations. The chapters on drug-related changes in gastrointestinal biopsies, eosinophilic diseases of the gastrointestinal tract, and breast implant-related lymphomas illustrate how careful morphological observation appropriately positioned in a clinical context continues to deliver new insight. In addition, when morphological observations open up multiple pathophysiological options, interpretations may be contested and these generate intense discussions of long duration, as exemplified in the chapter on minimally invasive thyroid neoplasms.

The other major ongoing development in our discipline is molecular genetic unravelling of disease mechanisms. This has become a major factor in the evolution of disease and most notably cancer classification. This is exemplified in the chapters on mesonephric and mesonephric-like carcinomas of the female genital tract, soft-tissue tumours with an epithelioid morphology, molecular biology of gliomas and switch/sucrose non-fermentable (SWI/SNF) complex deletions and NUT carcinomas in cancer pathology. How molecular genetic data impact on cancer classification is outlined in the chapters on papillary renal cell carcinomas and T- and natural killer (NK)-cell lymphomas involving the gastrointestinal tract.

We hope that our readers will profit from the insight provided by our authors and recognised scholars in the field. We continue to solicit comments from our readership. Do not hesitate to send us your reactions by email directly or through the Publisher.

Fred T Bosman
Ivan Damjanov

Editorial board

List of abbreviations

AFP	Alpha-fetoprotein	CNVs	Copy number variations
AH/EIN	Atypical hyperplasia/ endometrial intraepithelial neoplasia	CPIs	Checkpoint inhibitors
		CRINET	Cribriform neuroepithelial tumour
AI	Artificial intelligence	cTCR	Cytoplasmic T-cell receptor
ALCL	Anaplastic large cell lymphoma	CTLA-4	Cytotoxic T lymphocyte antigen 4
ALK	Anaplastic lymphoma kinase	D2-HG	D2-hydroxyglutarate
AMACR	Alpha-methylacyl-CoA racemase	DEC	Dyskeratotic epithelial cells
		DIPG	Diffuse intrinsic pontine gliomas
ARBs	Angiotensin-II receptor blockers	DIS	Dilated intercellular spaces
ASPS	Alveolar soft-part sarcoma	DLBCL	Diffuse large B-cell lymphoma
AT/RT	Atypical teratoid/rhabdoid tumours	DLGNT	Diffuse leptomeningeal glioneuronal tumour
ATP	Adenosine triphosphate	DNET	Dysembryoplastic neuroepithelial tumour
BAS	Bile-acid sequestrants		
BCH	Basal cell hyperplasia	EA	Eosinophil abscess
BET	Bromodomain	EA	Epithelioid angiosarcoma
BIA-ALCL	Breast implant associated anaplastic large cell lymphoma	EATL	Enteropathy-associated T-cell lymphoma
		ECP	Eosinophilic cationic protein
BIA	Breast implant associated	EGFR	Epidermal growth factor receptor
BP	Bisphosphonates		
cCD3	cytoplasmic CD3	EGIDs	Eosinophilic gastrointestinal diseases
ccRCC	Clear cell renal cell carcinoma	EHE	Epithelioid haemangioendothelioma
CCSST	Clear-cell sarcoma of soft tissue		
cIMPACT-NOW	Consortium to Inform Molecular and Practical Approaches to CNS Tumour Taxonomy	ENKTCL	Extranodal NK-/T-cell lymphoma
		EoC	Eosinophilic colitis
		EoD	Eosinophilic duodenitis
CIMP	CpG island methylator phenotypes	EoG	Eosinophilic gastritis
		EoI	Eosinophilic ileitis
CLL	Chronic lymphocytic leukaemia	EoJ	Eosinophilic jejunitis
		EoN	Eosinophilic enteritis
CMV	Cytomegalovirus	EoO	Eosinophilic oesophagitis
CNS	Central nervous system		

EoOHSS	Eosinophilic oesophagitis histologic scoring system
EPO	Eosinophil peroxidase
ERDF	European Regional Development Fund
ES	Epithelioid sarcoma
ESES	European Society of Endocrine Surgeons
ESL	Eosinophil surface layering
ESRD	End-stage renal disease
EZH2	Enhancer of zeste homolog-2
FATWO	Female adnexal tumour of probable Wolffian origin
FCT	Foundation for Science and Technology
FGP	Fundic gland polyps
FIGO	International Federation of Gynaecology and Obstetrics
FNA	Fine-needle aspiration
FNCLCC	Fédération Nationale des Centres de Lutte Contre le Cancer
FN	Field number
FT-UMP	Follicular tumour of uncertain malignant potential
FTC	Follicular thyroid carcinomas
FVPTC	Follicular variant of papillary thyroid carcinoma
GAVE	Gastric antral vascular ectasia
GFAP	Glial fibrillary acidic protein
GI	Gastrointestinal
GMS	Gömöri methenamine silver
GNT-KinF-A	Glioneuronal tumour kinase-fused
GORD	Gastro-oesophageal reflux disease
GSCs	Glioma stem cells
GvHD	Graft-versus-host disease
H&E	Haematoxylin and eosin

HAIC	Hepatic arterial infusion chemotherapy
HHV-8	Human herpesvirus-8
HIF-1α	Hypoxia-inducible factor-1 alpha
HNF-1β	Hepatocyte nuclear factor-1-beta
HPFs	High-power fields
HPRC	Hereditary papillary renal carcinoma syndrome
SEF-LGFMS	Sclerosing epithelioid fibrosarcoma-low-grade fibromyxoid sarcoma
IBD	Inflammatory bowel disease
IDH	Isocitrate dehydrogenase
IDHmut	*IDH*-mutant
IDHwt	*IDH*-wildtype
IELs	Intraepithelial lymphocytes
IHC	Immunohistochemistry
IL-10	Interleukin-10
irAE	Immune-related adverse events
ISCIII	Instituto de Salud Carlos III
LAD	Lymphadenopathy
LBCL	Large B-cell lymphoma
LC	Lanthanum carbonate
LGFMS	Low-grade fibromyxoid sarcoma
LOH	Loss of heterozygosity
LPD	Lymphoproliferative disorder
LPF	Lamina propria fibrosis
MBP	Major basic protein
MCC	Microcrystalline cellulose
MC	Microscopic colitis
MEITL	Monomorphic epitheliotropic intestinal T-cell lymphoma
MGMT	O^6-methylguanine-DNA-methyltransferase
MI-FTC	Minimally invasive follicular thyroid carcinoma
MLA	Mesonephric-like adenocarcinoma

MMF	Mycophenolate mofetil	PPIs	Proton-pump inhibitors
MPA	Mycophenolic acid	PRCC	Papillary renal cell carcinomas
MSS	Microsatellite stable		
MVP	Microvascular proliferation	PRNRP	Papillary renal neoplasm with reverse polarity
NEC	Not Elsewhere Classified		
NF	Nuclear factor	PR	Progesterone receptors
NGS	Next generation sequencing	PTC	Papillary thyroid carcinoma
		PTN	Pleiotrophin
NIFTP	Non-invasive follicular thyroid neoplasm with papillary-like nuclear features	PXA	Pleomorphic xanthoastrocytoma
		RCC	Renal cell carcinomas
		RCD	Refractory coeliac disease
NOS	Not otherwise specified	RMC	Renal medullary carcinoma
NPC	Neural precursor	sALCL	Systemic ALCL
NSAIDs	Non-steroidal anti-inflammatory drugs	SBA	Surface epithelial alteration
		SCCOHT	Small cell carcinoma of the ovary, hypercalcaemic type
NSCLC	Non-small cell lung carcinoma		
NSE	Neuron-specific enolase	SCC	Squamous cell carcinoma
NSHL	Nodular sclerosis Hodgkin lymphoma	SEF	Sclerosing epithelioid fibrosarcoma
NSMP	No specific molecular profile	SEGA	Subependymal giant cell astrocytoma
NST	No special type	SIRT	Selective internal radiation therapy
ODS	Oesophagitis dissecans superficialis		
		SLE	Sprue-like enteropathy
OFMT	Ossifying fibromyxoid tumour	SMA	Smooth muscle actin
		SPS	Sodium polystyrene sulphonate
OPC	Oligodendrocyte-progenitor		
		sTCR	Surface T-cell receptor
OR/ER	Oestrogen receptors	SWI/SNF	Switch/sucrose non-fermenting
OS	Overall survival		
PAS	Periodic acid Schiff reaction	T-LPD	T-cell lymphoproliferative disorder
PC-ALCL	Primary cutaneous ALCL		
PCR	Polymerase chain reaction	t-SNE	t-distributed stochastic neighbour embedding
PD-1	Programmed cell death 1		
PD-L1	Programmed cell death ligand 1	TCGA	The Cancer Genome Atlas
		TCR	T-cell receptor
PDGFRA	Platelet-derived growth factor receptor alpha	TCS	teratocarcinosarcoma
		TGF-β	Transforming growth factor-beta
PGE2	Prostaglandin E-2		
PI3K	Phosphoinositide 3-kinases	TME	Tumour microenvironment
PMC	Pseudomembranous colitis	TMZ	Temozolomide
		TNF	Tumour necrosis factor

TRB	T-cell receptor beta	VEGF	Vascular endothelial growth factor
TRG	T-cell receptor gamma		
UC	Ulcerative colitis	WDT-UMP	Well-differentiated tumour of uncertain malignant potential
UMP	Uncertain malignant potential		
UMP	Uncertain malignant potential	WDT	Well differentiated tumour
		WI-FTC	Widely invasive follicular thyroid carcinoma
US-FDA	United States Food and Drug Administration		
		ZNF	Zinc finger
VEGFR	Vascular endothelial growth factor receptor	α-KG	Alpha-ketoglutarate
		α-KGDDs	Alpha-KG-dependent dioxygenases

Contents

Chapter 1

Pathobiology, morphology and clinical significance of minimally invasive thyroid neoplasms

Paula Soares, José Manuel Cameselle-Teijeiro, Elisabete Teixeira, Antónia Póvoa, João Magalhães, Isabel Amendoeira, Manuel Sobrinho-Simões

INTRODUCTION

In this chapter, we review the concept, histopathology and clinical significance of "minimally invasive thyroid carcinomas". In addition, tumours with uncertain malignant potential (UMP) and non-invasive follicular thyroid neoplasm with papillary-like nuclear

Paula Soares BSc PhD, IPATIMUP—Instituto de Patologia e Imunologia Molecular da Universidade do Porto; Cancer Signaling and Metabolism, i3S—Instituto de Investigação e Inovação em Saúde; Departament of Pathology, Faculdade de Medicina da Universidade do Porto, Porto, Portugal
Email: psoares@ipatimup.pt (for correspondence)

José Manuel Cameselle-Teijeiro MD PhD, Department of Pathology, Clinical University Hospital, Galician Healthcare Service (SERGAS); School of Medicine, University of Santiago de Compostela, Santiago de Compostela, Spain
Email: josemanuel.cameselle@usc.es

Elisabete Teixeira MSc, IPATIMUP—Instituto de Patologia e Imunologia Molecular da Universidade do Porto; Cancer Signaling and Metabolism, i3S—Instituto de Investigação e Inovação em Saúde; Departament of Pathology, Faculdade de Medicina da Universidade do Porto, Porto, Portugal
Email: eteixeira@ipatimup.pt

Antónia Póvoa MD PhD, IPATIMUP—Instituto de Patologia e Imunologia Molecular da Universidade do Porto; Cancer Signaling and Metabolism, i3S—Instituto de Investigação e Inovação em Saúde; Department of General Surgery, Centro Hospitalar de Vila Nova de Gaia/Espinho (CHVNG/E), Vila Nova de Gaia, Portugal
Email: antonia.povoa@chvng.min-saude.pt

João Magalhães MD, IPATIMUP—Instituto de Patologia e Imunologia Molecular da Universidade do Porto; Cancer Signaling and Metabolism, i3S—Instituto de Investigação e Inovação em Saúde; Departament of Pathology, Faculdade de Medicina da Universidade do Porto, Porto, Portugal; Department of Pathology, Centro Hospitalar de São João, Porto, Portugal
Email: jmamag@gmail.com

Isabel Amendoeira MD, IPATIMUP—Instituto de Patologia e Imunologia Molecular da Universidade do Porto; Departament of Pathology, Faculdade de Medicina da Universidade do Porto; Department of Pathology, Centro Hospitalar de São João, Porto, Portugal
Email: iamendoeira@ipatimup.pt

Manuel Sobrinho-Simões MD, PhD, IPATIMUP—Instituto de Patologia e Imunologia Molecular da Universidade do Porto; Cancer Signaling and Metabolism, i3S—Instituto de Investigação e Inovação em Saúde; Departament of Pathology, Faculdade de Medicina da Universidade do Porto, Porto, Portugal
Email: ssimoes@ipatimup.pt

features (NIFTP) are addressed in the context of encapsulated/well circumscribed follicular patterned tumours.

Initially, when the concept of minimally invasive carcinomas was created, it was restricted to follicular thyroid carcinomas (FTC), which were separated into minimally and widely invasive follicular thyroid carcinomas (MI-FTC and WI-FTC, respectively). Once the importance of angioinvasion was recognised, the category of angioinvasive follicular carcinoma was created. This was further subdivided into limited angioinvasive and extensively angioinvasive follicular carcinoma.

Until the second decade of 21st century, the diagnosis of follicular variant of papillary thyroid carcinoma (FVPTC) was made when the nuclear features were those of papillary thyroid carcinoma (PTC), regardless of the growth pattern (encapsulated/well circumscribed or infiltrative), and the presence or absence of invasion signs. More recently, the concept of minimally invasive thyroid carcinomas was expanded towards the inclusion of cases of encapsulated FVPTC in the group of minimally invasive thyroid carcinomas regardless of the nuclear features, as well as oncocytic carcinoma.

IMPORTANCE OF INVASION

The concept of neoplastic invasion in thyroid tumour diagnosis to distinguish follicular thyroid adenomas (follicular adenomas) from follicular carcinomas was introduced by Graham in 1914 [1]. In fact, Graham referred to capsular penetration and/or vascular invasion as major diagnostic features, and these findings were reinforced in subsequent studies in the following 20 years [2] (**Figure 1.1**). The concept of invasion in the diagnosis of follicular tumours was supported in 1929 by Coller [3] and subsequently by Warren [4]. Years later, several studies further expanded the concept to oncocytic (Hürthle cell) carcinoma as another example of invasive follicular patterned thyroid neoplasm [5] (**Figure 1.1**).

Remarkably, the concept of invasion as essential diagnostic parameter was for many years only applied to encapsulated follicular patterned tumours, without recognising the importance of invasion in papillary thyroid carcinomas (PTC). By definition, these have papillary or mixed papillary-follicular architecture and lack encapsulation. Other more recent concepts are minimal invasion, in terms of its identification and definition of the degree of invasion, and the most recent subdivision of angioinvasion (invasion of blood vessels) into limited and extensive vascular invasion [6].

The focus on cancer features that substantiate the diagnostic and prognostic meaning of invasion by thyroid neoplastic cells joins together pathogenesis and diagnosis, in view of the notion that the most important characteristic of any malignant neoplasm is invasiveness, e.g. growth that does not respect tissue frontiers. Evaluation of the presence and degree of invasion in encapsulated/well-circumscribed tumours is crucial to understand the biology of follicular patterned thyroid neoplasms and to classify these lesions by separating the group of low-risk neoplasms, which includes NIFTP, follicular tumour of uncertain malignant potential (FT-UMP) and well-differentiated tumour of uncertain malignant potential (WDT-UMP), from minimally invasive thyroid neoplasms. When adequate and reproducible histopathological guidelines are generally used, this provides relevant information regarding prognosis and treatment. Regarding thyroid tumours, invasion needs to be specified according to site: into the capsule of the tumour, into the peritumoural thyroid parenchyma, and into lymphatic vessels and blood vessels.

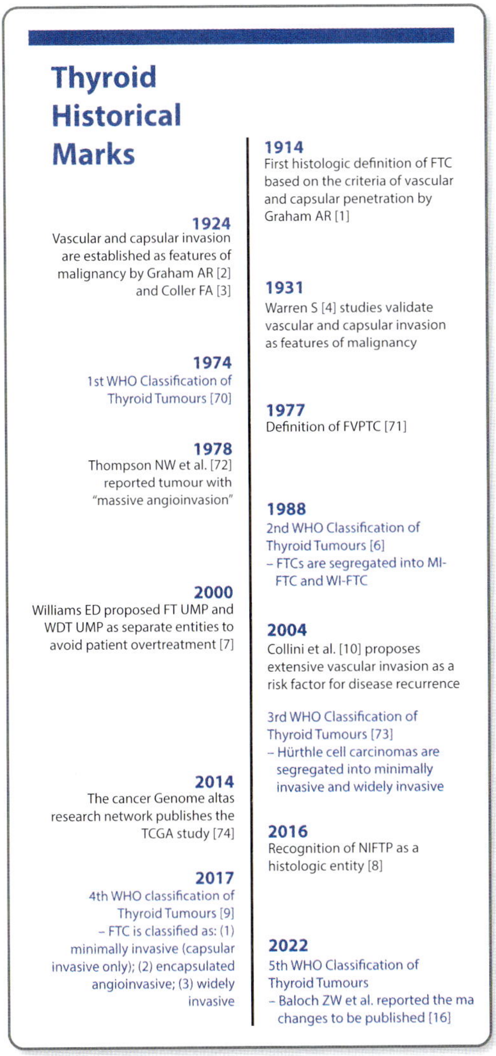

Figure 1.1 Timeline of most relevant thyroid historical marks. This timeline was built based on the following studies [1–10,16,70–75].

FT, follicular tumour; FTC, follicular thyroid carcinoma; FVPTC, follicular variant of papillary thyroid carcinoma; MI-FTC, minimally invasive follicular thyroid carcinoma; NIFTP, non-invasive follicular thyroid neoplasms with papillary-like nuclear features; TCGA, The Cancer Genome Atlas; UMP, uncertain malignant potential; WDT, well-differentiated tumour; WI-FTC, widely invasive follicular thyroid carcinoma

Thyroid Historical Marks

1914
First histologic definition of FTC based on the criteria of vascular and capsular penetration by Graham AR [1]

1924
Vascular and capsular invasion are established as features of malignancy by Graham AR [2] and Coller FA [3]

1931
Warren S [4] studies validate vascular and capsular invasion as features of malignancy

1974
1st WHO Classification of Thyroid Tumours [70]

1977
Definition of FVPTC [71]

1978
Thompson NW et al. [72] reported tumour with "massive angioinvasion"

1988
2nd WHO Classification of Thyroid Tumours [6]
– FTCs are segregated into MI-FTC and WI-FTC

2000
Williams ED proposed FT UMP and WDT UMP as separate entities to avoid patient overtreatment [7]

2004
Collini et al. [10] proposes extensive vascular invasion as a risk factor for disease recurrence

3rd WHO Classification of Thyroid Tumours [73]
– Hürthle cell carcinomas are segregated into minimally invasive and widely invasive

2014
The cancer Genome altas research network publishes the TCGA study [74]

2016
Recognition of NIFTP as a histologic entity [8]

2017
4th WHO classification of Thyroid Tumours [9]
– FTC is classified as: (1) minimally invasive (capsular invasive only); (2) encapsulated angioinvasive; (3) widely invasive

2022
5th WHO Classification of Thyroid Tumours
– Baloch ZW et al. reported the ma changes to be published [16]

In practice, a frequently encountered problem is the presence of questionable signs of capsular and/or vascular invasion in encapsulated, follicular patterned neoplasm without nuclear features of PTC, which has led to the category of tumours with UMP. This tangentially also addresses the concept of NIFTP [7–9].

Taken together, this approach results in a spectrum of clinicopathological entities of encapsulated tumours, ranging from NIFTP with an (extremely) low risk of malignancy, through the questionably invasive and minimally invasive thyroid neoplasms, to the highly aggressive extensively angioinvasive carcinomas [10]. The relevance of this detailed spectrum is the prognostic significance of the used terminology.

The concepts of widely invasive carcinoma and of any type of extrathyroidal neoplastic invasion are beyond the scope of this chapter. The same applies to invasion of intratumoural blood vessels, which lacks clinical significance [11]. We will, however, briefly address the pathobiology and clinical significance of invasion of lymphatic vessels by classic PTC.

HISTOPATHOLOGY OF FOLLICULAR PATTERNED NEOPLASMS

Histopathology of encapsulated (capsular and/or venous) invasive, follicular-patterned neoplasms

The fourth edition of the WHO thyroid tumour classification highlighted invasiveness rather than nuclear features as a key feature to define the malignant nature and prognosis of well-differentiated follicular cell neoplasms [9]. Accordingly, invasive encapsulated follicular variants of PTC, FTC, and oncocytic carcinoma are subdivided into the following three histopathological subtypes:

1. Minimally invasive (encapsulated tumours showing only capsular invasion)
2. Encapsulated angioinvasive (encapsulated tumours with venous invasion regardless of whether or not there is capsular invasion)
3. Widely invasive (overtly invasive tumours often accompanied by venous invasion).

Tumour capsular invasion is defined as the complete transgression of the thickness of the tumour fibrous capsule, generally accompanied by expansion of the invasive tongue of the tumour in the form of a mushroom or shark fin (**Figure 1.2**) [9,12]. When capsular invasion does not affect the entire thickness of the capsule, additional sections are necessary to confirm (or exclude) capsular invasion. When one or more tumour nodules adjacent to the capsule of a tumour are observed, sharing a similar microscopic appearance, it is also necessary to perform additional sections to exclude in-depth continuity between any of the nodules and the main tumour, which would provide evidence of capsular invasion [9,12].

Of note, often tumour capsular invasion actually represents capsular-vascular invasion (**Figure 1.3**). Capsular invasion usually occurs in areas of lesser resistance of the tumour capsule, at the point of penetration of the vein that drains the tumour. The cleavage plane between the tumour capsule and the venous wall constitutes an area prone to tumour herniation akin to capsular invasion, and facilitates tumour venous invasion (**Figure 1.4**). In contrast, spread via lymphatic vessels to regional lymph nodes is a very common

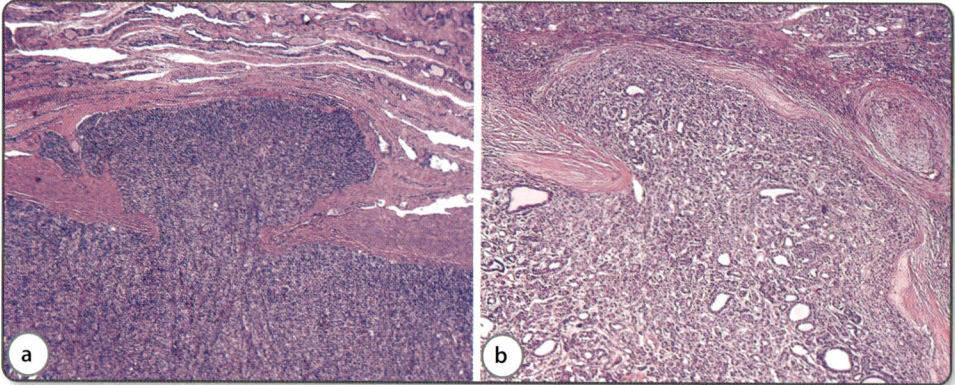

Figure 1.2 Minimally invasive follicular thyroid carcinoma (capsular invasion only). In thyroid carcinomas that show only capsular invasion, tumour cells invade the entire thickness of the tumour capsule, often with mushroom-shaped (a) or shark-fin growth (b).

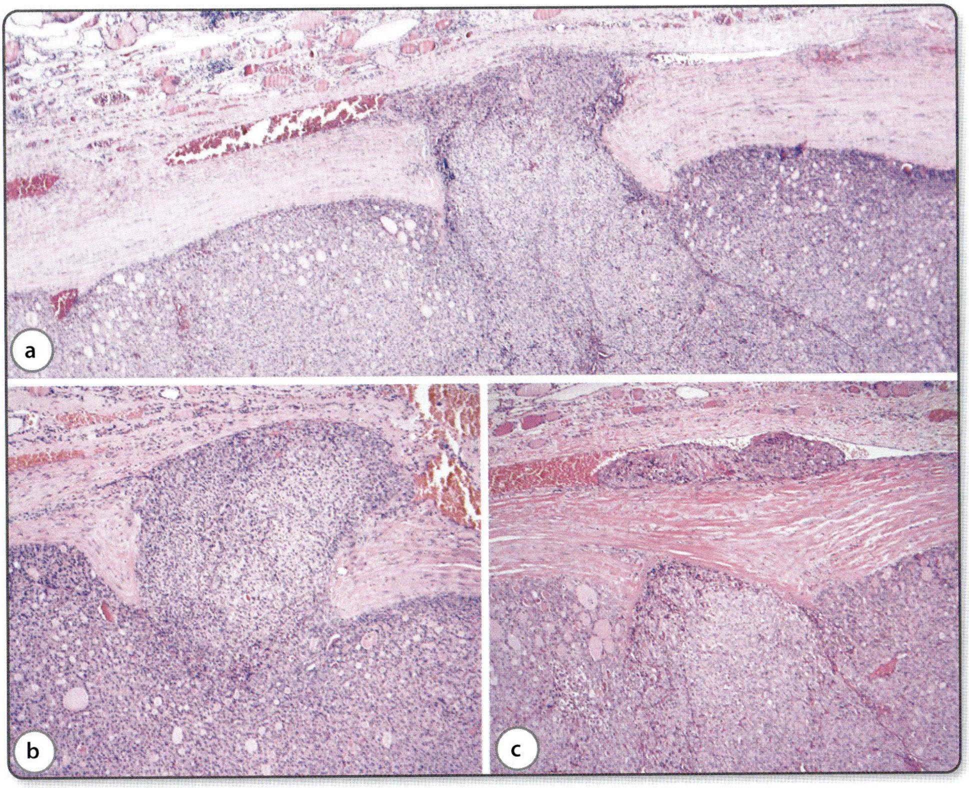

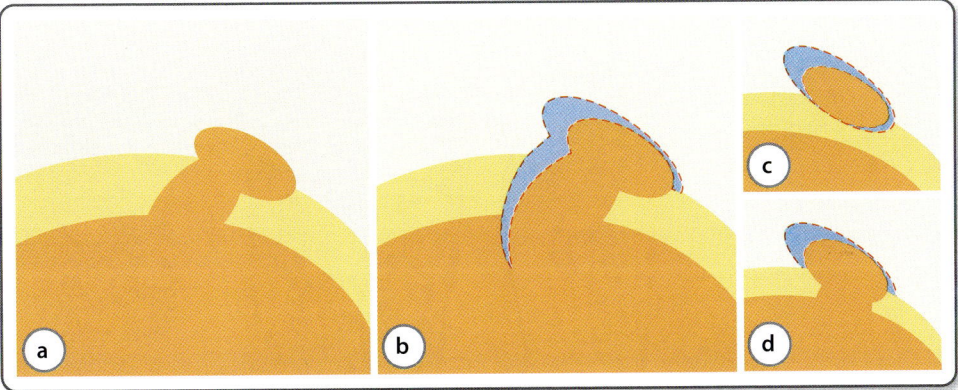

Figure 1.3 Angioinvasive encapsulated thyroid follicular carcinoma. This tumour initially presented with a focus of capsular invasion (a). Deeper sections of the same focus of suspected vascular invasion showed intimate relationship with adjacent veins (b) and finally genuine vascular invasion (c).

Figure 1.4 Schematic representation of capsular-vascular invasion in thyroid carcinoma. As in the case of figure 1.3, it is very common for capsular invasion to actually represent capsular-vascular invasion (a). Capsular invasion usually occurs in areas of lesser resistance of the tumour capsule at the point of penetration of the vein that drains the tumour (b). These foci of vascular invasion lined by the endothelium of the adjacent vein may represent preinvasive stages (c and d).

Tumour: brown; tumour capsule: yellow; vein lumen: blue; endothelial cells: red.

presentation of PTC and most of its subtypes that can be associated with recurrence, but not with patient mortality [13,14]. For this reason, identifying tumour venous invasion requires the application of strict criteria [9,12]. For the diagnosis of venous invasion only veins inside or outside the tumour capsule may be considered. Furthermore, confirmation of genuine venous invasion also requires that the tumour embolus adheres to the vascular wall and/or is lined by endothelium [12,15,16] **(Figure 1.5)**. When the tumour embolus is accompanied by fibrin and/or has infiltrated into the vascular wall the risk of distant metastases increases [11], which is consistent with the notion that some tumour emboli only covered by endothelium may represent a preinvasive stage [17]

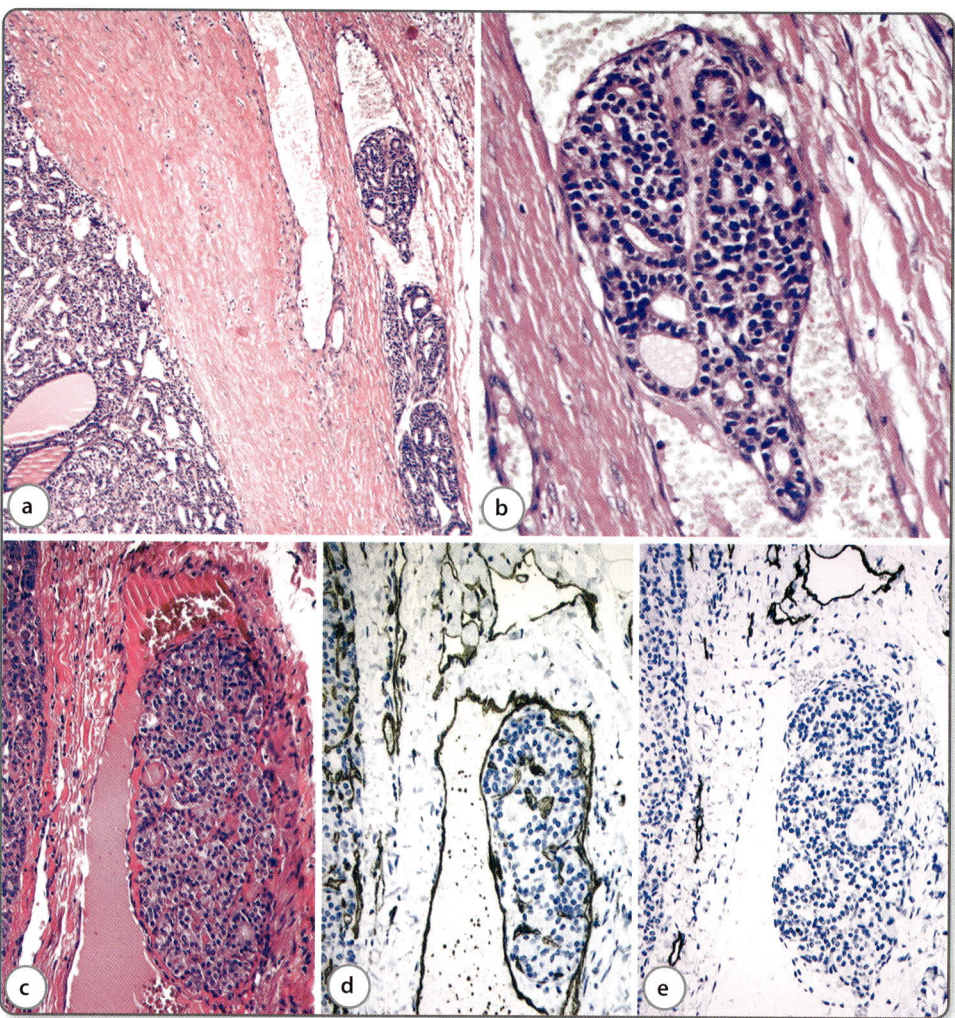

Figure 1.5 Angioinvasive encapsulated follicular carcinoma. The diagnosis of venous invasion is only applicable to veins inside or outside (a) the tumour capsule. The confirmation of genuine venous invasion also requires that the tumour thrombus be adhered to the vascular wall and/or lined by endothelium (b). Distant metastases in follicular carcinoma (c) occur through the veins which are positive for CD31 (d) and negative for lymphatic endothelial markers (D2-40) (e).

(**Figure 1.4**). It is important to stress that the presence of tumour plugs in subcapsular venous vessels does not count as blood vessel invasion.

Particular care must be taken not to confuse capsular invasion with artefacts secondary to capsule rupture after biopsy with a needle [18], or due to artefactual V-shaped folding of the tumour capsule (turned into itself) at the edge of a tissue section [19]. Reactive proliferations of endothelial cells projecting into the vascular lumen, intravascular papillary endothelial hyperplasia (Masson-like haemangioma) or Kaposi sarcoma-like endothelial proliferations may mimic vascular invasion by the tumour [12,20]. Although intravascular endothelial hyperplasia is more common in malignant thyroid tumours [21,22], it can also occur in follicular adenoma and adenomatous goitre [23,24] (**Figure 1.6**). Of note, while distant metastases in follicular carcinoma occur through veins [25], intravascular endothelial hyperplasia usually occurs in lymphatic vessels [22] (**Figure 1.5**). Cell groups trapped in the capsule with retraction artefact but devoid of endothelium can mimic angioinvasion. Immunostaining for vascular markers, particularly CD31 and/or ERG, and in case of need a marker for lymphatic vessels such as podoplanin (also known as D2-40), may help to establish whether the focus of tumour cells is covered by endothelial cells or to confirm that they are in a blood vessel lumen [12,16,25,26]. The presence of individual tumour cells in the vascular lumen neither adherent to the wall nor covered by endothelial cells is not true vascular invasion [12,15].

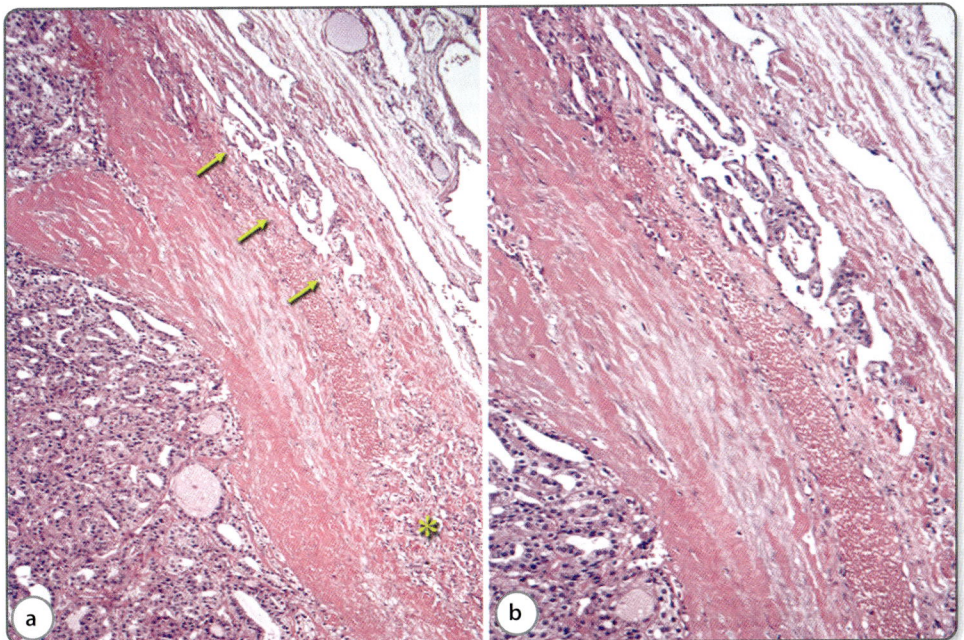

Figure 1.6 Intravascular endothelial hyperplasia. Intravascular endothelial hyperplasia is more common in malignant thyroid tumours but can also occur in benign tumours. Intravascular endothelial hyperplasia usually occurs in lymphatic vessels (a and b) and should not be confused with vascular invasion.

Histopathology of follicular patterned neoplasms with questionable capsular or vascular invasion

This category addresses tumours with follicular-cell nuclei (FT-UMP) or with equivocal (or even typical) nuclear features of PTC (WDT-UMP). We will also address NIFTP in this section as it belongs to the group of low-risk neoplasms. The concept of FT-UMP was created in 2000 when pathologists realised that sometimes it was not possible to decide whether or not there was capsular or vascular invasion in encapsulated follicular neoplasms (**Figure 1.7**). In parallel, for tumours of which the nuclear features of the neoplastic cells approached the appearance of PTC nuclei (large, clear and grooved) without fulfilling the criteria for typical PTC nuclei, the category of WDT-UMP was created.

The problem caused by classifying follicular patterned tumours as papillary carcinomas, exclusively based on the PTC-like appearance of the nuclei, was overtreatment of

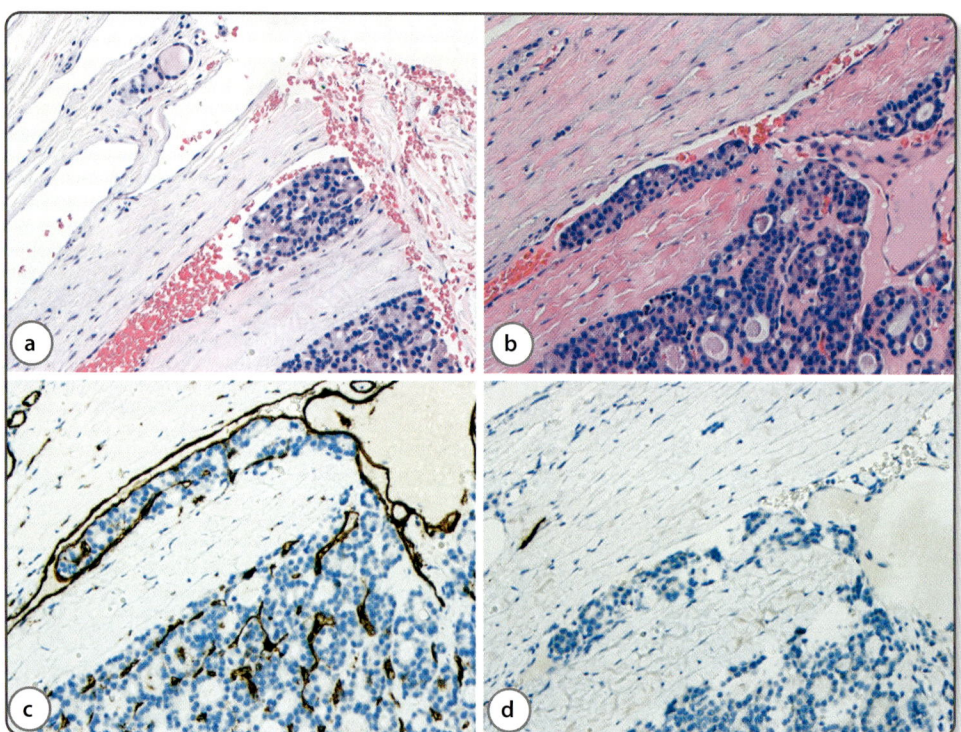

Figure 1.7 Follicular tumour of uncertain malignant potential (FT, UMP). (a) This tumour presented a focus of suggestive vascular invasion in a blood vessel in the capsule. However, there is not enough evidence to diagnose vascular invasion because the tumour plug was not lined by endothelial cells and there is not also a fibrin thrombus. This finding raises the possibility one is dealing with an artefact [haematoxylin and eosin (H&E)]. A thorough study was performed using numerous additional sections. (b) Just in one recut we observed an image suggestive of vascular invasion in the capsule of the tumour (H&E). (c and d) The confirmation of vascular invasion requires the presence of endothelial cells lining the blood vessel and the neoplastic cells using CD31 and D2-40, respectively. In this particular case, we were not able to identify unequivocal signs of vascular invasion and we kept the diagnosis of FT, UMP based upon questionable vascular invasion.

patients with encapsulated/well-circumscribed tumours. In an attempt to avoid this, the aforementioned WDT-UMP category was created. A diagnosis of WDT-UMP implies close follow-up after hemithyroidectomy, instead of total thyroidectomy plus radioiodine therapy, provided there are no signs of invasion. Follow-up of patients with encapsulated, non-invasive, follicular patterned tumours displaying PTC nuclei demonstrated that their prognosis is excellent, regardless of the type of surgery **(Figure 1.8)**. In contrast, infiltrative (predominantly) follicular patterned PTC carries a worse prognosis as it follows a natural history similar to that of classic PTC, with frequent lymph node metastases. Recently, Ito et al (2022) described distant recurrences in 1% of patients with a radioiodine-avid lesion classified as FT-UMP, with questionable capsular invasion but without vascular invasion [27]. They recommend re-examination of histological material in case of questionable capsular invasion and/or vascular invasion as well as long-term post-surgery active patient surveillance. Hysek et al (2019) reported a 5% recurrence rate of distant metastases in FT-UMP [28], suggesting that a fraction of these lesions may harbour malignant potential [28]. This finding once more emphasises the need for exhaustive examination of the surgical specimen.

The clinicopathological entity non-invasive follicular thyroid neoplasm with papillary-like nuclear features (with an uncomfortable acronym NIFTP) was carved out from WDT-UMP and encapsulated, non-invasive FVPTC in 2016 [8]. Its definition lacks in precision and hence it is somewhat heterogeneous. As an example, there is no consensus as to the percentage of true papillae allowed in NIFTP: <1% papillae or no well-formed papillae at all [16]. This is important as a diagnosis of NIFTP should exclude any type of more aggressive neoplasm, notably classic PTC [29].

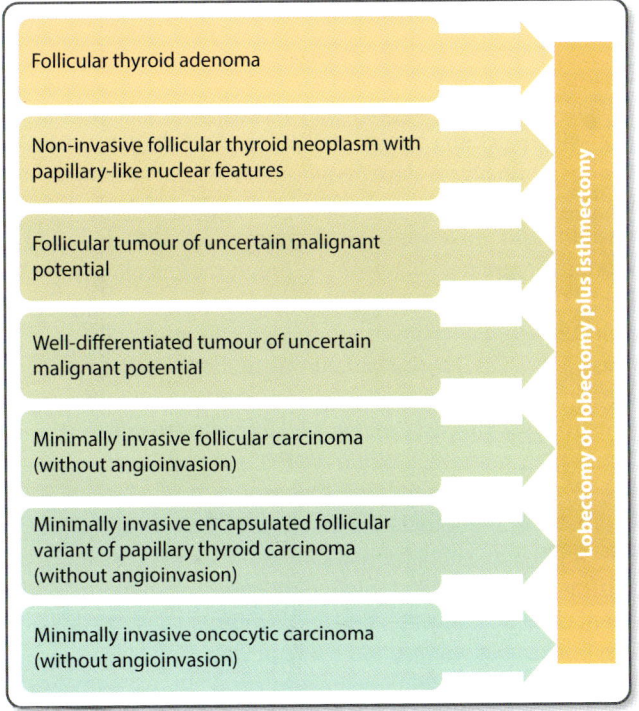

Figure 1.8 Thyroid tumours treated by lobectomy or lobectomy plus isthmectomy.

Follicular thyroid adenoma

Non-invasive follicular thyroid neoplasm with papillary-like nuclear features

Follicular tumour of uncertain malignant potential

Well-differentiated tumour of uncertain malignant potential

Minimally invasive follicular carcinoma (without angioinvasion)

Minimally invasive encapsulated follicular variant of papillary thyroid carcinoma (without angioinvasion)

Minimally invasive oncocytic carcinoma (without angioinvasion)

Lobectomy or lobectomy plus isthmectomy

The risk of lymph node metastasis remains a matter of debate. In two studies of NIFTP, with as criterium for papillae <1%, no nodal metastases were present at diagnosis [30,31] but lymph node status was not verified as in these studies prophylactic lymphadenectomy was not performed. In contrast, in NIFTP studies, using as criterium absence of papillae, Paniza et al (2019) did not find any metastasis at diagnosis [32] while Cho et al (2017) found micrometastases in central neck lymph nodes at diagnosis [33]. In several follow-up studies, no cases with residual or local/distant recurrent disease were reported, regardless of the used criterium for papillae (absence or <1%) [30,33,34]. Metastases at follow-up to regional lymph nodes [29,35] and distant metastases [29] were reported by few groups in cases with ≤1% papillary growth. A limiting factor of most of these studies is the question how exhaustively the specimens were studied regarding the presence of papillary structures, as a higher percentage of papillary structures would have supported a diagnosis of classic PTC.

Taken together, when strict criteria for a diagnosis of NIFTP are applied, metastases are not observed during follow-up [36]. Even large NIFTP (≥4 cm) show indolent behaviour [36] and have a very low recurrence rate [32] despite some isolated cases with biochemical persistence [34]. Nonetheless, the few cases with adverse outcome [29,35], argue against classification of NIFTP as a benign lesion, even when strict inclusion and exclusion criteria are applied [36].

The treatment of choice for NIFTP is hemithyroidectomy followed by clinical and radiologic surveillance [16]. Full thyroidectomy and radioactive iodine are not required treatments for this diagnostic category [33] and intense follow-up is not needed [32].

NEOPLASMS WITH MINIMAL CAPSULAR AND/OR VASCULAR INVASION

Definition

For intrathyroidal encapsulated follicular cell tumours, neoplasms with a very low risk of recurrence after a complete excision which includes benign (follicular adenoma), low-risk (FT-UMP, WDT-UMP, and NIFTP) and minimally invasive neoplasms (FTC, encapsulated FVPTC, and oncocytic carcinoma), hemithyroidectomy alone is curative (**Figure 1.8**) [37,41]. These subtypes guide risk stratification in terms of local recurrence, lymph node and distant metastases, which are important parameters determining prognosis and allowing individualised surgical strategies [42,43].

The category MI-FCT emerged in 1988, when FTC was subdivided into minimally invasive (MI-FTC) and widely invasive (WI-FTC) in the 2nd edition of the WHO Classification (1988) [6]. Data on prognosis and treatment of patients with minimally invasive thyroid neoplasms are mostly based on cases diagnosed according to this classification, which somewhat limits their relevance. While WI-FTCs are grossly invasive tumours infiltrating into blood vessels and/or adjacent thyroid tissue and often lack complete encapsulation, MI-FTC is more difficult to define. In the 1988 classification, MI-FCT includes neoplasms displaying limited or extensive angioinvasion, which goes beyond the current concept of minimally invasive thyroid carcinoma, defined by capsular invasion without vascular invasion. In current classifications, the presence of either capsular or vascular invasion separates benign from malignant tumours [44]. In view of the lacunar definition of MI-FCT, the prognostic significance of minimal invasion remains debatable [42].

This lack of clarity in diagnostic criteria resulted in their modification in subsequent years. Many studies, especially those prior to the 4th edition of WHO Classification (2017) [9] minimal invasion remained defined as capsular and/or vascular invasion, including minimal invasive tumors displaying <4 venous invasive foci [45,46]. In the 4th and 5th edition of the WHO Classification [9,16], a major change was introduced resulting into the subdivision of invasive encapsulated neoplasms into three categories:
1. Minimally invasive (classified as tumours with capsular invasion only)
2. Angioinvasive
3. Widely invasive

Prognostic factors

Although MI-FTC carries an overall good prognosis and is mostly considered to be an indolent tumour, some patients present with metastatic disease [46] and an aggressive clinical course [47–49]. In a cohort of 481 patients with 16 years of follow-up, disease-free survival of MI-FTC was similar to that of follicular adenoma (100% disease-free), with as implication that treatment might be the same for both entities [50]. However, a study on 195 MI-FTC patients reported distant metastases in about 8% of patients and half of these already presented distant metastases upon initial diagnosis [51].

An important question is which pathological variables, i.e. extent of capsular invasion, tumour size, and extent of angioinvasion, are predictive of the clinical course. In general, no significant association is found between capsular invasion and tumour recurrence [42,43,51–61].

Significance of tumour size is still debated: some studies reported that tumours >4 cm have an increased risk of recurrence [51,57,58], increased incidence of distant metastases and shorter distant metastases-free survival [55]. Another cohort comprising MI-FTC and WI-FTC showed that only tumour size (>4 cm) was an indicator of shorter disease-free survival [57]. Others did not find a significant association between tumour size and metastatic disease [59].

Recognition of venous invasion is particularly important, given that while disease-free survival at 40 months is 97% in minimally invasive carcinomas, it drops to 81 and 45% in encapsulated angioinvasive and widely invasive carcinomas, respectively [62,63]. Extensive angioinvasion (≥4 foci) has been reported as the most powerful risk factor for distant metastases [51,58,62,64].

Vascular invasion has consistently been associated with thyroid carcinoma prognosis and its presence has been included in the American Thyroid Association (ATA) guidelines for patient-risk assessment [44,61]. According to ATA guidelines, minimally invasive thyroid tumours are low-risk tumours with an expected recurrence rate of <1%, if an excellent response to treatment is achieved [61]. Patients with ≥4 foci of vascular invasion tumours have decreased recurrence-free survival [42,43,54]. When evaluating capsular and vascular invasion presence alone, no significant changes in patient prognosis were found; however, combined capsular and vascular invasion showed a significant impact on patient prognosis [54].

Taken together, the available data indicate that the risk of distant metastases and disease-specific mortality in MI-FTC increases with progression from capsular invasion alone to limited vascular invasion (<4 blood vessels) and afterwards to extensively invasive vascular invasion (≥4 blood vessels) [60].

Clinical variables also impact on the prognosis of MI-FTC, most notably older age which increases the risk of recurrent disease [53], decreases cancer-specific and distant metastasis-free survival [54–56], and is associated with distant recurrence [53]. Gender is not associated with outcome [42,52]. A study including 251 patients reported age as the most powerful prognostic factor but any association with vascular invasion and distant metastases was not found [55].

In encapsulated oncocytic carcinomas [65], it is the extent of vascular invasion rather than the mere presence of vascular invasion that denotes an aggressive behaviour [43,64], while extensive capsular invasion, gender, or age was not associated with a higher recurrence rate [43].

Treatment

MI-FTC diagnosis is as a rule established through histopathological study of the hemithyroidectomy specimen. The question to be answered is whether full thyroidectomy and radioiodine therapy are necessary, or postoperative surveillance suffices. Completion thyroidectomy is not uniformly recommended [50,53,56], particularly for minimally invasive (capsular invasion only) and <50 mm encapsulated, limited vascular invasive tumours (<4 vessels) [60]. The European Society of Endocrine Surgeons (ESES) recommends [42]:

- Hemithyroidectomy for:
  - Younger than 45-year-old patients with minimally invasive (capsule invasion only)
  - Less than 40-mm tumours, without vascular invasion, lymph node metastases or distant metastases.
- Thyroidectomy for:
  - Older than or equal to 45-year-old patients with ≥40 mm tumours with evidence of vascular invasion, lymph node metastases or distant metastases.
- Radioiodine therapy for:
  - Patients that underwent total thyroidectomy and whose tumours have extensive vascular invasion and/or lymph node metastases and/or distant metastases and/or recurrent disease [42,61].

Immunohistochemical and molecular markers in encapsulated neoplasms

We only briefly summarise the practical importance of molecular markers in low-risk malignant lesions (NIFTP, FT-UMP, and WDT-UMP) and minimally invasive carcinomas (**Figure 1.9**). All lesions with a *BRAF V600E* mutation, a *TERT* promoter mutation, or a mutation of *TP53* or *PIK3CA* should be considered as high risk [16,37–40]. Notably, morphologically low-risk lesions such as NIFTP, FT-UMP or WDT-UMP should not be classified as low-risk malignancy when any of these high-risk mutations are found (even though the clinical significance of these molecular findings remain to be clarified) [16].

In view of the importance of invasion in the pathobiology of low-risk thyroid neoplasms, much attention has been paid to expression of cell-adhesion (such as E-cadherin), cytoskeletal (vimentin) and extracellular matrix molecules (such as fibronectin, collagens and matrix metalloproteinases) or markers of epithelial-to-mesenchymal transition in the context of invasive capacity in thyroid tumours, by immunohistochemistry on human tissue specimens or in model systems. Most studies based upon human tissue specimens

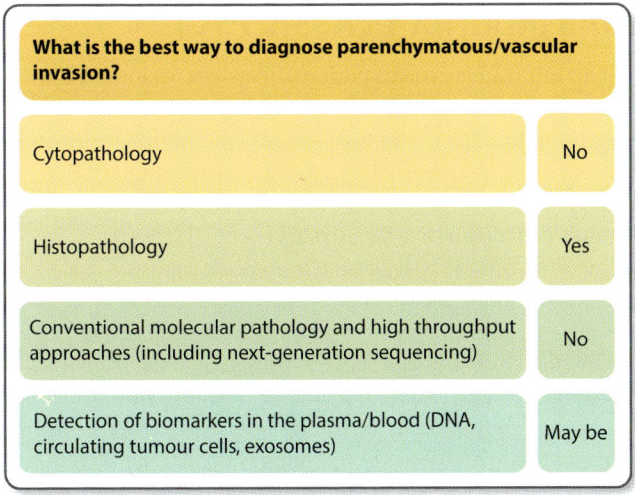

Figure 1.9 Ways to diagnose parenchymatous/vascular invasion.

(focusing on MI-FCT, WI-FTC minimally invasive FTC, FVPTC or oncocytic carcinoma) have not reported robust findings regarding expression of such proteins as helpful to establish capsular invasion or lymphatic/venous invasion [50,54,67–69]. The same holds true for MI-FCT studies [51,69]. Further studies in this field are required to better understand the role played by tumour microenvironment, including extracellular matrix and epithelial-mesenchymal transition, in the behaviour of encapsulated thyroid neoplasms.

ENCAPSULATED DIFFERENTIATED THYROID CARCINOMAS WITH HIGH-GRADE FEATURES

Encapsulated follicular cell-derived thyroid tumours (FTC, encapsulated FVPTC, and oncocytic carcinoma) usually carry a good prognosis [66,67], but occasionally they present so-called high-grade features, such as tumour necrosis and/or high-mitotic rate [66]. These tumours have been clustered in the newly created category of high-grade differentiated thyroid carcinomas [16], even though this category also contains highly invasive neoplasms.

The clinical importance of this new category remains to be clarified. Thompson et al performed a study comprising 130 patients with MI-FTC and segregated those patients in two-grade groups according to the histologic features large vessel invasion, extension into parenchyma, and tumour necrosis [68]; of the patients, 95 patients were classified as MI-FTC and the remaining 35 patients as "not low grade". No significant differences in prognosis were found between the two groups. Also Heffness et al found no significant differences in patient outcome based on the presence of necrosis or mitotic rate [52]. This was furthermore confirmed by Rivera et al [66] who reported that encapsulated, non-invasive follicular cell-derived thyroid tumours displaying high-grade features including extensive tumour necrosis had an indolent behaviour. In addition, tumours with high-grade features but lacking vascular invasion carried an excellent prognosis regardless of the presence of tumour necrosis. This suggests that high-grade features in a differentiated carcinoma, not accompanied by vascular invasion, are not predictive of aggressive tumour behaviour. However, this issue can only be resolved by long-term follow-up studies of such cases [66].

INFILTRATIVE TUMOURS (MAINLY CLASSIC PTC)

In case of a thyroid neoplasm with an infiltrative growth pattern, invasive carcinoma is the diagnosis and as a rule invasiveness is not graded unless extrathyroidal invasion and/ or invasion of venous vessels is encountered. The use of the category of minimal invasion is restricted to well-circumscribed/encapsulated follicular patterned neoplasms (FTC, FVPTC and oncocytic carcinoma).

The clinical significance of lymphatic invasion in infiltrative forms of PTC is an important point since lymphatic invasion and even regional lymph node metastases do not convey meaningful prognostic information. The umbrella term prognosis encompasses local recurrence, regional recurrence, as well as survival. In classic PTC lymph node metastases do not necessarily predict poor survival. Even in the presence of regional lymph node metastases, classic PTC often follows a (very) benign course in terms of mortality. In such cases, any attempt to grade lymphatic invasion using minimal invasion as a distinct category would be futile as histological confirmation of lymphatic invasion, regardless of the number and size of the lymphatic vessels, would immediately classify the case as lymphatic invasive [70–73].

It is important to emphasise that lymphatic invasion is difficult to establish in most cases of infiltrative PTC, regardless of the type of growth pattern [classic PTC and (predominantly) FVPTC] [74,75], even when using D2-40 immunohistochemistry, and as a rule this will not be mentioned in the pathology report. In case of dissemination of neoplastic cells and/or psammoma bodies throughout the thyroid parenchyma, lymphatic invasion might be mentioned in the report, even when not confirmed by D2-40 immunohistochemistry.

ACKNOWLEDGEMENTS

ET was supported by a PhD grant SFRH/BD/143458/2019 from the Foundation for Science and Technology (FCT). This article is partly supported by the project "Cancer Research on Therapy Resistance: From Basic Mechanisms to Novel Targets" – NORTE-01-0145-FEDER-000051, supported by Norte Portugal Regional Operational Programme (NORTE 2020), under the PORTUGAL 2020 Partnership Agreement, through the European Regional Development Fund (ERDF). Further funding (in part) by Programa Operacional Regional do Norte and co-funded by European Regional Development Fund under the project "The Porto Comprehensive Cancer Center" with the reference NORTE-01-0145-FEDER-072678 – Consórcio PORTO.CCC – Porto.Comprehensive Cancer Center Raquel Seruca. JMC-T was supported by grant no. PI19/01316 from Instituto de Salud Carlos III (ISCIII), State Research Agency and Ministry of Science and Innovation (Spain), co-funded by the European Union. The funders had no role in study design, data collection and analysis, decision to publish, or preparation of the manuscript.

Key points for clinical practice

Glossary

- *Invasion:* It is defined in the context of thyroid tumours by the infiltration by neoplastic cells of the surrounding (peritumoural) parenchyma, and/or lymphatic and blood vessels, and/or total penetration of the capsule whenever the tumour is encapsulated. The term "lymphovascular invasion", should be avoided, whenever possible, in order to keep lymphatic and blood vessels invasion separated.
- *Minimal invasion:* This term is used to define minimally invasive neoplasms. In the WHO classification of thyroid tumours (2017, 2023), the term is restricted to encapsulated, follicular patterned neoplasms demonstrating complete transcapsular penetration by the neoplastic cells without signs of vascular invasion. This includes minimally invasive follicular carcinoma, minimally invasive oncocytic carcinoma and minimally invasive follicular variant of papillary carcinoma.
- *Follicular adenoma:* Benign encapsulated, follicular/trabecular/solid neoplasm without nuclear features of papillary thyroid carcinoma and without signs of capsular and/or vascular invasion. This includes adenomas with papillary architecture which are often hyperfunctional (papillary adenoma, without nuclear features of papillary thyroid carcinoma) and oncocytic adenoma.
- *Non-invasive follicular thyroid neoplasm with papillary-like nuclear features (NIFTP)* encapsulated, follicular-patterned neoplasm with nuclear features of papillary thyroid carcinoma, without signs of capsular and/or vascular invasion.
- *Follicular tumour of uncertain malignant/potential (FT-UMP)* encapsulated, follicular-patterned neoplasm, with questionable signs of capsular and/or vascular invasion, without nuclear features of papillary thyroid carcinoma.
- *Well-differentiated tumour of uncertain malignant potential (WDT-UMP)* encapsulated, follicular-patterned neoplasm, with nuclear features of papillary thyroid carcinoma and questionable signs of capsular and/or vascular invasion.

What should not be called minimal invasion?

For the term minimal invasion to have full diagnostic and prognostic significance, its use should be strictly defined. The following situations clarify when the term should not be used.

- Incomplete transcapsular penetration and absence of signs of vascular invasion. This leads to a diagnosis of follicular adenoma, oncocytic adenoma or NIFTP (when the nuclei display PTC-like features).
- Questionable transcapsular penetration and/or questionable vascular invasion. This leads to a diagnosis of follicular tumour of uncertain malignant potential (FT-UMP) or, if the nuclei display PTC-like features, well-differentiated tumour of uncertain malignant potential (WDT-UMP).
- When invasion of capillaries and/or venous vessels by neoplastic cells is observed inside the tumour, or in a subcapsular location, this should not be considered minimal invasion, and the tumour under examination should be classified as benign.
- The presence of tumour plugs in subcapsular vessels does not count as vascular invasion. The putative biological meaning of this observation is unknown, but this histopathological feature does not carry clinical significance.
- When in an encapsulated, angioinvasive thyroid neoplasm less than four vessels are invaded, this is classified as limited vascular invasion, not as minimal vascular invasion.

- Regularly, several foci of extrathyroidal invasion by neoplastic cells may be found and these might show different degrees of invasion. In this context the least aggressive form is classified as microscopic extrathyroidal invasion, not as minimal invasion.
- Minimal invasion is not used for PTC with an infiltrative growth pattern, regardless of the tumour being a classic PTC or any subtype including follicular-patterned infiltrative PTC. This means that the term minimal invasion should not be used when dealing with a very small PTC (which was formerly classified as micro-PTC).

REFERENCES

1. Graham A. Malignant epithelial tumours of the thyroid with special reference to invasion of blood vessels. Surg Gynecol Obstet 1924; 39:781–790.
2. Graham A. Malignant tumours of the thyroid: Epithelial types. Ann Surg 1925; 82:30–44.
3. Coller FA. Adenoma and cancer of the thyroid: a study of their relation in ninety epithelial neoplasms of the thyroid. J Am Med Assoc 1929; 92:457–463.
4. Warren S. The significance of invasion of blood vessel in adenoma of the thyroid gland. Arch Pathol 1931; 11:255–7.
5. Goldstein NS, Czako P, Neill JS. Metastatic minimally invasive (encapsulated) follicular and Hurthle cell thyroid carcinoma: a study of 34 patients. Modern Pathol 2000; 13:123–130.
6. Hedinger C. Histological Classification of Thyroid Tumours. In: Hedinger C [Ed]. Histological Typing of Thyroid Tumours. Berlin, Heidelberg: Springer Berlin Heidelberg, 1988.
7. Williams ED. Guest Editorial: Two proposals regarding the terminology of thyroid tumors. Int J Surg Pathol. 2000; 8:181–183.
8. Nikiforov YE, Seethala RR, Tallini G, et al. Nomenclature revision for encapsulated follicular variant of papillary thyroid carcinoma: a paradigm shift to reduce overtreatment of indolent tumours. JAMA Oncol 2016; 2:1023–1029.
9. Lloyd R, Osamura R, Klöppel G, Rosai J. WHO classification of tumours of the thyroid gland. Lyon, France: International Agency for Research on Cancer (IARC), 2017.
10. Collini P, Sampietro G, Pilotti S. Extensive vascular invasion is a marker of risk of relapse in encapsulated non-Hürthle cell follicular carcinoma of the thyroid gland: a clinicopathological study of 18 consecutive cases from a single institution with a 11-year median follow-up. Histopathology 2004; 44:35–39.
11. Mete O, Asa SL. Pathological definition and clinical significance of vascular invasion in thyroid carcinomas of follicular epithelial derivation. Modern Pathol 2011; 24:1545–1552.
12. Cameselle-Teijeiro JM, Bella Cueto MR, Eloy C, et al. Tumores de la glándula tiroides. Propuesta para el manejo y estudio de las muestras de pacientes con neoplasias tiroideas. Rev Esp Patol. 2020; 53:27–36.
13. Leboulleux S, Rubino C, Baudin E, et al. Prognostic factors for persistent or recurrent disease of papillary thyroid carcinoma with neck lymph node metastases and/or tumour extension beyond the thyroid capsule at initial diagnosis. J Clin Endocrinol Metabol 2005; 90:5723–5729.
14. Hay ID, Johnson TR, Kaggal S, et al. Papillary thyroid carcinoma (PTC) in children and adults: comparison of initial presentation and long-term postoperative outcome in 4432 patients consecutively treated at the Mayo Clinic during eight decades (1936–2015). World J Surg 2018; 42:329–342.
15. Sobrinho-Simoes M, Eloy C, Magalhaes J, Lobo C, Amaro T. Follicular thyroid carcinoma. Modern Pathol 2011; 24:S10–S18.
16. Baloch ZW, Asa SL, Barletta JA, et al. Overview of the 2022 WHO classification of thyroid neoplasms. Endocrine Pathol 2022; 33:27–63.
17. Aida N, Yamada N, Asano G, Tanaka S. 3-D analysis of vascular and capsular invasion in thyroid follicular carcinoma. Pathol Int 2001; 51:425–430.

18. LiVolsi VA, Merino MJ. Worrisome histologic alterations following fine-needle aspiration of the thyroid (WHAFFT). Pathol Annu 1994; 29:99–120.
19. Rosai J, Kuhn E, Carcangiu M. Pitfalls in thyroid tumour pathology. Histopathology 2006; 49:107–120.
20. Cameselle-Teijeiro JM, Eloy C, Sobrinho-Simões M. Rare tumours of the thyroid gland: diagnosis and WHO classification. Berlin, Germany: Springer, 2018.
21. Tse L, Chan I, Chan J. Capsular intravascular endothelial hyperplasia: a peculiar form of vasoproliferative lesion associated with thyroid carcinoma. Histopathology 2001; 39:463–468.
22. Schmitz BA, Singh C, Gulbahce HE, Manivel JC, Pambuccian SE. Florid capsular and pericapsular papillary endothelial proliferation associated with poorly differentiated thyroid carcinoma. Int J Surg Pathol 2011; 19:110–112.
23. Sapino A, Papotti M, Macri L, Satolli MA, Bussolati G. Intranodular reactive endothelial hyperplasia in adenomatous goitre. Histopathology 1995; 26:457–462.
24. Papotti M, Arrondini M, Tavaglione V, Veltri A, Volante M. Diagnostic controversies in vascular proliferations of the thyroid gland. Endocr Pathol 2008; 19:175–183.
25. Lin X, Zhu B, Liu Y, Silverman JF. Follicular thyroid carcinoma invades venous rather than lymphatic vessels. Diagn Pathol 2010; 5:8.
26. Liu J, Tao L-I, Yu G-Y, et al. Diagnostic significance of CyclinD1 and D2-40 expression for follicular neoplasm of the thyroid. Pathol Res Pract 2022; 229:153739.
27. Ito Y, Hirokawa M, Hayashi T, et al. Clinical outcomes of follicular tumour of uncertain malignant potential of the thyroid: real-world data. Endocr J 2022: EJ21–0723.
28. Hysek M, Paulsson JO, Jatta K, et al. Clinical routine TERT promoter mutational screening of follicular thyroid tumours of uncertain malignant potential (FT-UMPs): a useful predictor of metastatic disease. Cancers 2019; 11:1443.
29. Parente DN, Kluijfhout WP, Bongers PJ, et al. Clinical safety of renaming encapsulated follicular variant of papillary thyroid carcinoma: is NIFTP truly benign? World J Surg 2018; 42:321–326.
30. Paja M, Zafón C, Iglesias C, Ugalde A, et al. Rate of non-invasive follicular thyroid neoplasms with papillary-like nuclear features depends on pathologist's criteria: A multicentre retrospective Southern European study with prolonged follow-up. Endocrine 2021; 73:131–140.
31. Sowder AM, Witt BL, Hunt JP. An update on the risk of lymph node metastasis for the follicular variant of papillary thyroid carcinoma with the new diagnostic paradigm. Head Neck Pathol 2018; 12:105–109.
32. de Jesus Paniza AC, Mendes TB, Viana MDB, et al. Revised criteria for diagnosis of NIFTP reveals a better correlation with tumour biological behavior. Endocr Connect 2019; 8:1529–1538.
33. Cho U, Mete O, Kim MH, Bae JS, Jung CK. Molecular correlates and rate of lymph node metastasis of non-invasive follicular thyroid neoplasm with papillary-like nuclear features and invasive follicular variant papillary thyroid carcinoma: the impact of rigid criteria to distinguish non-invasive follicular thyroid neoplasm with papillary-like nuclear features. Modern Pathol 2017; 30:810–825.
34. Rosario PW, Mourão GF, Nunes MB, Nunes MS, Calsolari MR. Noninvasive follicular thyroid neoplasm with papillary-like nuclear features. Endocrine-Related Cancer 2016; 23:893–897.
35. Kim MJ, Won JK, Jung KC, et al. Clinical characteristics of subtypes of follicular variant papillary thyroid carcinoma. Thyroid 2018; 28:311–318.
36. Zajkowska K, Kopczyński J, Góźdź S, Kowalska A. Noninvasive follicular thyroid neoplasm with papillary-like nuclear features: a problematic entity. Endocr Connect 2020; 9:R47–R58.
37. Póvoa AA, Teixeira E, Bella-Cueto MR, et al. Genetic determinants for prediction of outcome of patients with papillary thyroid carcinoma. Cancers 2021; 13:2048.
38. Penna GC, Vaisman F, Vaisman M, Sobrinho-Simões M, Soares P. Molecular Markers Involved in Tumourigenesis of Thyroid Carcinoma: Focus on Aggressive Histotypes. Cytogenetic Genome Res 2016; 150:194–207.
39. García-Rostán G, Costa AM, Pereira-Castro I, et al. Mutation of the PIK3CA gene in anaplastic thyroid cancer. Cancer Res 2005; 65:10199–207.
40. Nishida T, Nakao K, Hamaji M, Nakahara M-A, Tsujimoto M. Overexpression of p53 protein and DNA content are important biologic prognostic factors for thyroid cancer. Surgery 1996; 119:568–575.
41. Kakudo K, Bychkov A, Bai Y, et al. The new 4th edition World Health Organization classification for thyroid tumours, Asian perspectives. United States: Wiley Online Library; 2018.

42. Dionigi G, Kraimps JL, Schmid KW, et al. Minimally invasive follicular thyroid cancer (MIFTC) – a consensus report of the European Society of Endocrine Surgeons (ESES). Langenbeck's Arch Surg 2014; 399:165–184.

43. Ghossein RA, Hiltzik DH, Carlson DL, et al. Prognostic factors of recurrence in encapsulated Hurthle cell carcinoma of the thyroid gland. Cancer 2006; 106:1669–1676.

44. Xu B, Teplov A, Ibrahim K, et al. Detection and assessment of capsular invasion, vascular invasion and lymph node metastasis volume in thyroid carcinoma using microCT scanning of paraffin tissue blocks (3D whole block imaging): a proof of concept. Modern Pathol 2020; 33:2449–2457.

45. Poma AM, Giannini R, Piaggi P, et al. A six-gene panel to label follicular adenoma, low- and high-risk follicular thyroid carcinoma. Endocr Connect 2018; 7:124–132.

46. Lee Y-M, Park JH. A Case of Minimally Invasive Follicular Thyroid Carcinoma Relapsed as a Large Cervical Lymphadenopathy and Multiple Lung Metastases. J Endocr Surg 2020; 20:21–25.

47. Fozzatti L, Cheng SY. Tumour Cells and Cancer-Associated Fibroblasts: A Synergistic Crosstalk to Promote Thyroid Cancer. Endocrinol Metab (Seoul) 2020; 35:673–680.

48. Khoo ACH, Chen SL. A rare case of minimally invasive follicular thyroid cancer with intraluminal superior vena cava and right atrium metastases. World J Nucl Med 2019; 18:301–303.

49. Gao H, Wu S, Zhang X, Xie T. Minimally invasive follicular thyroid carcinoma mimicking pituitary adenoma: a case report. Int J Clin Experiment Pathol 2019; 12:3949.

50. Robinson A, Schneider D, Sippel R, Chen H. Minimally invasive follicular thyroid cancer: treat as a benign or malignant lesion? J Surg Res 2017; 207:235–240.

51. Lee Y-M, Sung T-Y, Yoon JH, Chung K-W, Hong SJ. Long term outcome of minimally invasive follicular thyroid carcinoma according to risk group stratification. J Endocr Surg 2018; 18:183–190.

52. Heffess CS, Thompson LD. Minimally invasive follicular thyroid carcinoma. Endocr Pathol 2001; 12:417–422.

53. Ito Y, Onoda N, Okamoto T. The revised clinical practice guidelines on the management of thyroid tumours by the Japan Associations of Endocrine Surgeons: Core questions and recommendations for treatments of thyroid cancer. Endocr J 2020; 67:669–717.

54. Stenson G, Nilsson I-L, Mu N, et al. Minimally invasive follicular thyroid carcinomas: prognostic factors. Endocrine 2016; 53:505–511.

55. Sugino K, Kameyama K, Ito K, et al. Outcomes and Prognostic Factors of 251 Patients with Minimally Invasive Follicular Thyroid Carcinoma. Thyroid 2012; 22:798–804.

56. Yamazaki H, Sugino K, Katoh R, et al. Outcomes for Minimally Invasive Follicular Thyroid Carcinoma in Relation to the Change in Age Stratification in the AJCC 8th Edition. Ann Surg Oncol 2021; 28:3576–3583.

57. Podda M, Saba A, Porru F, Reccia I, Pisanu A. Follicular thyroid carcinoma: differences in clinical relevance between minimally invasive and widely invasive tumours. World J Surg Oncol 2015; 13:193.

58. Ito Y, Hirokawa M, Masuoka H, et al. Prognostic factors of minimally invasive follicular thyroid carcinoma: Extensive vascular invasion significantly affects patient prognosis. Endocr J 2013; 60:637–642.

59. Ban EJ, Andrabi A, Grodski S, et al. Foilicular thyroid cancer: minimally invasive tumours can give rise to metastases. ANZ J Surg 2012; 82:136–139.

60. Daniels GH. Follicular thyroid carcinoma: a perspective. Thyroid 2018; 28:1229–1242.

61. Haugen BR, Alexander EK, Bible KC, et al. 2015 American Thyroid Association management guidelines for adult patients with thyroid nodules and differentiated thyroid cancer: the American Thyroid Association guidelines task force on thyroid nodules and differentiated thyroid cancer. Thyroid 2016; 26:1–133.

62. D'Avanzo A, Treseler P, Ituarte PH, et al. Follicular thyroid carcinoma: histology and prognosis. Cancer 2004; 100:1123–1129.

63. O'Neill CJ, Vaughan L, Learoyd DL, et al. Management of follicular thyroid carcinoma should be individualised based on degree of capsular and vascular invasion. Eur J Surg Oncol 2011; 37:181–185.

64. Xu B, Wang L, Tuttle RM, Ganly I, Ghossein R. Prognostic impact of extent of vascular invasion in low-grade encapsulated follicular cell-derived thyroid carcinomas: a clinicopathologic study of 276 cases. Hum Pathol 2015; 46:1789–1798.
65. Xu B, Ghossein R. Evolution of the histologic classification of thyroid neoplasms and its impact on clinical management. Eur J Surg Oncol 2018; 44:338–347.
66. Rivera M, Ricarte-Filho J, Patel S, et al. Encapsulated thyroid tumours of follicular cell origin with high grade features (high mitotic rate/tumour necrosis): a clinicopathologic and molecular study. Hum Pathol 2010; 41:172–180.
67. Liu J, Singh B, Tallini G, et al. Follicular variant of papillary thyroid carcinoma. Cancer 2006; 107:1255–1264.
68. Thompson LD, Wieneke JA, Paal E, et al. A clinicopathologic study of minimally invasive follicular carcinoma of the thyroid gland with a review of the English literature. Cancer 2001; 91:505–524.
69. Chow TL, Tam SW, Choi CY, Kwan WW. Hemithyroidectomy for low-risk follicular carcinoma of the thyroid: results from a regional hospital. Singapore Med J 2018; 59:311–315.
70. Hedinger C, Sobin LH. Histological typing of thyroid tumours – International Histological Classification of Tumours. Geneva, Switzerland: World Health Organization, 1974.
71. Chen K, Rosai J. Follicular variant of thyroid papillary carcinoma: a clinicopathologic study of six cases. Am J Surg Pathol 1977; 1:123–130.
72. Thompson NW, Brown J, Orringer M, Sisson J, Nishiyama R. Follicular carcinoma of the thyroid with massive angioinvasion: extension of tumour thrombus to the heart. Surgery 1978; 83:451–457.
73. DeLellis RA. Pathology and genetics of tumours of endocrine organs.France: IARC, 2004.
74. Cancer Genome Atlas Research Network. Integrated genomic characterization of papillary thyroid carcinoma. Cell 2014; 159:676–690.
75. Tallini G, Tuttle RM, Ghossein RA. The history of the follicular variant of papillary thyroid carcinoma. J Clin Endocrinol Metabol 2017; 102:15–22.

Chapter 2

Drug-related changes in gastrointestinal biopsies

Hanna Henzinger, Iva Brcic

INTRODUCTION

Gastrointestinal (GI) biopsies are among the most frequent types of specimen seen by pathologists in daily practice. A variety of histological findings can be encountered and the changes related to or induced by therapy with an ever-increasing number of novel drugs and therapeutic procedures are becoming very frequent. Symptoms can be mild to severe and in rare cases life-threatening; a correct diagnosis may lead to withdrawal of the causative drug and a relief of symptoms.

Various drug-associated mechanisms are involved in the pathogenesis of mucosal damage, resulting in different patterns of injury. These may include epithelial hyperplasia or degeneration, apoptosis, erosion, ulceration, fibrosis, necrosis, inflammatory infiltrates (most commonly eosinophils and lymphocytes) and deposition of pigments or crystals. In addition, drug fillers can be found in biopsy material.

In this chapter, we will review how various drugs cause mucosal damage of the tubal gut and describe the broad spectrum of histological changes that may be seen in GI biopsies. We will discuss these according to the most common site of GI tract involvement. We will emphasise clinical and histological features that may help practicing pathologists to identify drugs that might have been responsible for the encountered lesion.

DRUG-RELATED CHANGES OF THE UPPER GASTROINTESTINAL TRACT

Iatrogenic oesophagitis

Pill oesophagitis

Prolonged mucosal contact with a variety of drugs, e.g. potassium chloride (especially slow-release compounds), non-steroidal anti-inflammatory drugs (NSAIDs), antibiotics (i.e. tetracycline, doxycycline and clindamycin), oral iron supplements and bisphosphonates (BP)

Hanna Henzinger Medical student, Diagnostic & Research Institute of Pathology, Medical University of Graz, Graz, Austria
E-mail: hanna.henzinger@medunigraz.at

Iva Brcic MD PhD, Diagnostic & Research Institute of Pathology, Medical University of Graz, Neue Stiftingtalstraße, Graz, Austria
E-mail: iva.brcic@medunigraz.at (for correspondence)

may cause oesophageal injury, known as *pill* oesophagitis. The risk of pill oesophagitis is increased by disorders of oesophageal motility – either muscular or nervous – or oesophageal stenosis, both as a result of extended passage time of the drug through the oesophagus. Mucosal injuries are most common in the mid and distal oesophagus, especially around its natural point of constriction where the aortic arch crosses the oesophagus. Symptoms include odynophagia and retrosternal pain, which usually resolve after the provoking medication is discontinued. Endoscopically, iatrogenic oesophagitis presents with erosions and ulcerations. Occasionally, pill fragments can be found upon examination [1–3].

In oesophageal biopsies, apoptotic keratinocytes and occasionally even erosions and ulcerations can be seen, accompanied by an inflammatory infiltrate. These infiltrates usually contain only a few cells, but they may be also more cellular depending on the severity of injury. The inflammatory infiltrates may contain numerous eosinophils, suggesting reflux or eosinophilic oesophagitis. The differential diagnosis of pill oesophagitis includes also oesophageal lichen planus, which usually affects the proximal oesophagus [3,4].

Sloughing oesophagitis

In some patients, particularly those of high age and with multiple comorbidities and medications, endoscopy may show characteristic white sloughing membranes consisting of desquamated epithelial layers, typically in the middle and distal third of the oesophagus [5,6] **(Figure 2.1)**. This is known as sloughing oesophagitis, also referred to as exfoliative oesophagitis or oesophagitis dissecans superficialis (ODS). Symptoms are dysphagia, pain, and occasionally bleeding or regurgitation of mucosa [1]. There is also an association of sloughing oesophagitis with the intake of central nervous system depressants [7].

Histologically, the squamous epithelium appears two-toned **(Figure 2.1)**: an upper layer often detached from the mucosa and consisting of necrotic eosinophilic material that may be colonised by bacteria or yeasts and may show parakeratosis and an underlying basal zone which is oedematous, basophilic due to hyperplasia and often containing bullae and cysts [1,3].

Differential diagnosis includes fungal or viral infections that need to be to be ruled out. *Candida* oesophagitis has a similar endoscopic appearance with white plaques on the mucosal surface. It can be diagnosed by histological detection of fungal pseudohyphae, that can be facilitated by the use of special stains [e.g. Gömöri methenamine silver (GMS) or periodic acid Schiff reaction (PAS)]. Exfoliative oesophagitis has also been associated with heavy smoking, trauma, graft-versus-host disease (GvHD), coeliac disease and skin conditions such as bullous dermatoses [1,2]. Therefore, the correlation of histology with endoscopy supplemented by clinical data including history and symptoms are crucial for formulating the correct diagnosis and identifying the cause of patient's symptoms [6].

Bisphosphonate-associated oesophagitis

As previously mentioned, BPs such as alendronate and risedronate are common causes of iatrogenic oesophagitis, which affects 1.5% of patients treated with those drugs [8]. BPs inhibit osteoclast-mediated bone resorption and are often prescribed for osteoporosis, Paget's disease of bone and bone loss due to malignancies [9]. Nagano et al suggested that mucosal damage of the oesophagus is caused by BP-mediated production of mitochondrial superoxide [10].

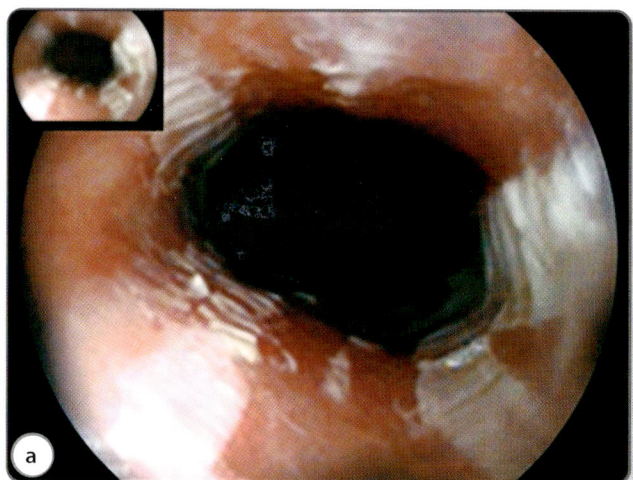

Figure 2.1 Oesophagitis dissecans superficialis. (a) Endoscopy showing large whitish stripes sloughing into the lumen of the oesophagus. (b) Histology shows an epithelial split above the basal zone, parakeratosis and "mummified" superficial layer resulting in a two-toned epithelium.

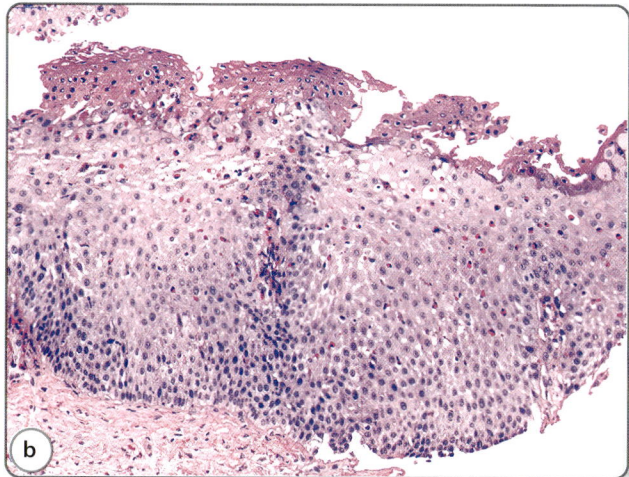

In BP-induced ulcerations, pale yellow, refractile crystals, which are believed to consist of cellulose (a pharmaceutical filler), may be found; these crystals are often surrounded by multinucleated giant cells [11–14]. In addition to oesophageal injury, BPs can, in rare cases, cause erosions and ulcers in the stomach and duodenum [15]. The ulcerogenic potential of BPs is elevated by concurrent intake of NSAIDs. Risedronate appears to be significantly less harmful to the GI tract than alendronate [16].

Iatrogenic gastritis

Reactive gastropathy

Reactive gastropathy, also known as reactive or chemical gastritis ("C-gastritis"), is one of the most common patterns of inflammation seen in gastric biopsies. Mucosal redness, oedema and friability, as well as erosions and ulcers may be seen endoscopically; however, gastroscopic findings are often inconspicuous [17]. The lesions are located in the antrum but may extend into the oxyntic mucosa as well. The mucosa is oedematous and hyperaemic with subepithelial telangiectasia. Foveolar glands are hyperplastic, elongated and contorted ("corkscrew-shaped") with cuboidal cells, mucin depletion and diffuse nuclear hyperchromasia **(Figure 2.2)**. Lamina propria shows proliferation of smooth muscle fibres and lacks inflammatory cell infiltrates [1,17–19]. Severe cases may show erosions and ulcerations **(Figure 2.2)** [14].

C-gastritis may be provoked by a variety of drugs, notably NSAIDs, but also corticosteroids and BPs among others [18,19]. Additional causes are bile reflux, alcohol abuse, portal hypertensive gastropathy and gastric antral vascular ectasia (GAVE) [1,2]. The pathogenesis depends on the aetiology; e.g. NSAIDs inhibit prostaglandin synthesis, which reduces mucosal blood flow and mucous secretion, rendering the mucosa vulnerable to injury [18]. Differential diagnoses include GAVE, *H. pylori* gastritis, and low-grade dysplasia.

In GAVE, similar to C-gastritis, foveolar hyperplasia, dilation of mucosal capillaries and increase of smooth muscle in the lamina propria can be observed in the antrum. The important diagnostic cue that distinguishes GAVE from reactive gastropathy is the presence of fibrin thrombi in dilated vessels. This morphological attribute is also responsible for the characteristic endoscopic appearance of GAVE described as "watermelon stomach" due to striking red stripes radiating from the pylorus [20].

In *H. pylori* gastritis, a band-like chronic and/or active inflammatory infiltrate is found underneath the surface epithelium. Bacterial organisms may be detected on the epithelial surface and in foveolae [1]. Some histological overlap of *H. pylori* gastritis and chemical gastropathy occurs, with moderate to severe inflammation as well as conspicuous foveolar hyperplasia [18,21]. In chronic cases, intestinal metaplasia and atrophy may occur **(Figure 2.2)** and occasionally dysplasia can develop.

Reactive gastropathy can be associated with other changes in the GI tract, such as ileitis and collagenous colitis. These findings may be due to common aetiology: NSAIDs, for example, are harmful to gastric mucosa but also to other parts of the GI tract, which will be elaborated later on in this chapter [22].

Gastric calcinosis

Gastric calcinosis is usually an incidental finding consisting of subepithelial extracellular basophilic crystalline aggregates in the gastric mucosa, predominantly in the antral area **(Figure 2.3)** [1,23]. Occasionally, oesophageal involvement has been described [24]. The crystalline deposits appear black on the von Kossa stain. They consist of calcium, phosphorus, aluminium and chlorine, and are surrounded by macrophages. Additionally, chemical gastropathy may coexist, exhibiting the typical histologic features already discussed [1,3,25]. By endoscopy, white plaques or nodules can be observed [23].

Gastric calcinosis may result from hypercalcaemia and/or hyperphosphataemia (e.g. related to chronic kidney disease or malignancy) or medications, most importantly aluminium-containing antacids and sucralfate. The presence of GC is significantly related to chronic renal failure and organ transplantation. Sucralfate and antacids are often taken by transplant patients [25,26], e.g. as prophylaxis for oral and intestinal mucositis after bone marrow transplantation [27]. Hence, GC has been reported in up to 33% of post-transplant gastric biopsies [25]. Crystalline aggregates need to be distinguished from iron gastropathy, resin deposition and gastric parasitosis [1,20].

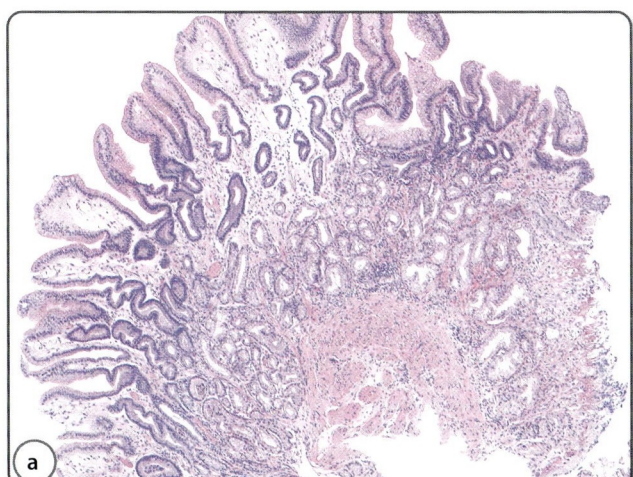

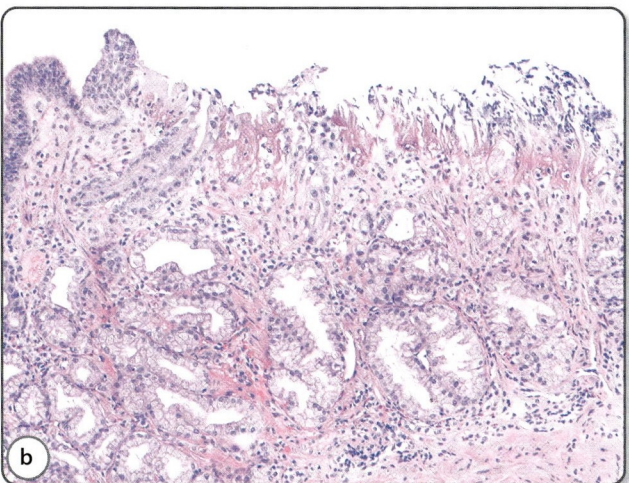

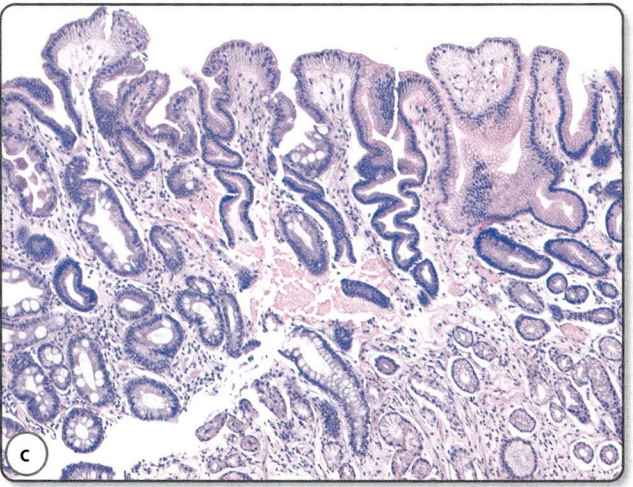

Figure 2.2 Reactive gastropathy. (a) Antral mucosa with "corkscrew-like" foveolar hyperplasia, reactive epithelial changes with mucin depletion, interfoveolar smooth muscle hyperplasia and erosion covered by fibrin. (b) Antral mucosa with erosion and (c) intestinal metaplasia.

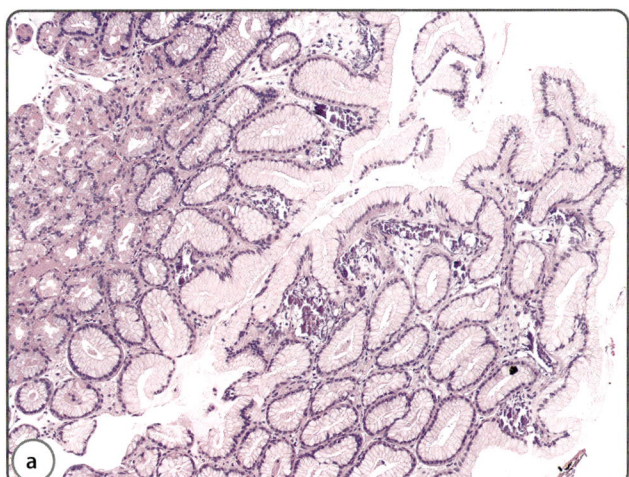

Figure 2.3 Gastric calcinosis. (a and b) Corpus mucosa with subepithelial extracellular basophilic crystalline aggregates.

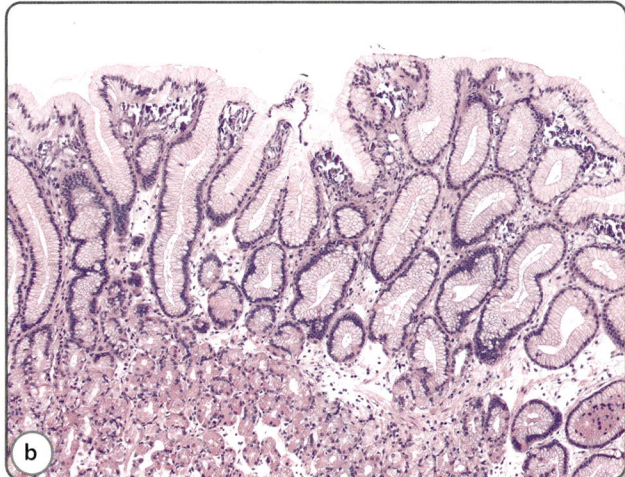

Proton pump inhibitor-associated gastropathy

Proton-pump inhibitors (PPIs), such as omeprazole, lansoprazole and pantoprazole, target the gastric acid pump – the H^+/K^+-ATPase in the cell membrane of parietal cells of the stomach – and suppress HCl secretion [28]. They are used for the treatment of gastro-oesophageal reflux disease (GORD) and Barrett's oesophagus, *H. pylori* eradication, peptic ulcer disease and Zollinger–Ellison syndrome, among others [29]. PPIs have a good safety profile; only 1–5% of patients report adverse drug reactions including abdominal pain, nausea and vomiting, constipation, diarrhoea, flatulence or headache [30].

Under the influence of PPIs, the gastric pH level rises, leading to increased gastrin secretion, which results in hypertrophy and hyperplasia of ECL cells and parietal cells. Histologically, PPI-induced alterations present as protrusion of voluminous parietal cells into the lumen of the oxyntic glands, giving the glands a serrated appearance (**Figure 2.4**). Furthermore, dilation of gastric glands and vacuolisation of parietal cells occurs often [3,31]. Chronic use of PPIs triggers the development of sporadic fundic gland polyps (FGP),

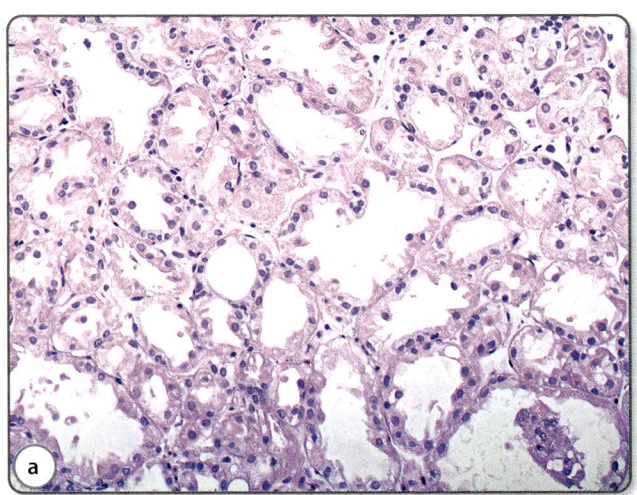

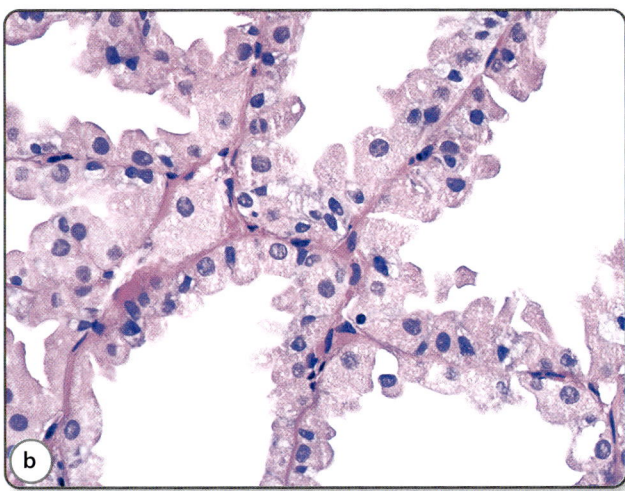

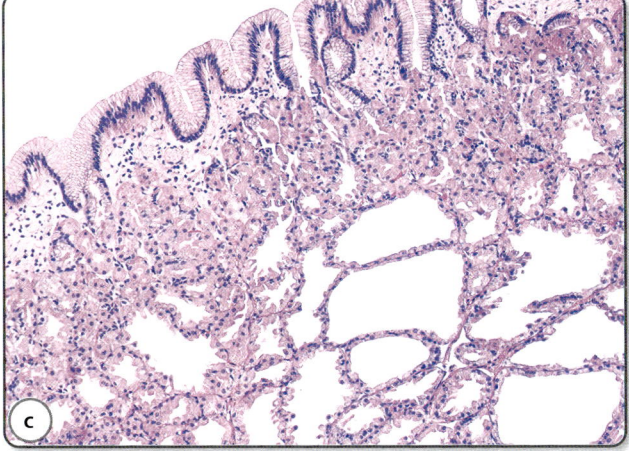

Figure 2.4 PPI effect: (a and b) Oxyntic mucosa shows dilated fundic glands lined by hypertrophic, hyperplastic parietal cells with luminal snout-like protrusions and prominent cytoplasmic vacuolisation. (c) Fundic gland polyp induced by PPIs: Polyp consists of dilated oxyntic glands with parietal cell hypertrophy and hyperplasia.

which are usually small and located in the gastric body and fundus. The development of FGP only depends on the duration of PPI use, and not on their dosage [32]. Histologically, FGPs consist of dilated oxyntic glands lined by chief, mucous and parietal cells **(Figure 2.4)**, the latter hypertrophic and hyperplastic [1]. Additionally, ECL cell hyperplasia due to hypergastrinaemia in patients with long-term PPI use may be a precursor lesion of gastric neuroendocrine neoplasia [33]. After discontinuation of PPI treatment, complete remission of PPI-induced changes has been reported [34].

PPIs, in particular lansoprazole, occasionally also induce microscopic colitis as will be discussed later on [35,36]. PPIs possibly play a role in the development of pseudomembranous colitis associated with antibiotics use, as discussed in the respective subchapter [37].

Iron gastropathy

In about 16% of people taking oral iron supplements, iron deposits are found in upper GI tract biopsies [38]. Iron deposits in the gastric mucosa occur in three distinct patterns which suggest different pathogenic mechanisms: extracellular iron aggregates are induced by oral iron supplements and may be accompanied by changes resembling reactive gastritis. Macrophages laden with iron, on the other hand, are rarely associated with iron pill intake, but result from prior inflammation or mucosal bleeding. Iron deposits in the epithelium of antral and fundic glands is rare and is related to systemic iron overload, e.g. due to multiple blood transfusions or in patients with haemochromatosis, or liver cirrhosis with portal hypertension [39].

Endoscopically, iron-induced injury may present as erythema or yellow-brown discolouration of the mucosa, as well as mucosal defects such as erosions or ulcers [40]. Furthermore, oral iron can also induce pill oesophagitis, as discussed before [41]. Mucosal abnormalities following iron pill administration may be seen within hours. Iron-induced injury and associated symptoms, including nausea and vomiting, epigastric pain or even melaena, disappear after discontinuation of the medication [1].

Microscopically, mucosal erosions contain brown-black granular or fibrillar crystalline material (refractile but non-polarisable), typically overlying the eroded epithelium. Iron depositions may be found in surface epithelium, lamina propria and glands **(Figure 2.5)**, and may be accompanied by giant cells [1,3,39]. Prussian blue stain may be used to enhance the visibility of iron accumulations **(Figure 2.5)**. It also helps in distinguishing iron from other mucosal deposits such as resins [Kayexalate, Sevelamer and bile-acid sequestrants (BAS)] or barium, which is rather golden yellow rather than brown in haematoxylin and eosin (H&E) stained sections [41]. Iron gastropathy may be confused with gastric calcinosis, but this differential diagnosis can be resolved by the subepithelial location of crystalline deposits in gastric calcinosis. Special von Kossa stain may be used to confirm the diagnosis since it stains the calcium-rich deposits black.

Lanthanum carbonate deposition

Lanthanum carbonate [(LC); Fosrenol] is a phosphate binder used for the treatment of hyperphosphataemia in patients with end-stage renal disease (ESRD). It is administered orally and prevents phosphate absorption in the GI tract, thus decreasing the levels of phosphate in plasma [42].

Lanthanum deposits in the GI tract were first described in 2015 [43]. They are most frequently encountered in the stomach, but also in the duodenum [44] and, in sporadic

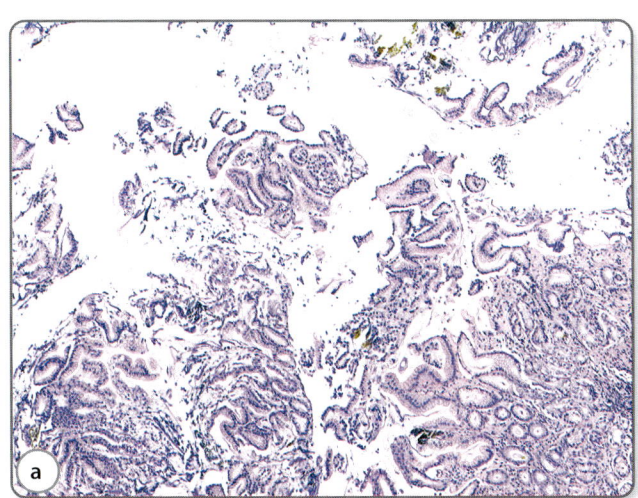

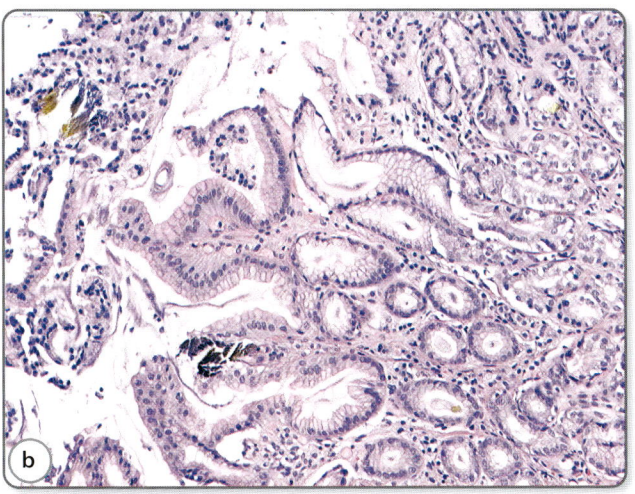

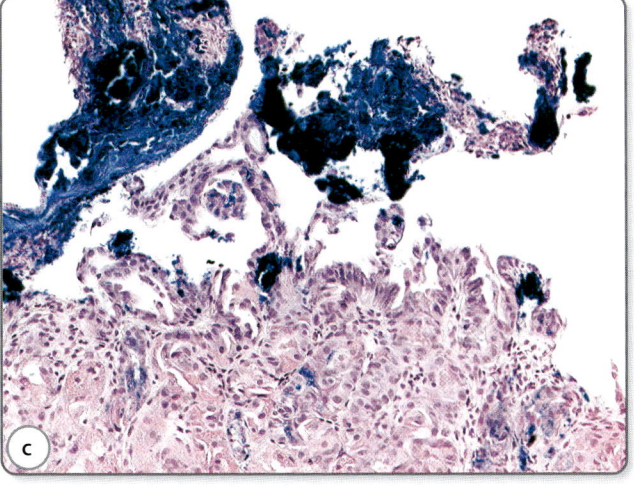

Figure 2.5 Iron gastropathy. (a and b) Antral iron deposits appear as brown to black fibrillar material within the eroded epithelium. (c) Distinct blue appearance of iron in Prussian blue stain.

cases, in the colon [45]. Ban et al found deposits in 71% of gastric and 30% of duodenal bulbus biopsies from patients with ESRD treated with lanthanum carbonate [46].

Coexistence of other pathologic changes in the stomach is common, such as intestinal metaplasia or foveolar hyperplasia. It has been suggested that disruption of the integrity of the gastric or duodenal epithelium increases the susceptibility of the mucosa to lanthanum deposition [46]. This hypothesis fits the observation that chronic renal failure leads to disruption of tight junctions in gastrointestinal epithelia [47].

Endoscopically, lanthanum deposits appear as white lesions [48,49]. The amount of lanthanum deposited depends on the total dose of lanthanum carbonate [50], with 3 months as the shortest reported time between start of LC therapy and a positive biopsy [51]. In most cases, lanthanum deposits are found within 2 years after onset of therapy [46]. At histological examination, the lanthanum deposits consisting of lanthanum and phosphorous appear as amphophilic and yellowish-brown to deep purple granules and rods within macrophages in the lamina propria. The deposits are refractile but non-birefringent under polarised light [46,52].

Lanthanum deposits in histiocytes may be confused with infections and other drug-induced gastrointestinal conditions, notably gastric calcinosis and iron gastropathy. The differential diagnosis in the latter cases can be aided by special stains: von Kossa stain, which is positive in GC but negative in lanthanum deposits, and Prussian blue, which only faintly stains lanthanum deposits in biopsies but is strongly positive in iron deposits [52].

Gastroduodenal ulceration from non-target seed distribution

In selective internal radiation therapy (SIRT), microspheres carrying the β-emitter [90]Yttrium are injected into the hepatic artery to target non-resectable liver metastases or hepatocellular carcinoma [23,53]. Normal liver cells derive most of their blood supply from the portal vein, but neoplasms receive their main blood supply through the hepatic artery, which allows for the [90]Yttrium to selectively target cancer cells and reduces the risk of radiation hepatitis [23,54]. However, microspheres may also be carried to other vessels and reach the stomach, duodenum or pancreas, inducing injuries in these organs. In the stomach, this complication affects 3–24% of SIRT treated patients [54,55]. Symptoms vary and include nausea and vomiting, abdominal pain, weight loss, diarrhoea or GI bleeding [54,55].

Microscopically, the pathognomonic feature of SIRT-related radiation injury is the presence of microspheres in the lamina propria and submucosa (**Figure 2.6**). The microspheres are jet black, round and consist of glass with a diameter of 20–30 μm or resin with a diameter of 20–40 μm [54,56]. In addition, signs of radiation gastritis may be present, including hyalinisation of the lamina propria with occasional ectatic vessels and cellular atypia in all layers of the mucosa (**Figure 2.6**) [23,57]. Persistent gastric ulcers that are non-responsive to antacid therapy also occur and are thought to develop due to chronic ischaemia resulting from radiation-induced vascular damage. In support of this hypothesis, mucosa with [90]Yttrium deposits shows decreased vascular density and vessels often show signs of damage [56]. Similar changes can also be encountered in biopsies from patients treated with hepatic arterial infusion chemotherapy (HAIC) for colon carcinoma. These changes may be confused with gastric dysplasia or early gastric carcinoma. Main diagnostic clues supporting the diagnosis of radiation damage include preservation of the architecture, accentuation of atypia in basal parts of the glands, low nuclear-cytoplasmic ratio, sparse mitoses, cytoplasmatic eosinophilia, and vacuolisation and atypia of endothelial cells and fibroblasts [58].

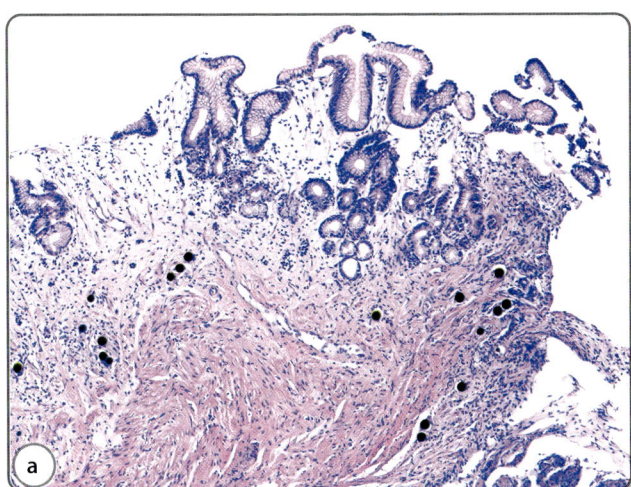

Figure 2.6 Selective internal radiation therapy. (a and b) Cardia biopsies with hyalinised lamina propria and dark purple 90Yttrium microspheres. (c and d) Antrum mucosa with lamina propria hyalinisation, focal loss of glands, reactive epithelial changes, prominent ectatic vessels and dark purple microspheres.
Continues overleaf

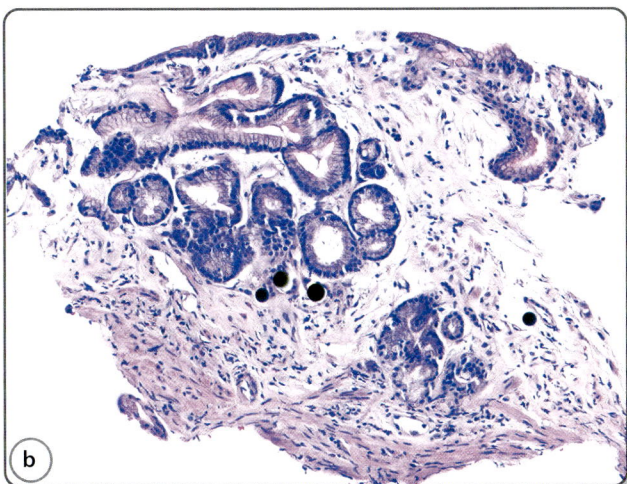

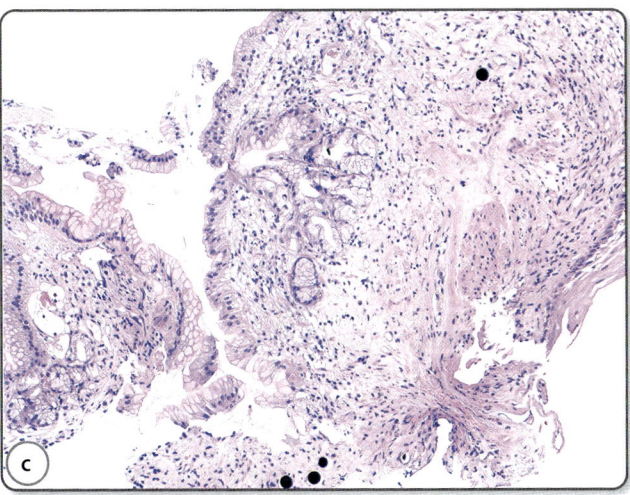

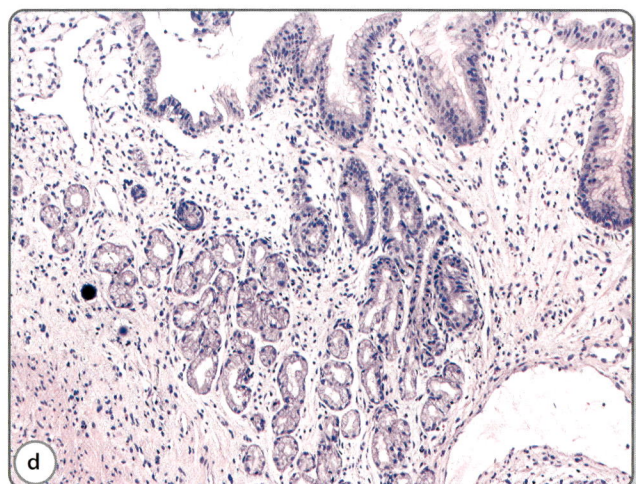

Figure 2.6 *Continued.*

DRUG-RELATED CHANGES OF THE LOWER GASTROINTESTINAL TRACT

Iatrogenic colitis

Microscopic colitis

Drug-induced microscopic colitis (MC) has been described in association with a variety of medications, including NSAIDs [59–61], SSRIs [61], lansoprazole [35,36], ranitidine [62], ticlopidine [63], flutamide, gold salts, bentazepam and carbamazepine [64].

The most common symptom is chronic diarrhoea, followed by weight loss and abdominal pain [59]. Usually, symptoms disappear and the mucosa returns to normal after cessation of the causative drug.

Endoscopic findings in MC are as a rule inconspicuous. Microscopically, MC is subdivided into collagenous colitis and lymphocytic colitis, which are most likely different stages in the development of the same condition. The prognosis and treatment do not differ between these two entities. Collagenous colitis has been associated in particular with NSAIDs and lansoprazole, while lymphocytic colitis has mostly been associated with ranitidine, ticlopidine or carbamazepine [65].

The main diagnostic feature is preserved architecture with an increased cell count in the lamina propria (**Figure 2.7**). The surface epithelium is often flattened and may be detached from the surface. In collagenous colitis, there is a distinct band of collagen beneath the epithelium, which is irregular and measures >10 μm in thickness (**Figure 2.7**). In lymphocytic colitis, this subepithelial collagen deposit is absent, while intraepithelial lymphocytosis is more pronounced, with >20 intraepithelial lymphocytes (IELs) per 100 epithelial cells (**Figure 2.8**).

The differential diagnoses include inflammatory bowel disease (which as a rule shows abnormal mucosal architecture), acute infectious colitis (which lacks IELs and a thick subepithelial collagen band), ischaemic colitis (which lacks IELs while ischaemic mucosal changes are prominent) and radiation colitis (which typically shows telangiectasia and atypia of fibroblasts and endothelial cells) [1,66].

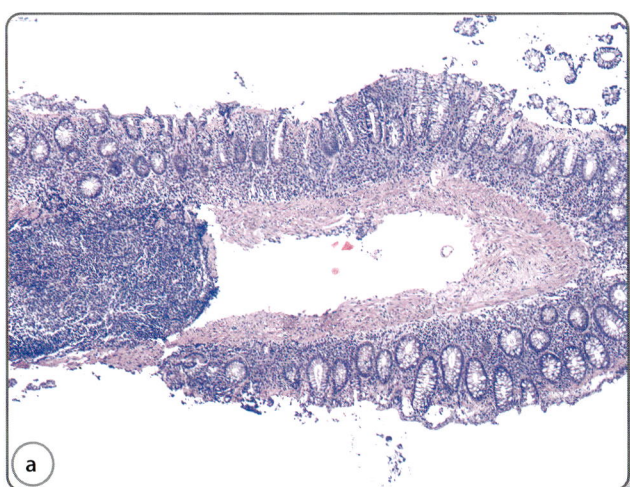

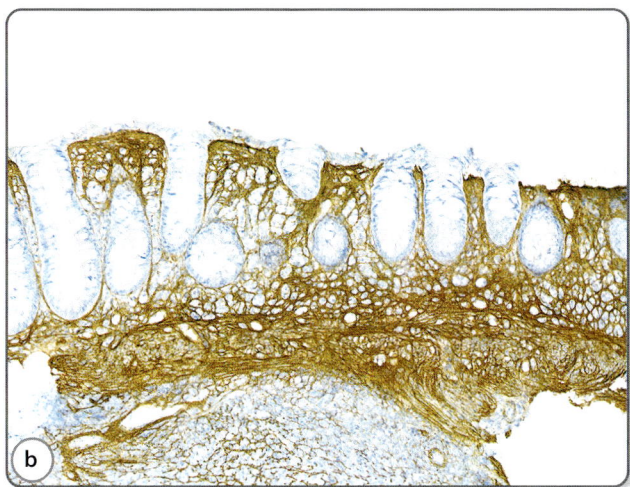

Figure 2.7 Collagenous colitis. (a) Subepithelial collagen is thickened and entraps fibroblasts and capillaries, the lamina propria is expanded by an inflammatory infiltrate, eosinophils are usually prominent. (b) Tenascin immunohistochemistry highlights the thick subepithelial collagen band.

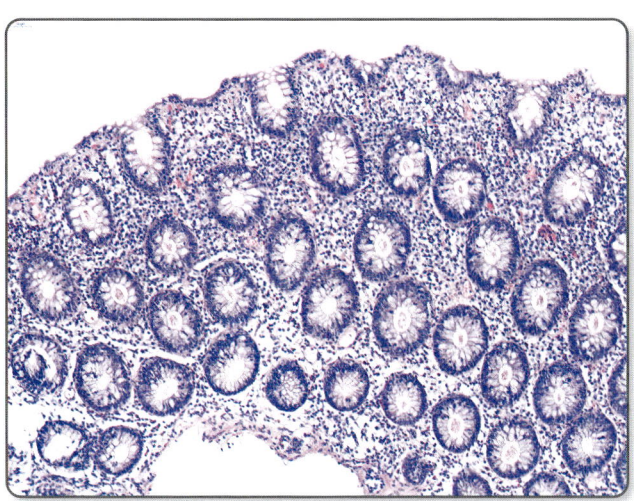

Figure 2.8 Lymphocytic colitis. Colon mucosa with preserved architecture, an increased cell count in the lamina propria, flattened surface epithelium and significant intraepithelial lymphocytosis.

Ischaemic colitis

Bowel ischaemia has been described in association with a variety of drugs. Pathogenetic mechanisms vary according to the drug: catecholamines, cocaine, digitalis and ergotamines induce vasospasm, which reduces intestinal blood flow [12,67,68]. Oestrogen and progesterone increase the risk of thrombosis, which may partially or totally occlude intestinal vasculature [69,70]. Diuretics reduce blood volume which will increase the risk of bowel ischaemia, especially if given in combination with the aforementioned drugs [12].

Patients with ischaemic colitis typically present with abdominal pain, hematochezia, emesis and fever [1,20]. Endoscopically, the mucosa appears pale and oedematous; in severe cases, petechiae, ulcerations and, occasionally, pseudomembranes can be seen [71].

Also, on histologic examination, pseudomembranes and haemorrhages are often observed and, depending on the aetiology, thrombi may be found in the small vessels [66]. The most important features of ischaemic colitis are withered crypts with necrosis at the surface but intact at the crypt base with oedema and haemorrhage and later on haemosiderin in the lamina propria (**Figure 2.9**). There are typically few if any

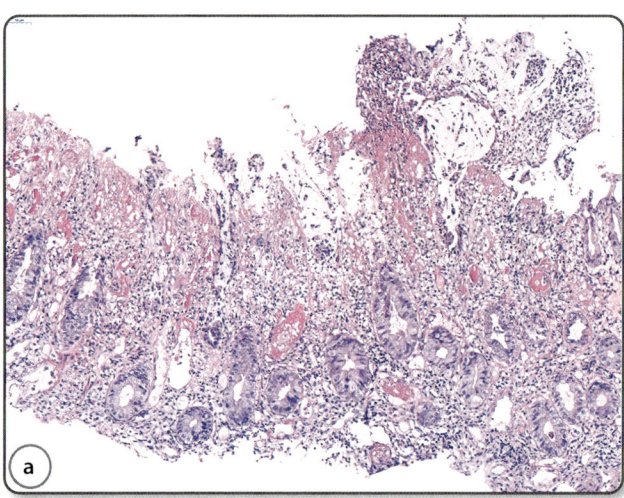

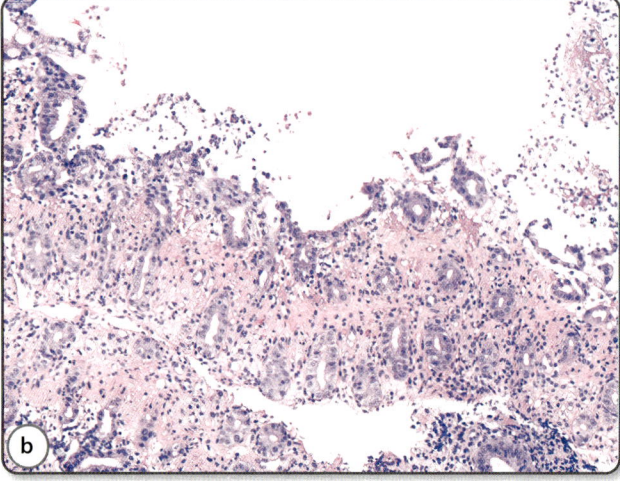

Figure 2.9 Ischaemic colitis. (a and b) Colon mucosa with withered crypts and necrosis at the upper part, scattered inflammatory cells, regenerative changes at the crypt base and hyalinisation of the lamina propria.

inflammatory infiltrates. Regenerative changes may be seen at the crypt base that might mimic dysplasia. In chronic cases, hyalinisation of the lamina propria develops [1,12].

Clinical history is always extremely important, as the cause of ischaemic changes found in the biopsy frequently cannot be determined based only on microscopic appearance. Differential diagnoses include infectious colitis due to *C. difficile* or enterohaemorrhagic *E. coli* and radiation colitis. The latter can be identified by the presence of hyalinised dilated vessels, and atypical fibroblasts and epithelial cells. Localisation in the right colon and presence of fibrin thrombi are hints for *E. coli* infection [1,66]. *C. difficile* colitis with pseudomembranes can be difficult to differentiate from ischaemic colitis but helpful features that support a diagnosis of pseudomembranous colitis are a diffuse process (ischaemia is typically localised) and absence of withered crypts, lamina propria haemorrhage and hyalinisation (further discussed later on). As a rule, pathogen detection is necessary for the confirmation of infection colitis.

Pneumatosis coli

Pneumatosis coli, also known as *pneumatosis cystoides intestinalis*, is a condition characterised by the presence of multiple gas cysts in the submucosa and/or subserosa of the bowel wall. The cysts are often surrounded by histiocytes, giant cells or eosinophils and may look like adipocytes [1]. Some patients present with abdominal symptoms, but most are asymptomatic. The disease is usually self-limiting but may be associated with pneumoperitoneum, which often requires invasive treatment [72]. Pneumatosis coli can develop secondary to infections and often has iatrogenic etiology [1], including endoscopy, surgery and medications. Drugs associated with pneumatosis coli are alpha-glucosidase inhibitors (miglitol, voglibose and acarbose, antidiabetic drugs inhibiting the degradation of carbohydrates into glucose in the GI tract [73,74] and sunitinib (a tyrosine-kinase inhibitor used to treat different kinds of cancer) [72]. Pneumatosis coli has also been reported following treatment with lactulose [75,76], immunosuppressants, steroids [77,78] and drugs associated with ischaemic colitis [1].

Melanosis coli

Melanosis coli is the microscopic finding of brown to black pigment in the mucosa of the colon or rectum. Endoscopically, this condition can present as a very dramatic brown discolouration of the bowel mucosa. Contrary to its name, the pigment is lipofuscin (not melanin) [79]. It is a product of the oxidation of unsaturated fatty acids in cell membranes of apoptotic colonic mucosal epithelium that accumulates in lamina propria macrophages [80]. Melanosis coli is most frequently associated with the use of anthranoid laxatives like senna or cascara sagrada, which directly induce apoptosis of the epithelial cells. Other factors that increase apoptosis of colonic epithelium may also lead to accumulation of lipofuscin in the mucosa [81].

On microscopic examination of rectal biopsies, melanosis coli has been found in over 70% of patients consuming anthranoid laxatives and over 25% of other patients with constipation [82]. Patients usually present with constipation, but the condition does not lead to any symptoms or adverse effects and usually resolves within a year (but often only weeks) after discontinuation of laxative use [1].

Macroscopically, brown to black discolourations occur in the whole colon (**Figure 2.10**), and occasionally the ileum, appendix or even regional lymph nodes may be involved. Small areas without discolouration, presumably because of underlying lymphoid follicles, result

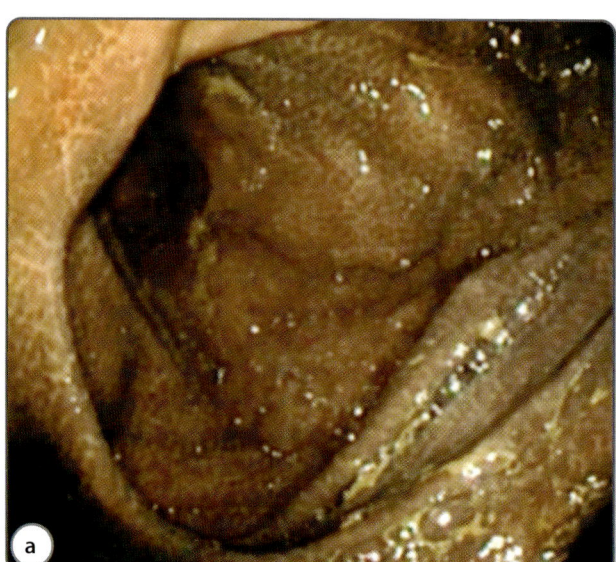

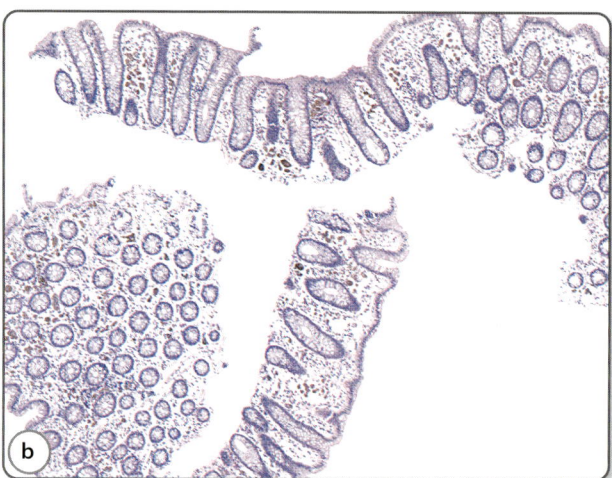

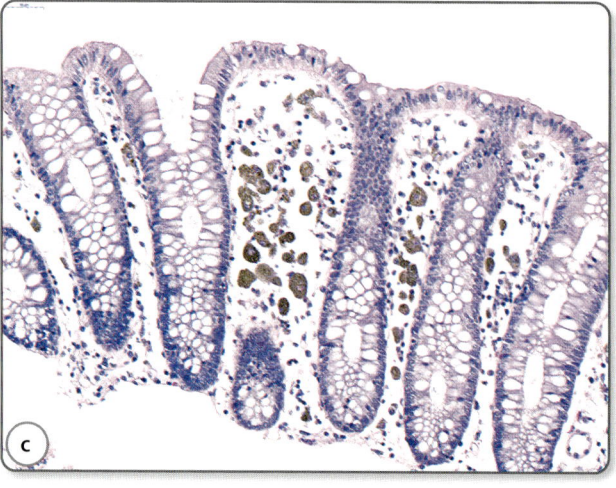

Figure 2.10 Melanosis coli. (a) Endoscopic image shows brown discolouration of the bowel mucosa. (b and c) Note the brown-black pigment in the macrophages.

in an appearance of a "starry sky". Increased epithelial apoptosis can also be found [80,81]. Such brown to black pigmentations correspond to lipofuscin-containing macrophages in the lamina propria and can sometimes be encountered in biopsies from an endoscopically normal colon (**Figure 2.10**) [1].

Differential diagnoses include iron depositions due to gastrointestinal bleeding or iron overload in patients with haemosiderosis or haemochromatosis; these are Prussian blue positive, while staining for fat component of lipofuscin (by Sudan Black B) is negative. Furthermore, tattoo ink or accumulations of actual melanin may mimic melanosis coli. Finally, brown bowel syndrome should be considered; in this condition the pigment responsible for the discolouration consists of lipofuscin but it is located in the smooth muscle of the entire GI tract, while the mucosa is normal [1].

Colonoscopy-related injuries

While colonoscopy itself may cause mechanical trauma to the colonic and rectal mucosa, chemical injury in the GI tract due to bowel preparation medications or endoscope disinfectant has also been described as an additional, be it lesser known complication of this procedure.

Glutaraldehyde

Glutaraldehyde 2% solution is used to disinfect endoscopes. It may induce ischaemic proctitis or colitis upon contact with the mucosa within 24–48 hours after colonoscopy. This can be prevented by properly rinsing endoscopes after disinfection or use of other disinfectant agents [3,83].

Sodium phosphate (OsmoPrep)

Sodium phosphate solution, a commonly prescribed oral bowel preparation before colonoscopy, may lead to focal active colitis characterised by a single focus or multiple foci of neutrophilic infiltration without any signs of chronic inflammation [23]. Other findings in the colon include increased crypt apoptosis (*apoptotic enteropathy*) as well as aphthoid lesions and erosions [84,85].

When administered in solid form, i.e. as a pill, sodium phosphate may induce – in addition to colonic injury – chemical gastritis mimicking gastric calcinosis and iron gastropathy. Deposits of sodium phosphate in the lamina propria are purple or black, <100 µm in diameter and von Kossa stain positive. Sodium phosphate-induced gastropathy can be distinguished from calcinosis using alizarine red stain, which is positive in calcinosis but does not stain sodium phosphate [86].

Angiotensin-II receptor blocker-associated enteropathy

Angiotensin-II receptor blockers (ARBs or sartans) are frequently used to treat hypertension [87]. In rare cases, sartans induce a severe gastrointestinal condition called "sprue-like enteropathy" (SLE) [88,89]. Most described cases of SLE are associated with the use of olmesartan, hence the name "olmesartan-associated enteropathy" is often used as a synonym for SLE; yet SLE has also been associated with irbesartan [90,91], telmisartan [92], losartan [93], valsartan [94], and eprosartan [95]. In our practice, we encountered a case of spure-like enteropathy associated with candesartan (**Figure 2.11**).

Patients present with diarrhoea and weight loss; additional symptoms may include nausea, vomiting, fatigue, abdominal pain and bloating. In duodenal biopsies, total to

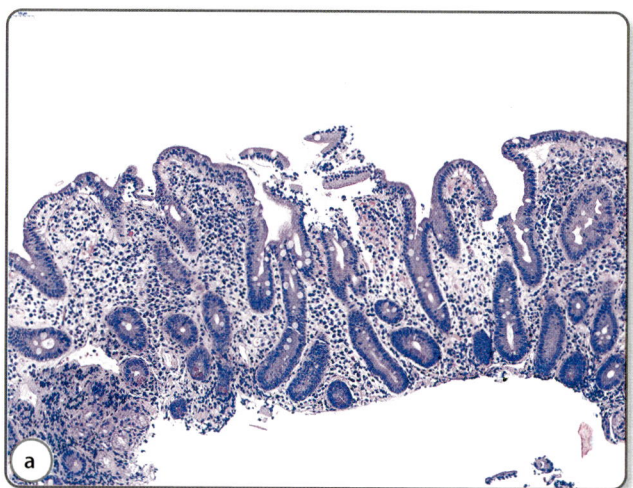

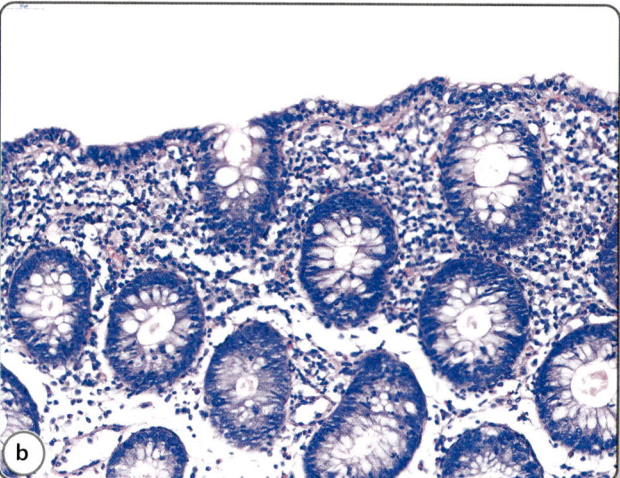

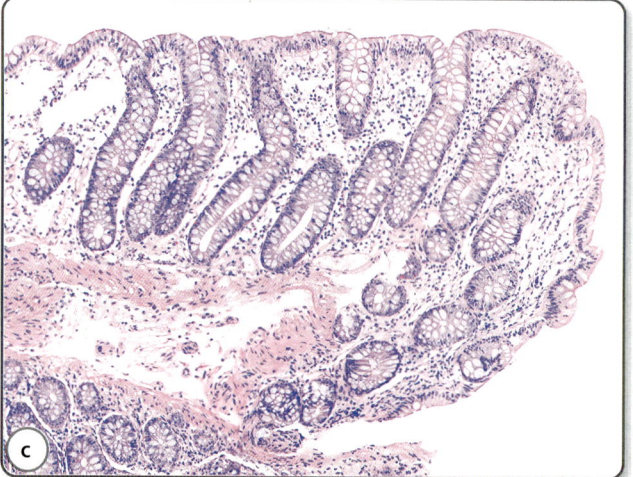

Figure 2.11 Sartans. (a) Case of candesartan-associated sprue-like enteropathy with villous blunting, crypt hyperplasia and intraepithelial lymphocytosis in a duodenal biopsy. (b) Intraepithelial lymphocytosis, flattened surface epithelium and focal active inflammation in the colon mucosa of the same patient. (c and d) Olmesartan-associated inflammation of the colon mucosa with intraepithelial lymphocytosis. (e and f) In comparison: Marsh 3b coeliac disease showing a higher degree of villous atrophy in the duodenum with significant intraepithelial lymphocytosis. *Continues opposite*

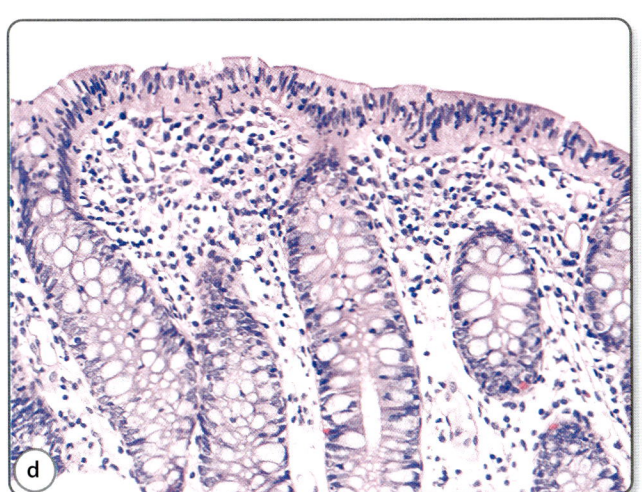

Figure 2.11 *Continued.*

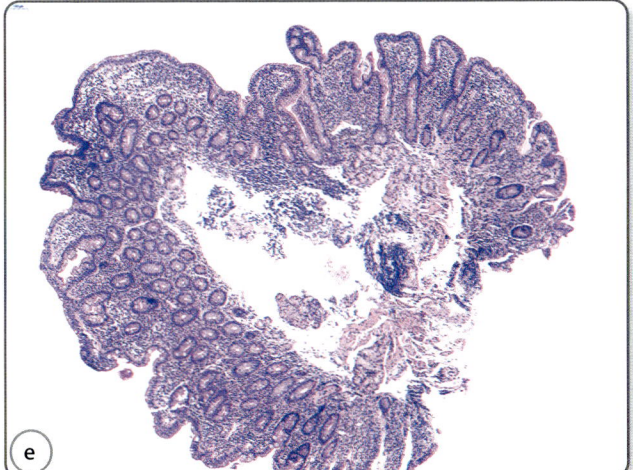

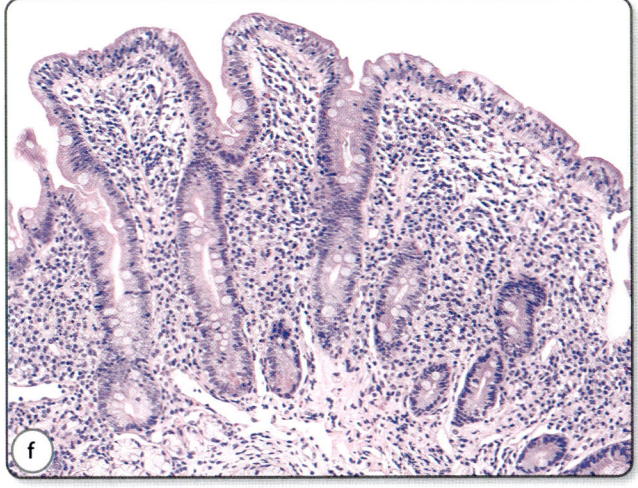

partial atrophy of villi is present in almost every case (**Figure 2.11**). Furthermore, an active inflammatory infiltrate can be seen and an increase of intraepithelial lymphocytes is present in two-thirds of cases (**Figure 2.11**) [88,96]. Sometimes, a thick band of collagen beneath the epithelial layer can be found, resembling collagenous sprue. Clinically and histologically, the condition resembles coeliac disease (**Figure 2.8**), but patients are older, tissue transglutaminase IgA is negative and a gluten-free diet has no effect [88]. Treatment with steroids and immunosuppressants augments symptoms [91]. The best therapy for SLE is discontinuation of ARB use. In addition, in one study 68% of the patients were HLA-DQ2 positive, which is significantly higher than the general population (which tends to be 25–30%), suggesting that people with this haplotype might be at a higher risk to develop severe adverse effects in the GI tract after ARB treatment [88].

In addition to coeliac disease and collagenous sprue, differential diagnoses for SLE include autoimmune enteropathy, tropical sprue, Crohn's disease and mycophenolate toxicity [97], which will be discussed later on. In addition to SLE, collagenous gastritis, ileitis and colitis have also been associated with sartan use in some cases, disappearing after stopping treatment with the drug [88,98]. A list of drugs causing small bowel intraepithelial lymphocytosis with or without villous atrophy mimicking coeliac disease is shown in **Box 2.1**.

Pancreatic enzyme replacement with methacrylic acid

Children with cystic fibrosis receiving pancreatic enzyme replacement containing methacrylic acid have been reported to develop fibrosing colonopathy. The severity varied from localised strictures in the right colon to stenoses affecting the entire colon with cobblestone appearance. Histologically, biopsies showed active or chronic inflammation, interruption of the muscularis mucosae, submucosal fibrosis and a thick muscularis propria. Presumably, these changes are caused by an allergic reaction to methacrylic acid, which is supported by the finding of an increased number of eosinophils and mast cells in biopsies and the absence of fibrosing colonopathy in patients treated with newer pancreatic enzyme preparations without the allergenic compound [99–101].

Intravenous cyclosporin

Cyclosporin inhibits the production of cytokines that regulate T-cell activation, especially IL-2 [102]. It is used as treatment for a variety of autoimmune diseases and may be indicated to treat steroid-refractory ulcerative colitis (UC) [103].

Box 2.1 Drugs causing small bowel intraepithelial lymphocytosis with or without villous atrophy mimicking coeliac disease.

- Check-point inhibitors (e.g. ipilimumab, ipilimumab/nivolumab, pembrolizumab)
- Angiotensin-II receptor blockers (e.g. olmesartan, valsartan, candesartan)
- Idelalisib
- Non-steroidal anti-inflammatory drugs
- Proton pump inhibitors (e.g. lansoprazole)
- Ticlopidine
- Histamine H2-receptor antagonists (e.g. ranitidine, cimetidine)

In colectomy specimens of patients with UC, histological changes such as epithelial regeneration and villous transformation were more often seen and more severe in patients treated with intravenous cyclosporin prior to surgery than in patients who received only intravenous corticosteroids.

Lack of maturation of epithelial cells towards the upper levels of the crypts following intravenous cyclosporin therapy needs to be differentiated from dysplasia: the cytoplasmic-to-nuclear ratio is higher compared to dysplasia and there is at least some level of nuclear maturation towards the surface [104].

Idelalisib

Idelalisib selectively inhibits the delta isoform of oncogenic phosphoinositide 3-kinase (PI3K), which is almost exclusively expressed in haematopoietic cells. This drug is approved for the treatment of relapsed or refractory chronic lymphocytic leukaemia (CLL) and certain types of non-Hodgkin lymphoma (i.e. follicular lymphoma and small lymphocytic lymphoma) [105,106].

The most commonly reported side effect of idelalisib is watery diarrhoea, affecting up to 46% of patients and 20% to a severe degree [107]. When diarrhoea occurs early on after starting the treatment this might not be taken as drug toxicity and can be treated symptomatically. However, late-onset diarrhoea is usually a sign of idelalisib-induced enterocolitis and requires termination of the treatment [106,108].

Microscopically, the features of idelalisib-induced colitis include apoptosis of colonic epithelial cells, an increased number of intraepithelial lymphocytes, neutrophilic inflammatory infiltrate and crypt abscesses, as well as distortion of crypt architecture and, in some cases, dilated and damaged crypts with luminal debris (**Figure 2.12**) [107,109]. In addition, idelalisib induces alterations in the small bowel that may resemble coeliac disease with villous atrophy, intraepithelial lymphocytosis and crypt apoptosis.

Important differential diagnoses to keep in mind when evaluating biopsies in this setting are, in addition to coeliac disease, GvHD, bacterial or cytomegalovirus (CMV) infection, autoimmune enteropathy, inflammatory bowel disease and toxicity of other drugs such as mycophenolate, which will be discussed later [109].

Iatrogenic enterocolitis

NSAID-associated enterocolitis

Non-steroidal anti-inflammatory drugs are known to induce a variety of pathologic changes throughout the entire GI tract, and we have already discussed most of them, notably pill oesophagitis, reactive gastropathy and several forms of colitis, including microscopic, ischaemic and focal active colitis. NSAID-induced erosions and ulcers are very common and can be present in any part of the GI tract (**Figure 2.13**) [14]. In the colon, these ulcers are typically right sided; in the stomach, ulcers are usually located in the antrum, while erosions are found mostly in the corpus [12].

In the small intestine, villous atrophy and intraepithelial lymphocytosis have been associated with NSAID exposure; the combination of these findings in the duodenum can mimic coeliac disease [14,110]. In general, NSAID-induced changes display rather little inflammation, probably due to the drugs' anti-inflammatory properties [13].

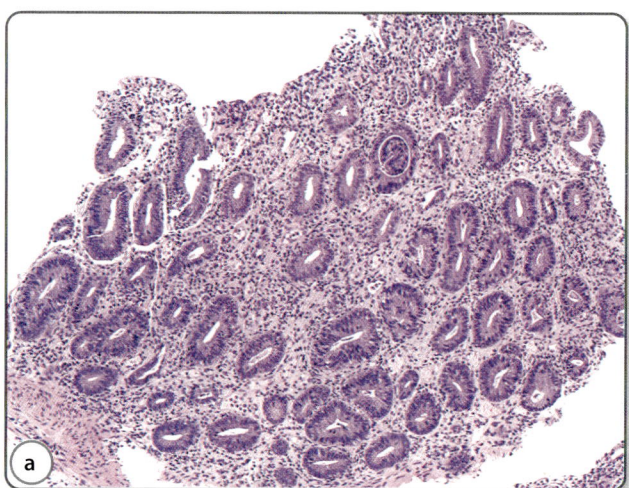

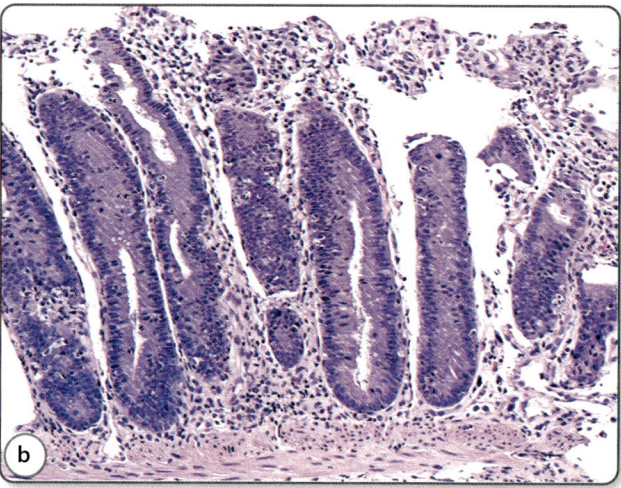

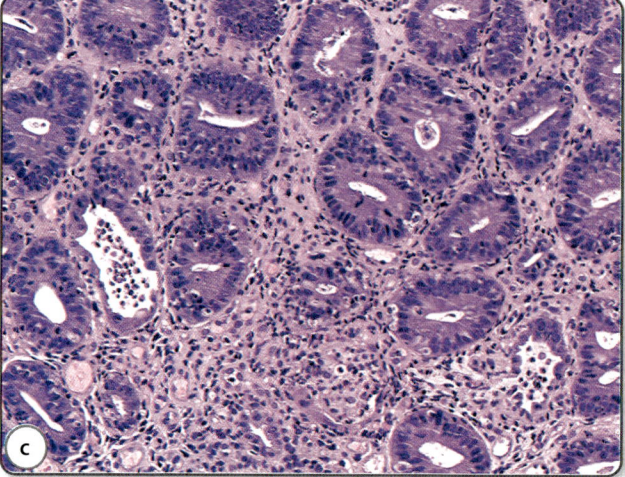

Figure 2.12 Idelalisib-associated colitis. (a to c) Colon biopsies showing increased number of intraepithelial lymphocytes and apoptosis of epithelial cells, accompanied by active inflammatory infiltrate and some damaged crypts.

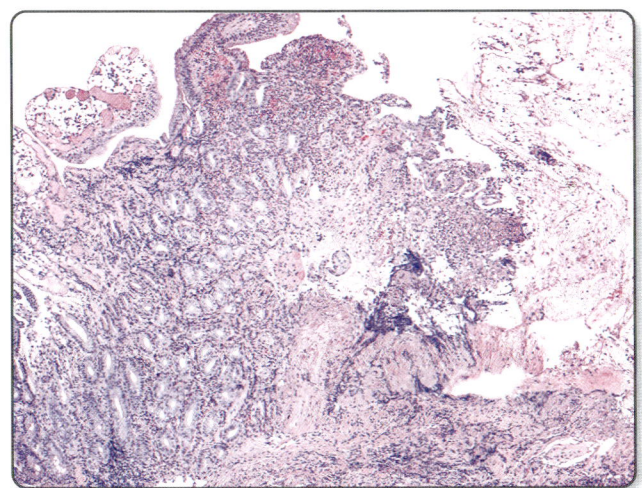

Figure 2.13 Duodenal ulcer associated with non-steroidal anti-inflammatory drug use.

Diaphragm disease

Diaphragm disease is defined by the presence of multiple circular stenoses in the small bowel, usually of short length, and affects up to 2% of long-term NSAID users. In some cases, it occurred 2 months after onset of NSAID therapy. Patients present with symptoms such as bowel obstruction and gastrointestinal bleeding [111,112].

The diaphragms are of different height and width and consist of mucosa, muscularis mucosae and submucosa. The tips of the diaphragms are often ulcerated and the mucosal parts surrounding these ulcers show architectural distortion, villous atrophy and reactive epithelial changes (hyperplasia with basophilia and an increased number of mitoses). Although there is no severe inflammatory infiltrate, an accumulation of mononuclear cells, neutrophils and eosinophils is present at the diaphragm tips. Focal inflammation and villous atrophy may also occur in the mucosa between the diaphragms [113,114].

Resin-associated lesions

Resins are orally administered drugs that bind other molecules in the GI tract, impeding their absorption. Depositions of resin crystals, such as kayexalate, sevelamer and BASs, have been described in all parts of the GI tract, often in association with inflammation, ischaemia and necrosis or stromal fibrosis and mucosal defects. In the case of kayexalate, it has been proven that the resin directly causes these changes [13].

Sodium polystyrene sulphonate [(SPS), kayexalate] is administered *per os* or as an enema, and exchanges sodium ions with potassium during its GI transit, leading to increased faecal potassium excretion in patients with hyperkalaemia due to chronic kidney failure [115]. SPS is usually administered in a sorbitol suspension, a combination that causes ischaemia and necrosis in the intestine, especially the colon and ileum [116,117]. The mortality of this severe adverse effect is around 30% and although previously believed to be primarily caused by sorbitol, cases of bowel ischaemia have also been described following exposure to sorbitol-free SPS preparations [118]. Furthermore, kayexalate causes mucosal injuries in the upper GI tract [119].

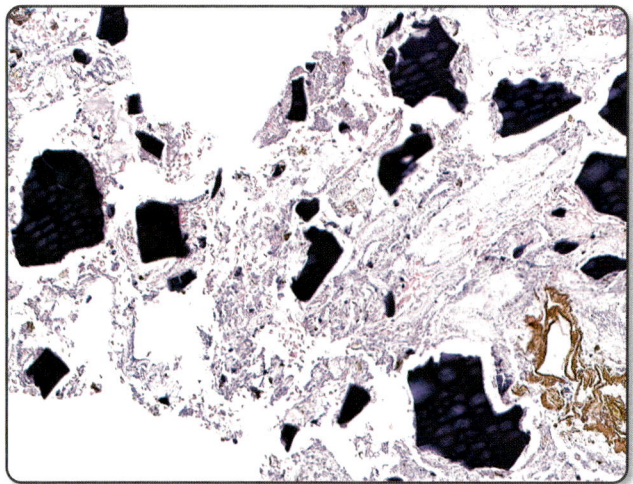

Figure 2.14 Kayexalate crystals: Note the purple colour with "fish-scale-like" appearance.

Sodium polystyrene sulphonate crystals are 10–200 μm in size, lightly basophilic in colour, refractile and non-polarisable, have a mosaic or fish-scale pattern and an angulated shape **(Figure 2.14)**. The crystals are usually found on the surface of the ischaemic mucosa or within ulcerations or debris, but presence of kayexalate crystals without any associated pathology is also possible [119].

Sevelamer, like SPS, is a cation-exchange resin used in patients with chronic kidney failure. It binds dietary phosphate in the GI tract, lowering serum phosphate levels. Depositions of sevelamer crystals are most frequently found in the colon but can also occur in the oesophagus and small bowel [120]. Sevelamer has been associated with gastrointestinal mucosal injury and inflammation **(Figure 2.12)** and a causative relation has been suggested [121].

Just like SPS, sevelamer crystals are non-polarisable and have a fish-scale pattern **(Figures 2.12 and 2.15)**. The centre of the crystals is of pink colour, while the periphery is yellow. Sevelamer depositions embedded within GI injury change their colour to red or brown [120].

Bile-acid sequestrant-associated lesions

Cholestyramine, colesevelam and colestipol are all BASs used to treat dyslipidaemia. BAS exchange chloride ions with bile acids, interrupting enterohepatic circulation which leads to a decrease in serum cholesterol.

Crystals of all three types of BASs look the same in histology sections: they are eosinophilic, polygonal structures that lack the fish-scale appearance of kayexalate and sevelamer. Although BAS depositions may occur in inflamed or damaged tissue, they do not harm the gastrointestinal mucosa directly. Yet, identifying BAS correctly is important, as they may be confused with other resins [122].

The use of different stains can help in the differentiation: while BAS is grey or pink in PAS stain, SPS is magenta and sevelamer is purple [120]. In slides stained according to Ziehl–Neelsen for acid fast bacilli, BAS is yellow, SPS is black and sevelamer is magenta. [122].

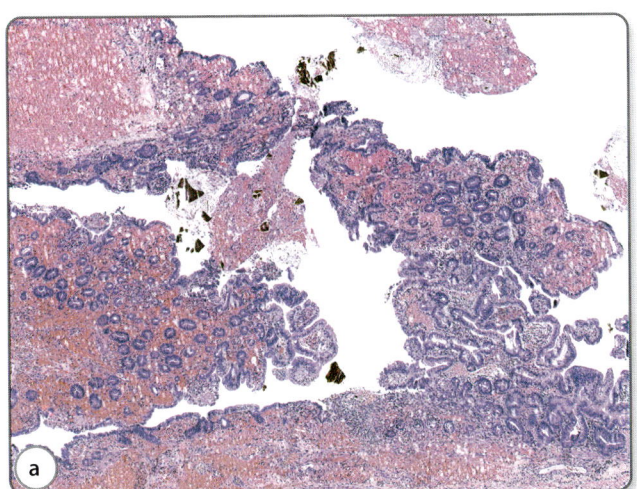

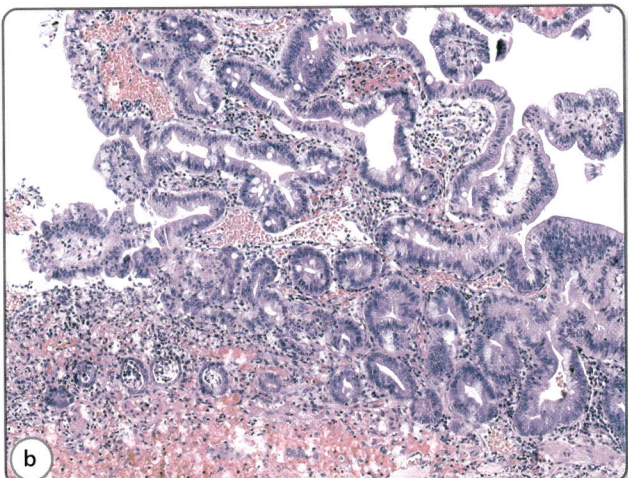

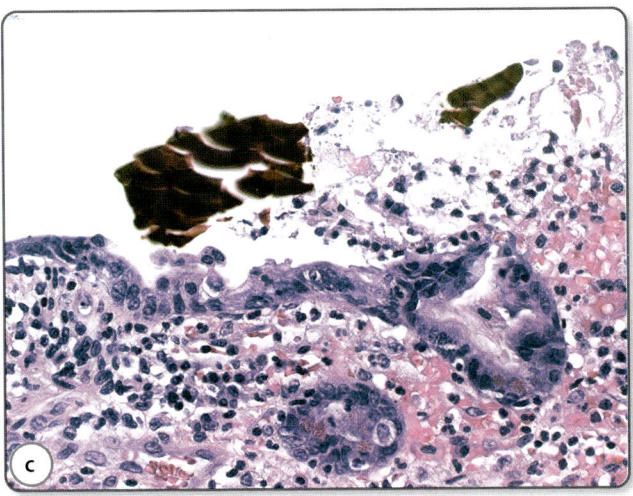

Figure 2.15 Sevelamer crystals and associated mucosal injury. (a) Colon resection with mucosal injury, regenerative epithelial changes and haemorrhage with necrotic debris and sevelamer crystals in lumen. (b) Higher power showing regenerative changes of the epithelium. (c) Characteristic two-toned crystals with "fish scales".

Pill stabiliser (filler)-associated lesions

Pill stabilisers or fillers [crospovidone and microcrystalline cellulose (MCC)] are inactive substances incorporated into medications to facilitate drug delivery. They are common, biologically inert, and most frequently found in the small bowel (they can, however, be found in any specimen from the GI tract – also in biopsies without pathological changes). Crospovidone is non-birefringent, coral-shaped and pink in the centre, surrounded by purple colour (**Figure 2.16**). In contrast, MCC is birefringent, clear and crystals have a matchstick shape (**Figure 2.16**) [123].

Antibiotics-associated lesions

Use of antibiotics can disrupt the normal protective bowel flora through overgrowth of pathogenic micro-organisms and result in a spectrum of histological changes.

Penicillin derivatives occasionally cause bloody diarrhoea 2–7 days after onset of therapy; this is a symptom of acute antibiotic-associated colitis that is often caused by *Klebsiella oxytoca* infection. This form of haemorrhagic colitis is localised mainly in the right colon and endoscopy shows oedema, haemorrhage and, in some cases, defects of the colonic mucosa [124,125].

The microscopic picture of this entity has similarities with ischaemic colitis and focal active colitis, as hyalinisation of the lamina propria, neutrophilic infiltration with cryptitis and mucosal haemorrhage are seen. In addition, haemorrhage in the lamina propria, increased number of apoptotic bodies and reactive atypia of epithelial cells with micropapillary protrusions with loss of goblet cells is observed (**Figure 2.17**). Discontinuation of penicillin usually leads to complete recovery [124,126].

Pseudomembranous colitis (PMC) is a well-known form of antibiotics-associated colitis named after the distinct endoscopic appearance of yellow-whitish plaques on the surface of the colon mucosa. It is most commonly caused by *Clostridioides difficile* infection following treatment with broad-spectrum antibiotics [127,128].

Pseudomembranous colitis is the most severe form of *C. difficile* infection with symptoms ranging from diarrhoea and abdominal pain to fever and blood in the stool [129]. Three different microscopic patterns reflecting different severity of inflammation have been described by Price et al [128]. In the first and mildest form, inflammation is limited to the epithelium between glands and the adjacent lamina propria. The second pattern is characterised by disrupted colonic glands with epithelial debris, mucus and fibrin exudate at the top, forming pseudomembranes (**Figure 2.18**). In the third form, complete mucosal necrosis with thick pseudomembranes at the surface is seen (**Figure 2.18**).

While *C. difficile* infection is the most common cause of PMC and should therefore always be excluded before looking at other causes, similar morphology can also occasionally be seen in collagenous colitis (as described earlier), *Behçet's* disease, ischaemic colitis, IBD and other infections such as those caused by *Salmonella*, *Shigella*, *S. aureus*, *E. coli*, or cytomegalovirus [127,130].

Upper GI tract injuries can be induced by oral antibiotics such as mentioned before, including tetracycline, doxycycline and clindamycin especially in the context of pill oesophagitis and chemical gastropathy.

Doxycycline has an exceptional position among the drugs associated with these injuries, as it causes distinct vascular changes. Xiao et al [131] reported two patients with epigastric pain following oral doxycycline therapy: both patients were diagnosed with reactive gastropathy, but biopsies showed superficial necrosis and vascular degeneration

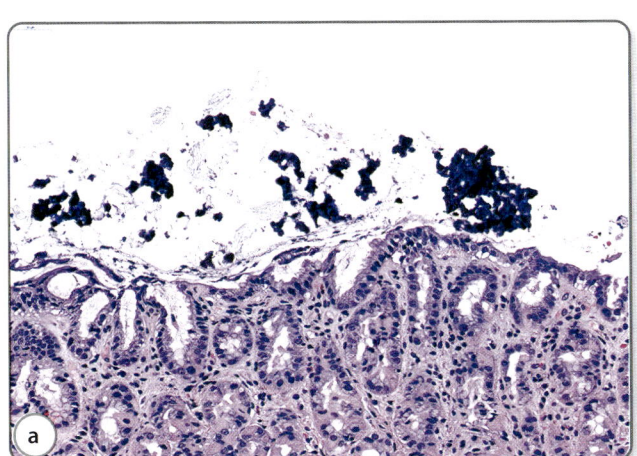

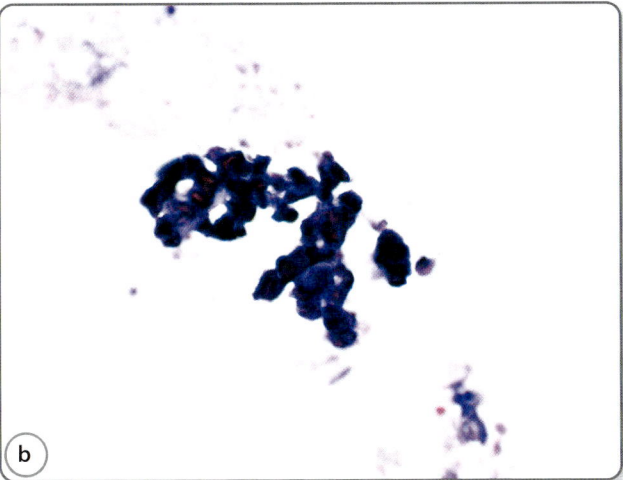

Figure 2.16 Crospovidone deposits. (a and b) Coral-shaped crystals with a pink centre and purple margin. (c) MCC deposits: Clear, matchstick-shaped crystals.

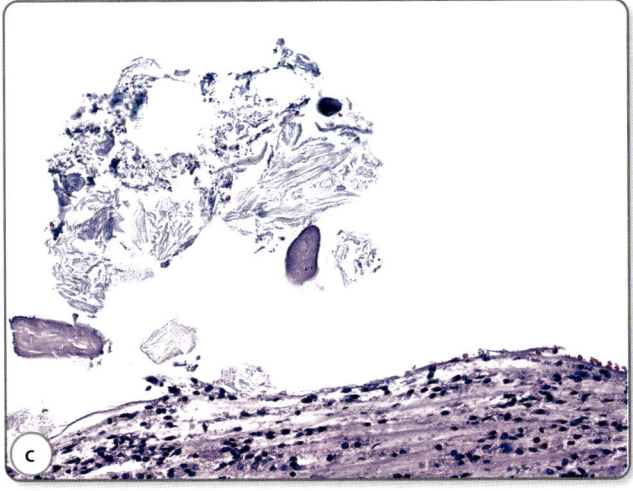

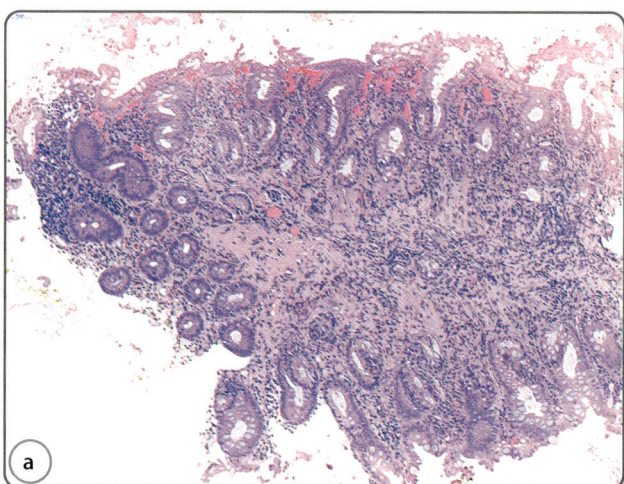

Figure 2.17 Haemorrhagic colitis due to *Klebsiella oxytoca* infection. (a to c) Increased apoptosis and reactive atypia of colonic epithelial cells with micropapillary protrusions and loss of goblet cells, lamina propria haemorrhage and moderate inflammation. Courtesy of Prof G Gorkiewicz, Medical University of Graz.

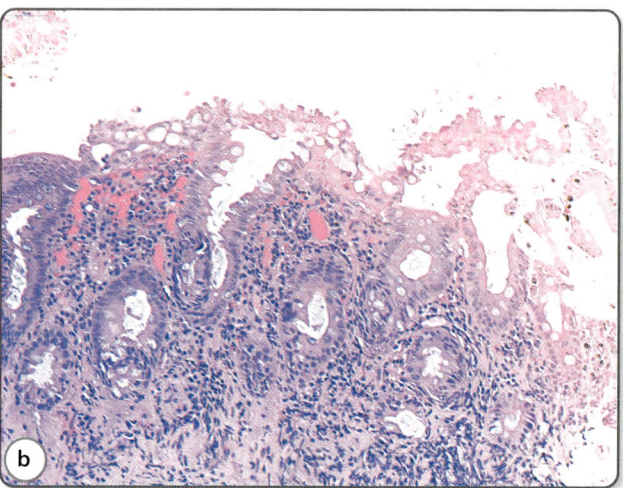

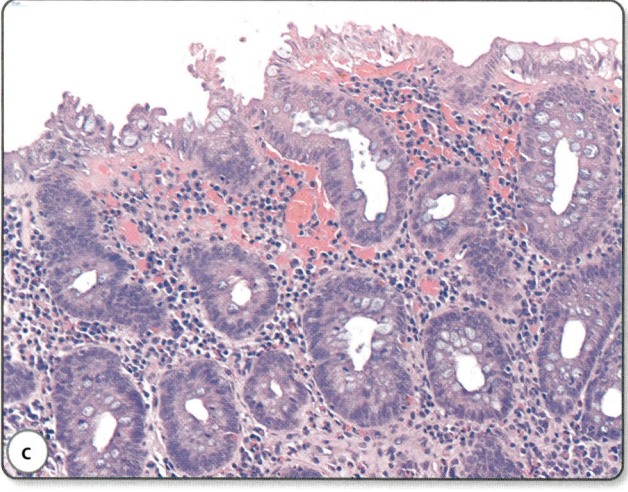

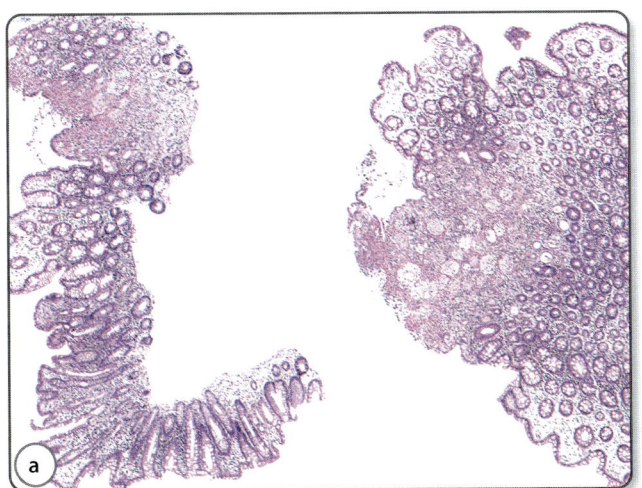

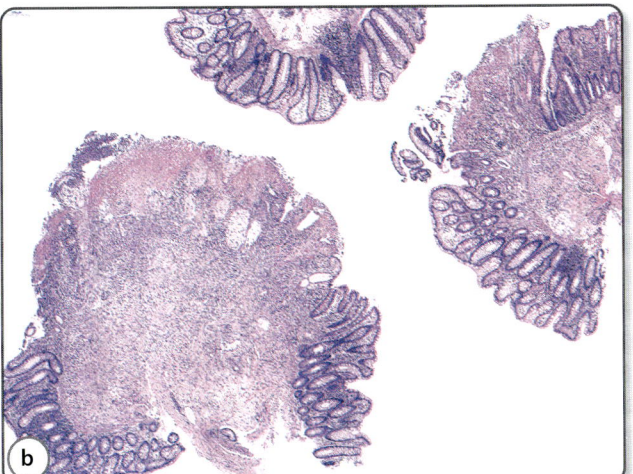

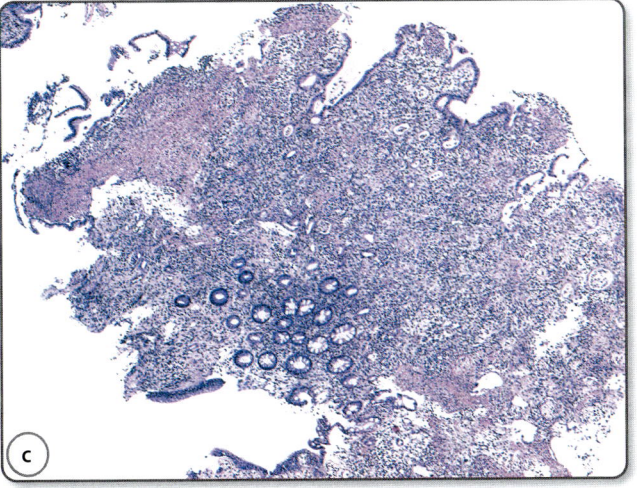

Figure 2.18 Pseudomembranous colitis. (a and b) Colon mucosa with focally disrupted colonic glands with epithelial debris, mucus and fibrin exudate forming pseudomembranes on top. (c) Acute colitis with ischaemic mucosal changes, eruptive volcano like lesions and fibrinopurulent exudate on the mucosal surface. (d) Higher power showing desquamation of the epithelium and pseudomembranes composed of fibrin and abundant cellular debris.
Continues overleaf

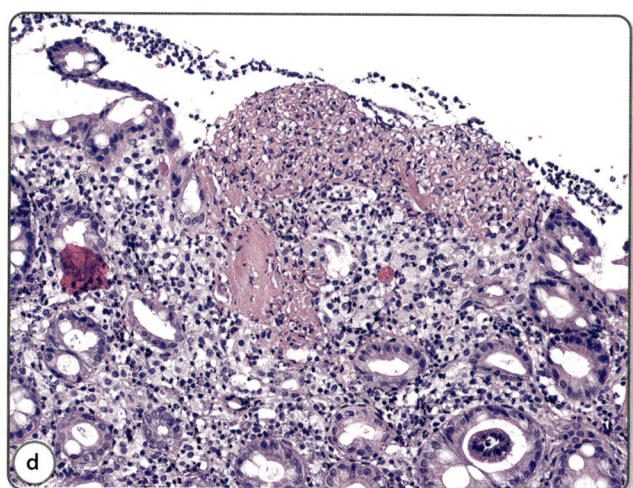

Figure 2.18 *Continued.*

with microthrombi. The symptoms ceased when doxycycline was discontinued. Medlicott et al [132] also reported two patients, whose oesophageal biopsies following suspected oesophagitis revealed oedematous zones resembling halos around submucosal arterioles. These halos contained reactive lymphocytes. Since these microscopic findings may be reminiscent of vasculitis or, in the stomach, of GAVE and portal hypertensive gastropathy, it is important to think of the possibility of doxycycline-induced injury [133].

Clofazimine-associated lesions

Clofazimine, a medication used for the treatment of leprosy, can lead to crystal storing histiocytosis in the intestinal mucosa accompanied by abdominal pain. Crystals are bright red in frozen sections and clear in standard sections, birefringent under polarised light and surrounded by histiocytes and sometimes plasma cells [134].

Mycophenolate-associated lesions

Mycophenolate is the prodrug of mycophenolic acid (MPA), inhibitor of inosine monophosphate dehydrogenase, an enzyme essential in the de novo purine synthesis of lymphoid cells. It is an effective immunosuppressant drug that is used for the treatment of autoimmune disorders and the prevention of graft rejection after solid organ and stem-cell transplantation. Mycophenolate is available as mycophenolate mofetil [(MMF), CellCept; absorbed in the stomach] and mycophenolate sodium (absorbed in the intestine).

Even though mycophenolate is a relatively specific inhibitor of lymphocyte proliferation, the gastrointestinal mucosa is frequently affected by toxicity, especially in patients with decreased kidney function or when high doses are used. Patients present with various abdominal symptoms, most commonly watery diarrhoea, and endoscopy may show erythema, congestion or mucosal defects [14,135]. In the colon, four different histologic patterns of mycophenolate toxicity have been described:
- *IBD-like pattern*, characterised by architectural distortion and occasional loss of crypts, crypt abscesses, mucin depletion, Paneth cell metaplasia and an inflammatory infiltrate in the lamina propria that is usually milder than in IBD.

- *Ischaemia-like pattern,* showing little to no inflammation in the lamina propria, but atrophy and loss of crypts accompanied by mucin depletion.
- *Self-limited colitis-like pattern*, characterised by the presence of neutrophils within an abundant inflammatory infiltrate in the lamina propria and in crypt epithelium (cryptitis).
- *GvHD-like pattern,* showing pronounced apoptosis in the crypt bases with preservation of the architecture and a lamina propria free of significant inflammation **(Figure 2.19)** [136]. Affected crypts often appear dilated and/or damaged, lined by thin eosinophilic epithelium and the crypt lumen may contain eosinophilic debris [137].

Similar histological changes can be found in CMV infection and GvHD, therefore, it is important to rule out these diseases in the post-transplant setting. Of note, CMV infection can occur in patients under mycophenolate therapy, and to distinguish between these two causes can be difficult (if not impossible) **(Figure 2.20)**. Proposed findings to discriminate mycophenolate colitis from GvHD include that >15 eosinophils per 10 high power fields is

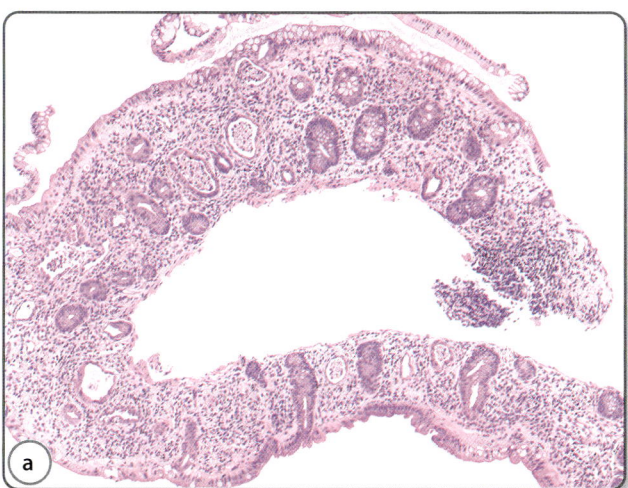

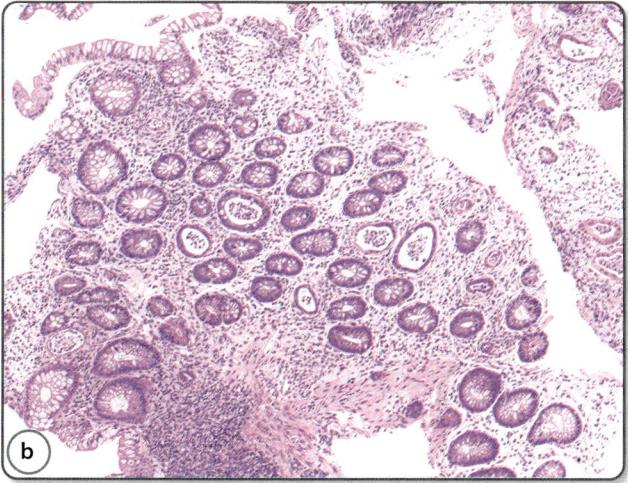

Figure 2.19 Mycophenolate-induced colitis. (a to d) Colon mucosa with increased inflammatory infiltrate (in particular eosinophils), focally attenuated epithelium with mucin depletion, abundant crypt abscesses and apoptosis. *Continues overleaf*

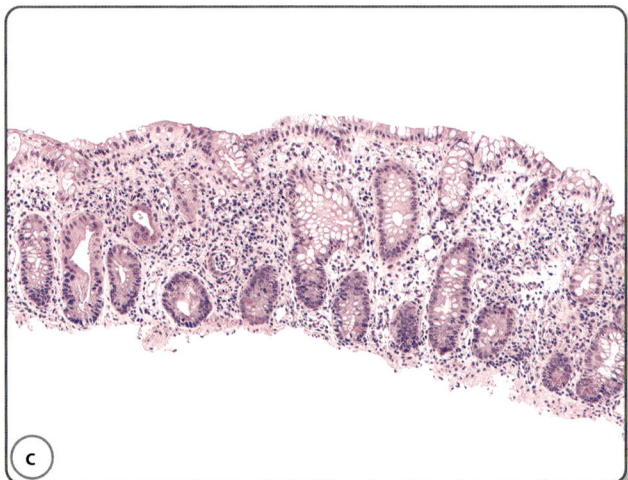

Figure 2.19 *Continued.*

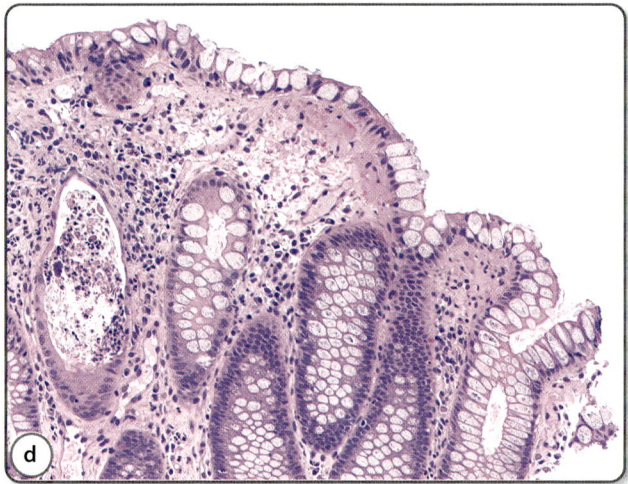

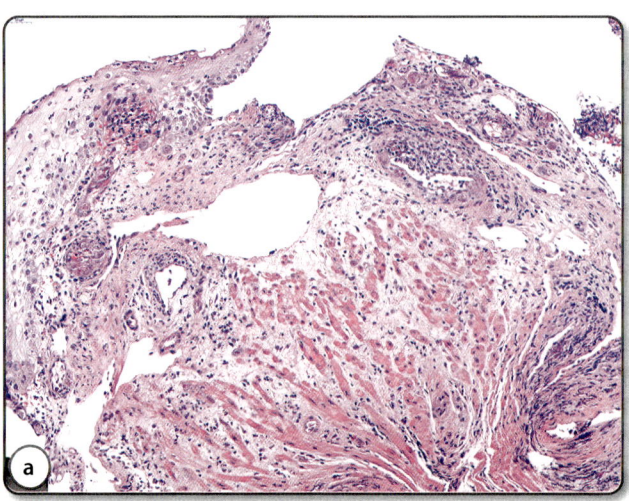

Figure 2.20 CMV infection associated with injury in oesophagus and antrum. (a and b) Ulcerated oesophageal mucosa with endothelial and epithelial cells with viral cytoplasmic inclusions. (c) Antrum mucosa with dense inflammatory infiltrate with prominent eosinophils, apoptosis and viral cytoplasmic inclusions in the antral glands. (d) Immunohistochemistry showing CMV inclusions in antral glands. *Continues opposite.*

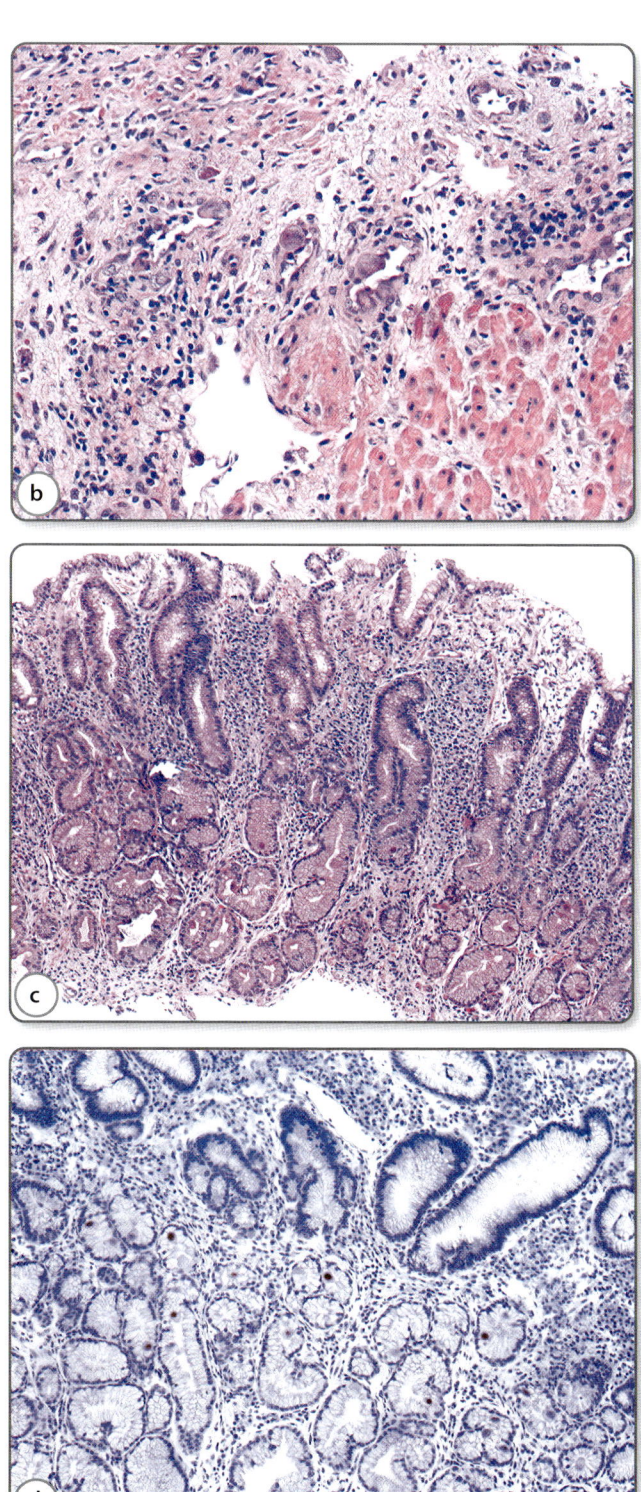

Figure 2.20 *Continued.*

more likely to be mycophenolate-induced while the presence of apoptotic microabscesses and endocrine nests favours GvHD [138]. The most common differential diagnoses in eosinophilic pattern of injury throughout the GI tract are listed in **Box 2.2**.

In the upper GI tract, mycophenolate toxicity leads to increased epithelial apoptosis similar to mild GvHD as well as a spectrum of findings such as reactive changes, inflammation and mucosal defects. The list of drugs, infections and conditions that can cause apoptotic pattern of injury throughout the GI tract is summarised in **Box 2.3**. Furthermore, gastritis and ballooning degeneration of parietal cells of the stomach, chronic peptic duodenitis and even coeliac-resembling alterations in the duodenum have been associated with MMF intake. All of these changes disappear after dosage reduction or cessation of mycophenolate [139].

Lesions associated with chemotherapy

Gastrointestinal complications and symptoms like diarrhoea, nausea and emesis are well known side effects of chemotherapy. The histological changes can be found anywhere in the GI tract. Since chemotherapy induces apoptosis or necrosis of cells with a high

---

Box 2.2 List of the most common differential diagnoses in eosinophilic pattern of injury throughout the gastrointestinal tract.

- Medications
- Reflux oesophagitis
- Allergy
- Idiopathic eosinophilic oesophagitis/gastritis/gastroenteritis/colitis
- Parasites
- Cytomegalovirus
- Neoplasia [e.g. systemic mastocytosis, Langerhans cell histiocytosis, hodgkin lymphoma, inflammatory fibroid polyp (small bowel)]
- Inflammatory bowel disease
- Vasculitis
- Connective tissue disorders (like scleroderma, systemic lupus erythematosus)

Box 2.3 List of drugs, infections and conditions that can cause apoptotic pattern of injury throughout the gastrointestinal tract.

- Non-steroidal anti-inflammatory drugs
- Mycophenolate [e.g. MMF (CellCept), mycophenolate sodium]
- Cytomegalovirus
- Graft-versus-host disease
- Immune mediated diseases (e.g. autoimmune enteropathy, common variable immunodeficiency)
- Allograft rejection

proliferation rate, the gastrointestinal epithelium can be damaged, which may result in erosions or ulcerations. The epithelial cells are eosinophilic, an increased count of apoptotic bodies occurs along with necrotic material in the lumen of the frequently widened crypts or glands [14,140]. Furthermore, some chemotherapeutic drugs induce cellular atypia that can be suggestive of dysplasia. However, despite the presence of distinct nucleoli, nuclear enlargement and hyperchromasia, these cells still have abundant cytoplasm and little to no mitoses are found [14].

Due to loss of epithelial integrity and depletion of immune cells, chemotherapy also increases the susceptibility to gastrointestinal infections [140]. Neutropenic enterocolitis, also known as typhlitis, is a severe and life-threatening complication that primarily affects the caecum and terminal ileum and is characterised, as the name suggests, by a low blood count of neutrophils. The histologic findings in the bowel wall are drastic, including infiltration of bacteria and fungi, necrosis, haemorrhage, ulcerations and sometimes even perforation [141].

Taxanes and colchicine

Taxanes like docetaxel and paclitaxel have an exceptional position among chemotherapeutic agents, as they cause specific histologic alterations. Their antitumour effect is derived from interference with the mitotic spindle, causing mitotic arrest during metaphase [142]. Colchicine is a drug with an almost similar mechanism of action, as it inhibits microtubule polymerisation, and leads to the same histologic changes; however, it is not an antineoplastic drug and is nowadays mainly used for the treatment of gout [143].

Both taxanes and colchicine increase the number of mitotic figures, especially ring mitoses, and apoptosis seen in areas with a high proliferation rate **(Figures 2.21 and 2.22)** [144,145]. *Colchicine* mainly affects the antrum (foveolar neck regions) and the small bowel (duodenal crypt bases). Colchicine-induced changes occur only when the drug is present in toxic doses, mostly in patients with renal failure. In addition to ring mitoses and increased apoptosis, pseudostratification of the epithelium and gastric or duodenal erosions can be the result of colchicine toxicity [144].

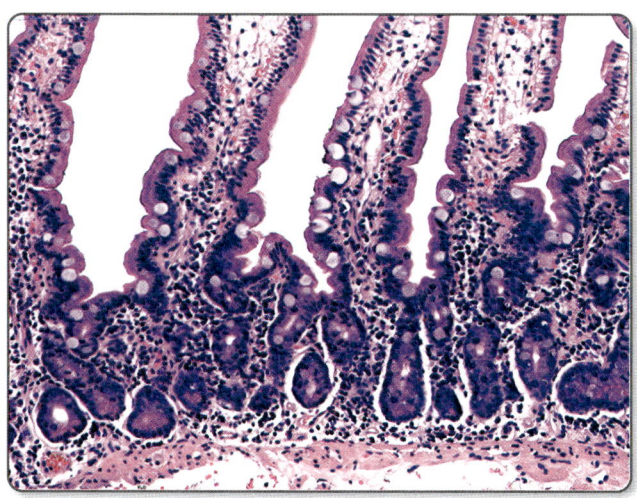

Figure 2.21 Taxane-induced changes in the duodenum: Note the prominent ring mitoses.

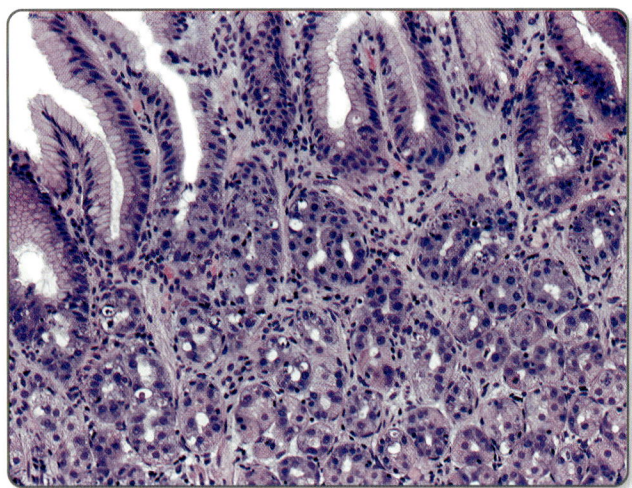

Figure 2.22 Colchicine-induced changes. Antrum mucosa with preserved architecture and numerous ring mitotic figures and apoptosis.

In contrast, ring mitoses in biopsies after *taxane* intake are usually most pronounced in the oesophagus and do not represent a sign of toxicity [145]. However, in severe cases, taxanes lead to necrosis and ulceration of the epithelium [146], with gastrointestinal necrosis affecting about 2% of patients receiving paclitaxel [147].

Colchicine and taxane-induced alterations may be confused with dysplasia in some cases, especially when changes due to taxanes are present in Barrett's oesophagus. The absence of hyperchromasia and pleomorphism of nuclei exclude this possibility [145].

Lesions associated with checkpoint inhibitors

Immune checkpoint inhibitors (CPIs) are a newer class of antitumoural drugs that induce a T-cell mediated immune response against cancer cells. CPIs are antibodies that target cytotoxic T lymphocyte antigen 4 (CTLA-4; ipilimumab), programmed cell death receptor 1 (PD-1; nivolumab, pembrolizumab and avelumab) or programmed cell death ligand 1 (PD-L1; atezolizumab) and are used for the treatment of advanced stage cancer such as malignant melanoma, non-small cell lung carcinoma and urothelial carcinoma.

In addition to their antitumoural efficacy, CPI-mediated immune dysregulation may induce adverse effects on the GI tract [148,149]. Diarrhoea and colitis occur in around 30% of patients receiving CPI treatment as immune-related adverse events (irAE) [150]. The median time between the start of therapy and onset of symptoms is 5–6 weeks for ipilimumab and 3–6 months for anti-PD-1 antibodies like nivolumab and pembrolizumab [151]. Ipilimumab leads to more severe side effects than nivolumab, and a combination of both holds the greatest risk for irAE [152].

Pathological changes are most commonly reported in the colon but can also be present in the stomach and small bowel. Colonoscopy and gross findings range from normal mucosa to erythema and friability with mild inflammatory changes to severe disease with mucosal defects, exudate, granularity and loss of vascularity [149,153,154]. Colon perforation following ipilimumab therapy has also been described [155].

Histologically, increase in IELs and epithelial cell apoptosis accompanied by abundant lamina propria inflammatory infiltration (lymphocytes, plasma cells, neutrophils and eosinophils) is found (**Figure 2.23**) [154]. Increase of IELs and apoptosis, together with

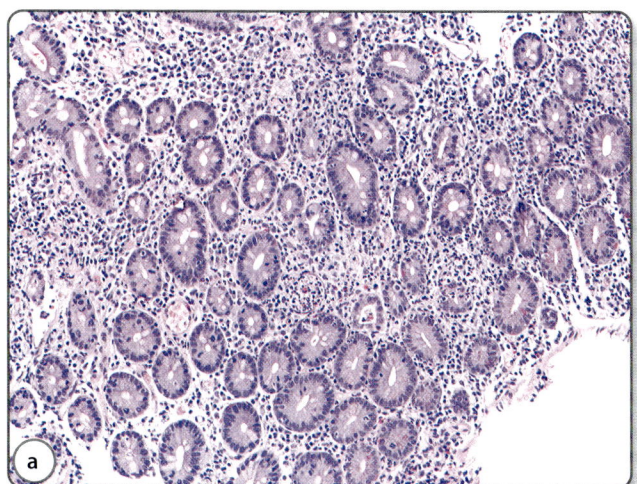

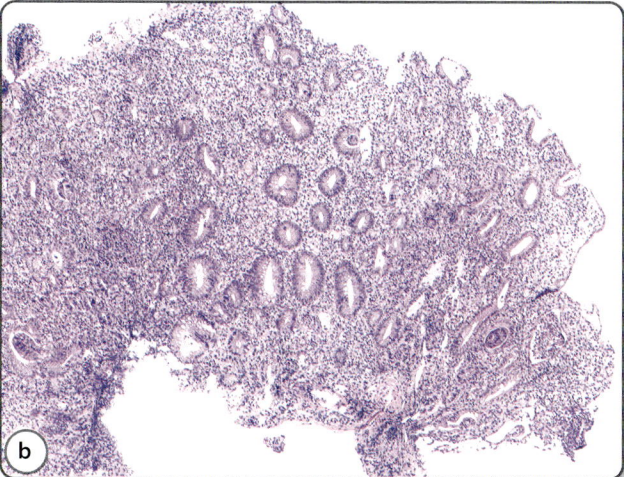

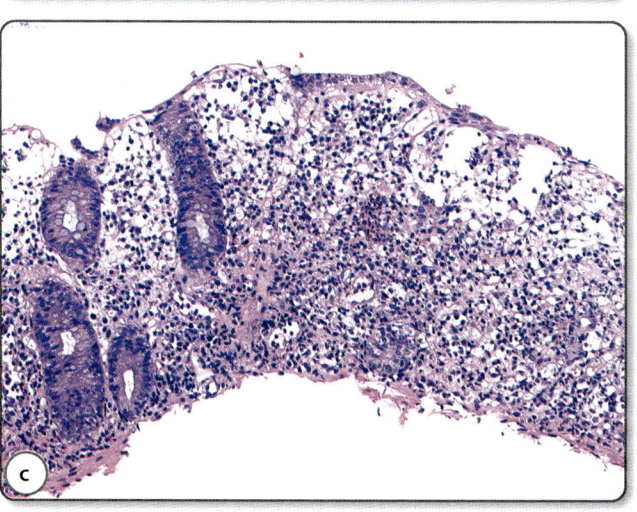

Figure 2.23 Ipilimumab-induced injury of the (a) duodenum and (b) colon with increased inflammation, intraepithelial lymphocytosis, prominent crypt apoptosis, focal cryptitis and crypt abscesses. (c) Colon mucosa with flattened surface epithelium, dense mixed inflammatory infiltrate and focal crypt loss. (d to f) Colectomy specimen with severe colitis after combined Ipilimumab – Nivolumab treatment showing ulceration and pseudopolypoid colon mucosa with abundant inflammatory infiltrate, cryptitis, crypt abscesses and erosions.
Continues overleaf

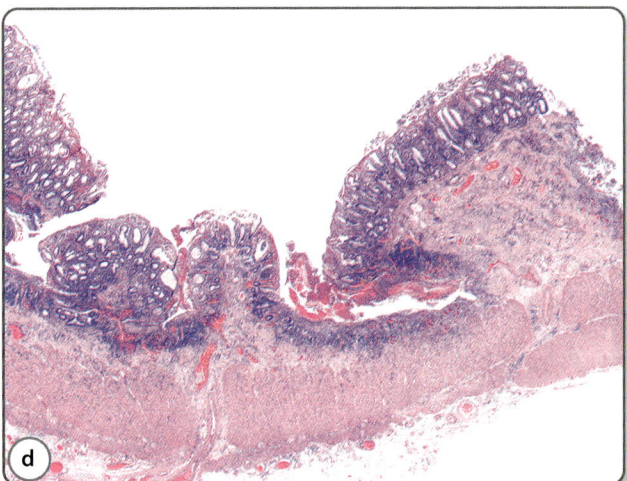

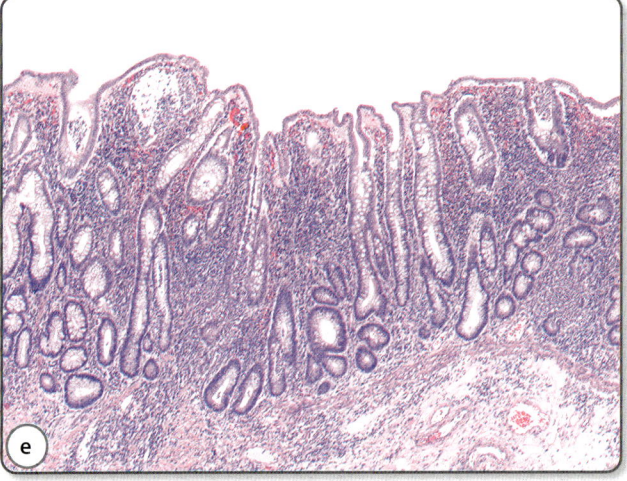

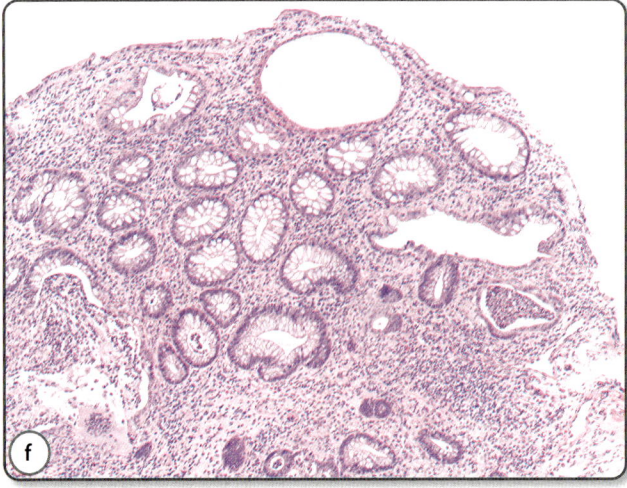

Figure 2.23 *Continued.*

architectural irregularity, focal inflammation and mucin depletion, have also been described in the stomach. In duodenal and ileal biopsies, villous blunting, mucosal defects, and – in the ileum – neutrophilic inflammation have been reported [156].

Neutrophilic inflammation with cryptitis and crypt abscesses is also commonly observed in colon affected by CPI toxicity (also known as "active colitis with apoptosis"). These findings are frequently accompanied by loss or atrophy of crypts with thinned epithelium and luminal debris following apoptosis (**Figure 2.21**), as seen in mycophenolate colitis. Occasionally, erosions and ulcers are seen [148,149,154].

Additionally, changes resembling lymphocytic colitis, including a high number of IELs, flattening of surface epithelium and a mononuclear cell infiltrate in the lamina propria, may be found [148]. Single cases of collagenous colitis following pembrolizumab and nivolumab therapy have been reported [157,158].

Considering the spectrum of histological changes and the fact that patients are immunocompromised, it is always important to rule out CMV infection by immunohistochemistry when evaluating biopsies from patients treated with CPIs. Histology can also mimic IBD or bacterial colitis. Lack of signs of chronicity usually rules out the former and increased apoptosis in the crypt bases argues against the latter. Other medications leading to similar histology are MMF, anti-tumour necrosis factor (anti-TNF) therapy, idelalisib, methotrexate and fluorouracil [148,153,159].

CONCLUSION

In everyday practice, the correct diagnosis of a wide spectrum of drug-induced changes seen in GI tract biopsies can be very challenging. Frequently, the histological changes are overlapping and different drugs may cause similar patterns of injury. Therefore, a multidisciplinary approach with good clinical-pathological correlation is of utmost importance for the correct diagnosis and optimal treatment of the patient. In some cases, multiple biopsies should be obtained for histologic analysis to rule out other causes. Typical patterns of drug-induced histological changes in GI biopsies are reactive and/or hyperplastic epithelial change, erosions, ulcerations, fibrosis, necrosis, lymphocytic and/or eosinophilic inflammatory infiltrate and apoptosis. A very concise finding allowing the identification of drug-induced injury is the presence of drug fillers, pigment or crystal deposits.

Key points for clinical practice

- A correct diagnosis is essential for a wide spectrum of drug-induced changes seen in GI biopsies, but this can be very challenging, as often the histological changes overlap.
- Multidisciplinary approach with good clinical-histopathological correlation is of utmost importance for the correct diagnosis and optimal treatment of the patient.
- Multiple biopsies should be obtained for histologic analysis to rule out other differential diagnoses.
- Patterns of histological changes found in GI biopsies are limited and frequently overlap.
- Different drugs may cause similar patterns of mucosal injury.

- Patterns of injury include reactive and/or hyperplastic epithelial change, erosions, ulcerations, fibrosis, necrosis, inflammatory infiltrate (most commonly eosinophils and lymphocytes) and apoptosis.
- Drug fillers, pigment or crystal deposits show typical histological features allowing their correct identification.

Conflicts of interest: All authors declare no conflicts of interest relevant to this work.

Source of funding: None declared.

REFERENCES

1. Greenson JK. Diagnostic Pathology: Gastrointestinal, 2nd Edition. Philadelphia: Elsevier, 2016.
2. Maguire A, Sheahan K. Pathology of oesophagitis. Histopathology 2012; 60:864–879.
3. De Petris G, Caldero SG, Chen L, et al. Histopathological changes in the gastrointestinal tract due to medications: an update for the surgical pathologist (part II of II). Int J Surg Pathol 2014; 22:202–211.
4. Katzka DA, Smyrk TC, Bruce AJ, et al. Variations in presentations of esophageal involvement in lichen planus. Clin Gastroenterol Hepatol 2010; 8:777–782.
5. Moawad FJ, Appleman HD. Sloughing esophagitis: a spectacular histologic and endoscopic disease without a uniform clinical correlation. Ann N Y Acad Sci 2016; 1380:178–182.
6. Hart PA, Romano RC, Moreira RK, Ravi K, Sweetser S. Esophagitis dissecans superficialis: Clinical, endoscopic, and histologic features. Dig Dis Sci 2015; 60:2049–2057.
7. Purdy JK, Appelman HD, McKenna BJ. Sloughing esophagitis is associated with chronic debilitation and medications that injure the esophageal mucosa. Mod Pathol 2012; 25:767–775.
8. Liberman UI, Hirsch LJ. Esophagitis and alendronate. N Engl J Med 1996; 335:1069–1970.
9. Drake MT, Clarke BL, Khosla S. Bisphosphonates: mechanism of action and role in clinical practice. Mayo Clin Proc 2008; 83:1032–1045.
10. Nagano Y, Matsui H, Shimokawa O, et al. Bisphosphonate-induced gastrointestinal mucosal injury is mediated by mitochondrial superoxide production and lipid peroxidation. J Clin Biochem Nutr 2012; 51:196–203.
11. Abraham SC, Cruz-Correa M, Lee LA, Yardley JH, Wu TT. Alendronate-associated esophageal injury: pathologic and endoscopic features. Mod Pathol 1999; 12:1152–1157.
12. Parfitt JR, Driman DK. Pathological effects of drugs on the gastrointestinal tract: a review. Hum Pathol 2007; 38:527–536.
13. De Petris G, Gatius Caldero S, Chen L, et al. Histopathological changes in the gastrointestinal tract due to drugs: an update for the surgical pathologist (part I of II). Int J Surg Pathol 2014; 22:120–128.
14. Kwak HA, Hart J. The many faces of medication-related injury in the gastrointestinal tract. Surg Pathol Clin 2017; 10:887–908.
15. de Groen PC, Lubbe DF, Hirsch LJ, et al. Esophagitis associated with the use of alendronate. N Engl J Med 1996; 335:1016–1021.
16. Graham DY. What the gastroenterologist should know about the gastrointestinal safety profiles of bisphosphonates. Dig Dis Sci 2002; 47:1665–1678.
17. Wolf EM, Plieschnegger W, Schmack B, et al. Evolving patterns in the diagnosis of reactive gastropathy: data from a prospective Central European multicenter study with proposal of a new histologic scoring system. Pathol Res Pract 2014; 210:847–854.
18. Genta RM. Differential diagnosis of reactive gastropathy. Semin Diagn Pathol 2005; 22:273–283.
19. Sobala GM, King RF, Axon AT, Dixon MF. Reflux gastritis in the intact stomach. J Clin Pathol 1990; 43:303–306.
20. Montgomery EAG, Whitney M, Epstein JI. Differential Diagnoses in Surgical Pathology: Gastrointestinal System. Philadelphia: Wolters Kluwer, 2015.
21. Leung WK, Yu J, To KF, et al. Apoptosis and proliferation in Helicobacter pylori-associated gastric intestinal metaplasia. Aliment Pharmacol Ther 2001; 15:1467–1472.

22. Maguilnik I, Neumann WL, Sonnenberg A, Genta RM. Reactive gastropathy is associated with inflammatory conditions throughout the gastrointestinal tract. Aliment Pharmacol Ther 2012; 36:736–743.

23. Arnold CAL-H, Dora M, Montgomery EA. Atlas of Gastrointestinal Pathology: A Pattern Based Approach to Non-Neoplastic Biopsies. Philadelphia: Wolters Kluwer, 2015.

24. Capper D, Jones DTW, Sill M, et al. DNA methylation-based classification of central nervous system tumours. Nature 2018; 555:469–474.

25. Greenson JK, Trinidad SB, Pfeil SA, et al. Gastric mucosal calcinosis. Calcified aluminum phosphate deposits secondary to aluminum-containing antacids or sucralfate therapy in organ transplant patients. Am J Surg Pathol 1993; 17:45–50.

26. Gorospe M, Fadare O. Gastric mucosal calcinosis: clinicopathologic considerations. Adv Anat Pathol 2007; 14:224–228.

27. Castagna L, Benhamou E, Pedraza E, et al. Prevention of mucositis in bone marrow transplantation: a double blind randomised controlled trial of sucralfate. Ann Oncol 2001; 12:953–955.

28. Sachs G, Shin JM, Briving C, Wallmark B, Hersey S. The pharmacology of the gastric acid pump: the H^+,K^+-ATPase. Annu Rev Pharmacol Toxicol 1995; 35:277–305.

29. Stedman CA, Barclay ML. Review article: comparison of the pharmacokinetics, acid suppression and efficacy of proton pump inhibitors. Aliment Pharmacol Ther 2000; 14:963–978.

30. McCarthy DM. Adverse effects of proton pump inhibitor drugs: clues and conclusions. Curr Opin Gastroenterol 2010; 26:624–631.

31. Nishi T, Makuuchi H, Weinstein WM. Changes in gastric ECL cells and parietal cells after long-term administration of high-dose omeprazole to patients with Barrett's esophagus. Tokai J Exp Clin Med 2005; 30:117–121.

32. Ally MR, Veerappan GR, Maydonovitch CL, et al. Chronic proton pump inhibitor therapy associated with increased development of fundic gland polyps. Dig Dis Sci 2009; 54:2617–2622.

33. Rais R, Trikalinos NA, Liu J, Chatterjee D. Enterochromaffin-like cell hyperplasia-associated gastric neuroendocrine tumors may arise in the setting of proton pump inhibitor use. Arch Pathol Lab Med 2022; 146:366–371.

34. Yasugi K, Haruma K, Kawanaka M, et al. Disappearance of gastric hyperplastic polyps after the discontinuation of proton pump inhibitor in a patient with liver cirrhosis. Case Rep Gastroenterol 2021; 15:202–209.

35. Thomson RD, Lestina LS, Bensen SP, et al. Lansoprazole-associated microscopic colitis: a case series. Am J Gastroenterol 2002; 97:2908–2913.

36. Umeno J, Matsumoto T, Nakamura S, et al. Linear mucosal defect may be characteristic of lansoprazole-associated collagenous colitis. Gastrointest Endosc 2008; 67:1185–1191.

37. Dial S, Delaney JA, Barkun AN, Suissa S. Use of gastric acid-suppressive agents and the risk of community-acquired Clostridium difficile-associated disease. JAMA 2005; 294:2989–2995.

38. Kaye P, Abdulla K, Wood J, et al. Iron-induced mucosal pathology of the upper gastrointestinal tract: a common finding in patients on oral iron therapy. Histopathology 2008; 53:311–317.

39. Marginean EC, Bennick M, Cyczk J, Robert ME, Jain D. Gastric siderosis: patterns and significance. Am J Surg Pathol 2006; 30:514–520.

40. Ji H, Yardley JH. Iron medication-associated gastric mucosal injury. Arch Pathol Lab Med 2004; 128:821–822.

41. Haig A, Driman DK. Iron-induced mucosal injury to the upper gastrointestinal tract. Histopathology 2006; 48:808–812.

42. Albaaj F, Hutchison AJ. Lanthanum carbonate (fosrenol): a novel agent for the treatment of hyperphosphataemia in renal failure and dialysis patients. Int J Clin Pract 2005; 59:1091–1096.

43. Makino M, Kawaguchi K, Shimojo H, et al. Extensive lanthanum deposition in the gastric mucosa: the first histopathological report. Pathol Int 2015; 65:33–37.

44. Iwamuro M, Tanaka T, Urata H, Kimoto K, Okada H. Lanthanum phosphate deposition in the duodenum. Gastrointest Endosc 2017; 85:1103–1104.

45. Goto K, Ogawa K. Lanthanum Deposition Is Frequently Observed in the Gastric Mucosa of Dialysis Patients With Lanthanum Carbonate Therapy: A Clinicopathologic study of 13 cases, including 1 case of lanthanum granuloma in the colon and 2 nongranulomatous gastric cases. Int J Surg Pathol 2016; 24:89–92.

46. Ban S, Suzuki S, Kubota K, et al. Gastric mucosal status susceptible to lanthanum deposition in patients treated with dialysis and lanthanum carbonate. Ann Diagn Pathol 2017; 26:6–9.

47. Vaziri ND, Yuan J, Nazertehrani S, Ni Z, Liu S. Chronic kidney disease causes disruption of gastric and small intestinal epithelial tight junction. Am J Nephrol 2013; 38:99–103.

48. Iwamuro M, Urata H, Tanaka T, et al. Lanthanum deposition corresponds to white lesions in the stomach. Pathol Res Pract 2018; 214:934–939.

49. Iwamuro M, Urata H, Tanaka T, et al. Frequent involvement of the duodenum with lanthanum deposition: A retrospective observational study. Intern Med 2019; 58:2283–2289.

50. Nishida S, Ota K, Hattori K, et al. Investigation of the clinical significance and pathological features of lanthanum deposition in the gastric mucosa. BMC Gastroenterol 2020; 20:396.

51. Yabuki K, Shiba E, Harada H, et al. Lanthanum deposition in the gastrointestinal mucosa and regional lymph nodes in dialysis patients: Analysis of surgically excised specimens and review of the literature. Pathol Res Pract 2016; 212:919–926.

52. Hoda RS, Sanyal S, Abraham JL, et al. Lanthanum deposition from oral lanthanum carbonate in the upper gastrointestinal tract. Histopathology 2017; 70:1072–1078.

53. Sato KT, Lewandowski RJ, Mulcahy MF, et al. Unresectable chemorefractory liver metastases: radioembolization with 90Y microspheres--safety, efficacy, and survival. Radiology 2008; 247:507–515.

54. Konda A, Savin MA, Cappell MS, Duffy MC. Radiation microsphere-induced GI ulcers after selective internal radiation therapy for hepatic tumors: an underrecognized clinical entity. Gastrointest Endosc 2009; 70:561–567.

55. Ogawa F, Mino-Kenudson M, Shimizu M, Ligato S, Lauwers GY. Gastroduodenitis associated with yttrium 90-microsphere selective internal radiation: an iatrogenic complication in need of recognition. Arch Pathol Lab Med 2008; 132:1734–1738.

56. Sun B, Lapetino SR, Diffalha SA, et al. Microvascular injury in persistent gastric ulcers after yttrium-90 microsphere radioembolization for liver malignancies. Hum Pathol 2016; 50:11–14.

57. Blesl A, Brcic I, Jaschke W, et al. Chronic gastric ulcer disease complicating selective internal radiation therapy (SIRT) in a patient with cholangiocellular carcinoma. Z Gastroenterol 2019; 57:1304–1308.

58. Petras RE, Hart WR, Bukowski RM. Gastric epithelial atypia associated with hepatic arterial infusion chemotherapy. Its distinction from early gastric carcinoma. Cancer 1985; 56:745–750.

59. Chande N, Driman DK, Reynolds RP. Collagenous colitis and lymphocytic colitis: patient characteristics and clinical presentation. Scand J Gastroenterol 2005; 40:343–347.

60. Giardiello FM, Hansen FC, 3rd, Lazenby AJ, et al. Collagenous colitis in setting of nonsteroidal antiinflammatory drugs and antibiotics. Dig Dis Sci 1990; 35:257–260.

61. Verhaegh BP, de Vries F, Masclee AA, et al. High risk of drug-induced microscopic colitis with concomitant use of NSAIDs and proton pump inhibitors. Aliment Pharmacol Ther 2016; 43:1004–1013.

62. Beaugerie L, Patey N, Brousse N. Ranitidine, diarrhoea, and lymphocytic colitis. Gut 1995; 37:708–711.

63. Berrebi D, Sautet A, Flejou JF, et al. Ticlopidine induced colitis: a histopathological study including apoptosis. J Clin Pathol 1998; 51:280–283.

64. Mahajan L, Wyllie R, Goldblum J. Lymphocytic colitis in a pediatric patient: a possible adverse reaction to carbamazepine. Am J Gastroenterol 1997; 92:2126–2127.

65. Ianiro G, Cammarota G, Valerio L, et al. Microscopic colitis. World J Gastroenterol 2012; 18:6206–6215.

66. Cerilli LA, Greenson JK. The differential diagnosis of colitis in endoscopic biopsy specimens: a review article. Arch Pathol Lab Med 2012; 136:854–864.

67. Boutros HH, Pautler S, Chakrabarti S. Cocaine-induced ischemic colitis with small-vessel thrombosis of colon and gallbladder. J Clin Gastroenterol 1997; 24:49–53.

68. Stillman AE, Weinberg M, Mast WC, Palpant S. Ischemic bowel disease attributable to ergot. Gastroenterology 1977; 72:1336–1337.

69. Zervoudis S, Grammatopoulos T, Iatrakis G, et al. Ischemic colitis in postmenopausal women taking hormone replacement therapy. Gynecol Endocrinol 2008; 24:257–260.

70. Deana DG, Dean PJ. Reversible ischemic colitis in young women. Association with oral contraceptive use. Am J Surg Pathol 1995; 19:454–462.
71. Dignan CR, Greenson JK. Can ischemic colitis be differentiated from C difficile colitis in biopsy specimens? Am J Surg Pathol 1997; 21:706–710.
72. Lee YS, Han JJ, Kim SY, Maeng CH. Pneumatosis cystoides intestinalis associated with sunitinib and a literature review. BMC Cancer 2017; 17:732.
73. Kojima K, Tsujimoto T, Fujii H, et al. Pneumatosis cystoides intestinalis induced by the alpha-glucosidase inhibitor miglitol. Intern Med 2010; 49:1545–1548.
74. Bischoff H. The mechanism of alpha-glucosidase inhibition in the management of diabetes. Clin Invest Med 1995; 18:303–311.
75. Goodman RA, Riley TR, 3rd. Lactulose-induced pneumatosis intestinalis and pneumoperitoneum. Dig Dis Sci 2001; 46:2549–2553.
76. Roy J, Kang M, Stern B, Riley T, Schreibman I. Lactulose-induced pneumatosis intestinalis following colonoscopy: a case report. Clin J Gastroenterol 2021; 14:1152–1156.
77. Ammons MA, Bauling PC, Weil R, 3rd. Pneumatosis cystoides intestinalis with pneumoperitoneum in renal transplant patients on cyclosporine and prednisone. Transplant Proc 1986; 18:1868–1870.
78. Arman Bilir O, Demir AM, Akcabelen YM, et al. Pneumatosis cystoides intestinalis: A rare complication after hematopoietic stem cell transplantation. Pediatr Transplant 2021; 25:e14136.
79. Li X, Zhou Y, Zhou S, et al. Histopathology of melanosis coli and determination of its associated genes by comparative analysis of expression microarrays. Mol Med Rep 2015; 12:5807–5815.
80. Benavides SH, Morgante PE, Monserrat AJ, Zarate J, Porta EA. The pigment of melanosis coli: a lectin histochemical study. Gastrointest Endosc 1997; 46:131–138.
81. Byers RJ, Marsh P, Parkinson D, Haboubi NY. Melanosis coli is associated with an increase in colonic epithelial apoptosis and not with laxative use. Histopathology. 1997; 30:160–164.
82. Badiali D, Marcheggiano A, Pallone F, et al. Melanosis of the rectum in patients with chronic constipation. Dis Colon Rectum 1985; 28:241–245.
83. Stein BL, Lamoureux E, Miller M, et al. Glutaraldehyde-induced colitis. Can J Surg 2001; 44:113–116.
84. McCarthy AJ, Lauwers GY, Sheahan K. Iatrogenic pathology of the intestines. Histopathology 2015; 66:15–28.
85. Driman DK, Preiksaitis HG. Colorectal inflammation and increased cell proliferation associated with oral sodium phosphate bowel preparation solution. Hum Pathol 1998; 29:972–978.
86. Matsukuma K, Gui D, Olson KA, et al. OsmoPrep-associated gastritis: A histopathologic mimic of Iron pill gastritis and mucosal calcinosis. Am J Surg Pathol 2016; 40:1550–1556.
87. Barreras A, Gurk-Turner C. Angiotensin II receptor blockers. Proc (Bayl Univ Med Cent) 2003; 16:123–126.
88. Rubio-Tapia A, Herman ML, Ludvigsson JF, et al. Severe spruelike enteropathy associated with olmesartan. Mayo Clin Proc 2012; 87:732–738.
89. Greywoode R, Braunstein ED, Arguelles-Grande C, Green PH, Lebwohl B. Olmesartan, other antihypertensives, and chronic diarrhea among patients undergoing endoscopic procedures: a case-control study. Mayo Clin Proc 2014; 89:1239–1243.
90. Malfertheiner P, Ripellino C, Cataldo N. Severe intestinal malabsorption associated with ACE inhibitor or angiotensin receptor blocker treatment. An observational cohort study in Germany and Italy. Pharmacoepidemiol Drug Saf 2018; 27:581–586.
91. Marthey L, Cadiot G, Seksik P, et al. Olmesartan-associated enteropathy: results of a national survey. Aliment Pharmacol Ther 2014; 40:1103–1109.
92. Mandavdhare HS, Sharma V, Prasad KK, et al. Telmisartan-induced sprue-like enteropathy: a case report and a review of patients using non-olmesartan angiotensin receptor blockers. Intest Res 2017; 15:419–421.
93. Negro A, Rossi GM, Santi R, Iori V, De Marco L. A case of severe sprue-like enteropathy associated with losartan. J Clin Gastroenterol 2015; 49:794.
94. Herman ML, Rubio-Tapia A, Wu TT, Murray JA. A Case of severe sprue-like enteropathy associated with valsartan. ACG Case Rep J 2015; 2:92–94.
95. Maier H, Hehemann K, Vieth M. Celiac disease-like enteropathy due to antihypertensive therapy with the angiotensin-II receptor type 1 inhibitor eprosartan. Cesk Patol 2015; 51:87–88.

96.   Ianiro G, Bibbo S, Montalto M, et al. Systematic review: Sprue-like enteropathy associated with olmesartan. Aliment Pharmacol Ther 2014; 40:16–23.
97.   Burbure N, Lebwohl B, Arguelles-Grande C, et al. Olmesartan-associated sprue-like enteropathy: a systematic review with emphasis on histopathology. Hum Pathol 2016; 50:127–134.
98.   Cyrany J, Vasatko T, Machac J, et al. Letter: telmisartan-associated enteropathy - is there any class effect? Aliment Pharmacol Ther 2014; 40:569–570.
99.   Pawel BR, de Chadarevian JP, Franco ME. The pathology of fibrosing colonopathy of cystic fibrosis: a study of 12 cases and review of the literature. Hum Pathol 1997; 28:395–399.
100. Bakowski MT, Prescott P. Patterns of use of pancreatic enzyme supplements in fibrosing colonopathy: implications for pathogenesis. Pharmacoepidemiol Drug Saf 1997; 6:347–358.
101. Prescott P, Bakowski MT. Pathogenesis of fibrosing colonopathy: the role of methacrylic acid copolymer. Pharmacoepidemiol Drug Saf 1999; 8:377–384.
102. Russell G, Graveley R, Seid J, al-Humidan AK, Skjodt H. Mechanisms of action of cyclosporine and effects on connective tissues. Semin Arthritis Rheum 1992; 21:16–22.
103. Hyde GM, Thillainayagam AV, Jewell DP. Intravenous cyclosporin as rescue therapy in severe ulcerative colitis: time for a reappraisal? Eur J Gastroenterol Hepatol 1998; 10:411413.
104. Hyde GM, Jewell DP, Warren BF. Histological changes associated with the use of intravenous cyclosporin in the treatment of severe ulcerative colitis may mimic dysplasia. Colorectal Dis 2002; 4:455–458.
105. Yang Q, Modi P, Newcomb T, Queva C, Gandhi V. Idelalisib: First-in-class PI3K delta inhibitor for the treatment of chronic lymphocytic leukemia, small lymphocytic leukemia, and Follicular lymphoma. Clin Cancer Res 2015; 21:1537–1542.
106. Coutre SE, Barrientos JC, Brown JR, et al. Management of adverse events associated with idelalisib treatment: expert panel opinion. Leuk Lymphoma 2015; 56:2779–2786.
107. Weidner AS, Panarelli NC, Geyer JT, et al. Idelalisib-associated colitis: Histologic findings in 14 patients. Am J Surg Pathol 2015; 39:1661–1667.
108. De Petris G, De Marco L, Lopez JI. Drug-induced gastrointestinal injury (DIGI). Updates, reflections and key points. Pathologica 2017; 109:97–109.
109. Louie CY, DiMaio MA, Matsukuma KE, et al. Idelalisib-associated Enterocolitis: Clinicopathologic features and distinction From other enterocolitides. Am J Surg Pathol 2015; 39:1653–1660.
110. Kakar S, Nehra V, Murray JA, Dayharsh GA, Burgart LJ. Significance of intraepithelial lymphocytosis in small bowel biopsy samples with normal mucosal architecture. Am J Gastroenterol 2003; 98:2027–2033.
111. Wang YZ, Sun G, Cai FC, Yang YS. Clinical features, diagnosis, and treatment strategies of gastrointestinal diaphragm disease associated with nonsteroidal anti-inflammatory drugs. Gastroenterol Res Pract 2016; 2016:3679741.
112. Maiden L, Thjodleifsson B, Seigal A, et al. Long-term effects of nonsteroidal anti-inflammatory drugs and cyclooxygenase-2 selective agents on the small bowel: a cross-sectional capsule enteroscopy study. Clin Gastroenterol Hepatol 2007; 5:1040–1045.
113. De Petris G, Lopez JI. Histopathology of diaphragm disease of the small intestine: a study of 10 cases from a single institution. Am J Clin Pathol 2008; 130:518–525.
114. Lang J, Price AB, Levi AJ, et al. Diaphragm disease: pathology of disease of the small intestine induced by non-steroidal anti-inflammatory drugs. J Clin Pathol 1988; 41:516–526.
115. Bridgeman MB, Shah M, Foote E. Potassium-lowering agents for the treatment of nonemergent hyperkalemia: pharmacology, dosing and comparative efficacy. Nephrol Dial Transplant 2019; 34:iii45–iii50.
116. McGowan CE, Saha S, Chu G, Resnick MB, Moss SF. Intestinal necrosis due to sodium polystyrene sulfonate (Kayexalate) in sorbitol. South Med J 2009; 102:493–497.
117. Rashid A, Hamilton SR. Necrosis of the gastrointestinal tract in uremic patients as a result of sodium polystyrene sulfonate (kayexalate) in sorbitol: an underrecognized condition. Am J Surg Pathol 1997; 21:60–69.
118. Harel Z, Harel S, Shah PS, et al. Gastrointestinal adverse events with sodium polystyrene sulfonate (kayexalate) use: a systematic review. Am J Med 2013; 126:264, e9–e24.

119. Abraham SC, Bhagavan BS, Lee LA, Rashid A, Wu TT. Upper gastrointestinal tract injury in patients receiving kayexalate (sodium polystyrene sulfonate) in sorbitol: clinical, endoscopic, and histopathologic findings. Am J Surg Pathol 2001; 25:637–644.

120. Swanson BJ, Limketkai BN, Liu TC, et al. Sevelamer crystals in the gastrointestinal tract (GIT): a new entity associated with mucosal injury. Am J Surg Pathol 2013; 37:1686–1693.

121. Yuste C, Merida E, Hernandez E, et al. Gastrointestinal complications induced by sevelamer crystals. Clin Kidney J 2017; 10:539–544.

122. Arnold MA, Swanson BJ, Crowder CD, et al. Colesevelam and colestipol: novel medication resins in the gastrointestinal tract. Am J Surg Pathol 2014; 38:1530–1537.

123. Shaddy SM, Arnold MA, Shilo K, et al. Crospovidone and microcrystalline cellulose: A novel description of pharmaceutical fillers in the gastrointestinal tract. Am J Surg Pathol 2017; 41:564–569.

124. Hogenauer C, Langner C, Beubler E, et al. Klebsiella oxytoca as a causative organism of antibiotic-associated hemorrhagic colitis. N Engl J Med 2006; 355:2418–2426.

125. Beaugerie L, Metz M, Barbut F, et al. Klebsiella oxytoca as an agent of antibiotic-associated hemorrhagic colitis. Clin Gastroenterol Hepatol 2003; 1:370–376.

126. Youn Y, Lee SW, Cho HH, et al. Antibiotics-associated hemorrhagic colitis caused by Klebsiella oxytoca: Two case reports. Pediatr Gastroenterol Hepatol Nutr 2018; 21:141–146.

127. Farooq PD, Urrunaga NH, Tang DM, von Rosenvinge EC. Pseudomembranous colitis. Dis Mon 2015; 61:181–206.

128. Price AB, Davies DR. Pseudomembranous colitis. J Clin Pathol 1977; 30:1–12.

129. Surawicz CM, McFarland LV. Pseudomembranous colitis: causes and cures. Digestion 1999; 60:91–100.

130. Tang DM, Urrunaga NH, von Rosenvinge EC. Pseudomembranous colitis: Not always Clostridium difficile. Cleve Clin J Med 2016; 83:361–366.

131. Xiao SY, Zhao L, Hart J, Semrad CE. Gastric mucosal necrosis with vascular degeneration induced by doxycycline. Am J Surg Pathol 2013; 37:259–263.

132. Medlicott SA, Ma M, Misra T, Dupre MP. Vascular wall degeneration in doxycycline-related esophagitis. Am J Surg Pathol 2013; 37:1114–1115.

133. Shih AR, Lauwers GY, Mattia A, Schaefer EA, Misdraji J. Vascular Injury Characterizes doxycycline-induced upper gastrointestinal tract mucosal injury. Am J Surg Pathol 2017; 41:374–381.

134. Sukpanichnant S, Hargrove NS, Kachintorn U, et al. Clofazimine-induced crystal-storing histiocytosis producing chronic abdominal pain in a leprosy patient. Am J Surg Pathol 2000; 24:129–135.

135. Behrend M. Adverse gastrointestinal effects of mycophenolate mofetil: aetiology, incidence and management. Drug Saf 2001; 24:645–663.

136. Selbst MK, Ahrens WA, Robert ME, et al. Spectrum of histologic changes in colonic biopsies in patients treated with mycophenolate mofetil. Mod Pathol 2009; 22:737–743.

137. Parfitt JR, Jayakumar S, Driman DK. Mycophenolate mofetil-related gastrointestinal mucosal injury: variable injury patterns, including graft-versus-host disease-like changes. Am J Surg Pathol 2008; 32:1367–1372.

138. Star KV, Ho VT, Wang HH, Odze RD. Histologic features in colon biopsies can discriminate mycophenolate from GVHD-induced colitis. Am J Surg Pathol 2013; 37:1319–1328.

139. Nguyen T, Park JY, Scudiere JR, Montgomery E. Mycophenolic acid (cellcept and myofortic) induced injury of the upper GI tract. Am J Surg Pathol 2009; 33:1355–1363.

140. Boussios S, Pentheroudakis G, Katsanos K, Pavlidis N. Systemic treatment-induced gastrointestinal toxicity: incidence, clinical presentation and management. Ann Gastroenterol 2012; 25:106–118.

141. Xia R, Zhang X. Neutropenic enterocolitis: A clinico-pathological review. World J Gastrointest Pathophysiol 2019; 10:36–41.

142. Abal M, Andreu JM, Barasoain I. Taxanes: microtubule and centrosome targets, and cell cycle dependent mechanisms of action. Curr Cancer Drug Targets 2003; 3:193–203.

143. Leung YY, Yao Hui LL, Kraus VB. Colchicine--Update on mechanisms of action and therapeutic uses. Semin Arthritis Rheum 2015; 45:341–350.

144. Iacobuzio-Donahue CA, Lee EL, Abraham SC, Yardley JH, Wu TT. Colchicine toxicity: distinct morphologic findings in gastrointestinal biopsies. Am J Surg Pathol 2001; 25:1067–1073.

145. Daniels JA, Gibson MK, Xu L, et al. Gastrointestinal tract epithelial changes associated with taxanes: marker of drug toxicity versus effect. Am J Surg Pathol 2008; 32:473–477.
146. Hruban RH, Yardley JH, Donehower RC, Boitnott JK. Taxol toxicity. Epithelial necrosis in the gastrointestinal tract associated with polymerized microtubule accumulation and mitotic arrest. Cancer 1989; 63:1944–1950.
147. Seewaldt VL, Cain JM, Goff BA, et al. A retrospective review of paclitaxel-associated gastrointestinal necrosis in patients with epithelial ovarian cancer. Gynecol Oncol 1997; 67:137–140.
148. Chen JH, Pezhouh MK, Lauwers GY, Masia R. Histopathologic features of colitis due to immunotherapy with anti-PD-1 antibodies. Am J Surg Pathol 2017; 41:643–654.
149. Gupta A, De Felice KM, Loftus EV, Jr., Khanna S. Systematic review: colitis associated with anti-CTLA-4 therapy. Aliment Pharmacol Ther 2015; 42:406–417.
150. Prieux-Klotz C, Dior M, Damotte D, et al. Immune checkpoint inhibitor-induced colitis: Diagnosis and management. Target Oncol 2017; 12:301–308.
151. Geukes Foppen MH, Rozeman EA, van Wilpe S, et al. Immune checkpoint inhibition-related colitis: symptoms, endoscopic features, histology and response to management. ESMO Open 2018; 3:e000278.
152. Larkin J, Chiarion-Sileni V, Gonzalez R, et al. Combined nivolumab and ipilimumab or monotherapy in untreated melanoma. N Engl J Med 2015; 373:23–34.
153. Karamchandani DM, Chetty R. Immune checkpoint inhibitor-induced gastrointestinal and hepatic injury: pathologists' perspective. J Clin Pathol 2018; 71:665–671.
154. Verschuren EC, van den Eertwegh AJ, Wonders J, et al. Clinical, endoscopic, and histologic characteristics of ipilimumab-associated colitis. Clin Gastroenterol Hepatol 2016; 14:836–842.
155. Mitchell KA, Kluger H, Sznol M, Hartman DJ. Ipilimumab-induced perforating colitis. J Clin Gastroenterol 2013; 47:781–785.
156. Oble DA, Mino-Kenudson M, Goldsmith J, et al. Alpha-CTLA-4 mAb-associated panenteritis: a histologic and immunohistochemical analysis. Am J Surg Pathol 2008; 32:1130–1137.
157. Baroudjian B, Lourenco N, Pages C, et al. Anti-PD1-induced collagenous colitis in a melanoma patient. Melanoma Res 2016; 26:308–311.
158. Janela-Lapert R, Bouteiller J, Deschamps-Huvier A, Duval-Modeste AB, Joly P. Anti-PD-1 induced collagenous colitis in metastatic melanoma: a rare severe adverse event. Melanoma Res 2020; 30:603–605.
159. Karamchandani DM, Chetty R. Apoptotic colopathy: a pragmatic approach to diagnosis. J Clin Pathol 2018; 71:1033–1040.

Chapter 3

Eosinophilic diseases of the gastrointestinal tract

Robert M Genta, Shelby D Melton, Kevin O Turner

INTRODUCTION

Eosinophilic gastrointestinal diseases (EGIDs) are chronic inflammatory conditions characterised by persistent gastrointestinal (GI) symptoms and elevated levels of activated eosinophils in the GI tract [1]. In recent years, these conditions have garnered increasing attention from both researchers and clinicians. As eosinophilic oesophagitis (EoO) continues to solidify itself as a widely recognised condition with published diagnostic criteria and therapeutic guidelines [2–4], some have shifted their focus to the rest of the GI tract.

Historically, increased eosinophils in the stomach, small intestine, and colon have been viewed as a curiosity at best by the most pathologists and gastroenterologists. These conditions present with a constellation of non-specific symptoms (early satiety, nausea and vomiting, abdominal pain and cramping, bloating, and diarrhoea) that overlap with other common GI conditions, such as functional dyspepsia or irritable bowel syndrome. This broad-based clinical presentation, together with low disease awareness [5,6], perceived rarity, and the frequent absence of significant endoscopic findings [4,7] makes EGIDs an uncommon clinical suspicion. Pathologists have either completely ignored the findings or – when too obvious to leave unmentioned – may have reported them descriptively, such as "gastric mucosa with increased eosinophils," often listing parasites as a probable cause or suggesting the possibility of eosinophilic gastroenteritis. Since eosinophilic gastroenteritis had never been clearly defined, it was regarded as a non-actionable diagnosis by most clinicians. As a result, many patients face a long and frustrating delay with inappropriate care before the correct diagnosis is made [8].

In the past two decades, several studies have suggested that a subset of patients with dysfunctional dyspepsia, nausea, vomiting, and other symptoms also have increased

Robert M Genta MD, Departments of Pathology and Medicine, Baylor College of Medicine, Houston, TX, USA; Inform Diagnostics, TX, USA
E-mail: rmgenta@gastropath.com (for correspondence)

Shelby D Melton MD, Pathology and Laboratory Medicine Service, VA North Texas Health Care System, Dallas, TX, USA; Department of Pathology, UT Southwestern Medical Center, Dallas, TX, USA
E-mail: shelbyd.melton@va.gov

Kevin O Turner MD, Department of Pathology, University of Minnesota, Minneapolis, MN, USA
E-mail: turn0585@umn.edu

eosinophils in stomach and small intestine [9–11]. This has prompted those interested in such conditions to attempt to describe them further. Although a clear relationship between the magnitude of eosinophilic infiltrates and clinical manifestations has not been unequivocally demonstrated, an effort to quantify the eosinophils in the GI mucosa has been underway in an attempt to better characterise these eosinophilic conditions. The effort is spilling from the research to the clinical arena, and pathologists are requested with increasing frequency to quantify the eosinophil density not only in the oesophagus, where it is essentially expected, but also in the remainder of the GI tract.

The objective of this chapter is to present pathologists with state-of-the-art clinical and pathological information on EGIGs, and provide them the tools to incorporate the assessment of eosinophilia in the diagnosis of GI mucosal biopsies using a systematic approach to their evaluation, counting, and reporting.

THE EOSINOPHIL

Eosinophils are proinflammatory cells that are produced in the bone marrow and can be found in the blood and in tissue. The normal eosinophil range in peripheral blood is 0–450 eos/μL. In normal tissues, eosinophils are found in varying densities depending on the location. The lifecycle of an eosinophil involves approximately 8 days of maturation in the bone marrow, followed by up to 12 hours of circulation, and finally a 1- to 2-week life span in the tissues. Eosinophils have a characteristic appearance on haematoxylin and eosin (H&E) staining. They measure 12–17 μm in diameter and consist of a classic bilobate nucleus and myriad cytoplasmic granules that stain a characteristic pinkish red with H&E. The eosinophil granules contain proteins, including major basic protein (MBP), eosinophil peroxidase (EPO), eosinophilic cationic protein (ECP), and eosinophil-derived neurotoxin, as well as a several cytokines including transforming growth factor-beta1, vascular cell adhesion molecule, and phospho-SMAD2/3 [12–14]. Although an experienced pathologist rarely confuses eosinophils with other cells, it is important to recognise their differences from neutrophils, another acute inflammatory cell with a multilobate nuclei and cytoplasmic granules; these, however, are smaller and stain much lighter than eosinophil granules. Other structures that may histologically mimic eosinophils include Paneth cells and neuroendocrine cells within the glandular epithelium, but their granules are much larger than those found in the cytoplasm of eosinophils. Smooth muscle fibres cut at a certain angles and lymphocytes overlying red blood cells may also mimic eosinophils when observed at low power.

EOSINOPHILIC DISEASES OF THE GASTROINTESTINAL TRACT – TERMINOLOGY

In 2022, an International Consensus Group of gastroenterologists, pathologists, allergists, and researchers formed and used Delphi methods to standardise the nomenclature of EGIDs [15]. The group recognised that the widespread practice of using ambiguous terminology such as "eosinophilic gastroenteritis" was detrimental to the research and advancement of these conditions.

After deliberation, the group agreed on the following terms:

EGID – eosinophilic gastrointestinal diseases
EoO – eosinophilic oesophagitis
EoG – eosinophilic gastritis
EoN – eosinophilic enteritis
EoD – eosinophilic duodenitis
EoJ – eosinophilic jejunitis
EoI – eosinophilic ileitis
EoC – eosinophilic colitis

Eosinophilic gastroenteritis – Limited to stomach and small intestine, (*now historic term)

*The term eosinophilic gastroenteritis is being de-emphasized in favor of more specific naming conventions.

QUANTIFICATION OF EOSINOPHILS – TECHNICAL ASPECTS

A detailed set of guidelines on the assessment of eosinophils in the mucosa of GI tract can be found in a recently published topical primer, to which interested readers are referred [16]. A summary of these guidelines is provided below.

Oesophagus: Counting eosinophils within the squamous mucosa of the oesophagus is quite different from counting eosinophils in the remainder of the GI tract. This is because that in the normal oesophagus there are no resident inflammatory cells, including eosinophils. There are also no structures within the squamous epithelium other than squamous cells. This makes for a "clean background" in which to count eosinophils and, therefore, it is a fairly simple counting experience. The most effective strategy is to survey the specimen at low power, detect the areas with the highest eosinophil density, and then proceed to count eosinophils in one or more high-power fields (HPFs) in those areas.

Glandular mucosa of stomach, small intestine, and colon: A similar straightforward strategy cannot be easily applied to the remainder of the digestive tract, where the lamina propria of the normal mucosa is replete with inflammatory cells, including lymphocytes, plasma cells, mast cells, histiocytes, and variable numbers of eosinophils. In addition, there are many structures (not present in squamous mucosa) that interfere with the counting of individual cells, epithelial cells, glands, blood vessels, smooth muscle fibres, and stromal cells. In these locations, where counting can become more complex, it becomes crucial to develop a systematic approach.

Where to count?

When preparing to perform a count, the slide should be examined, and the number of levels and location of tissue fragment should be noted. The slides should then be examined on low-power and evaluated for stain quality and areas of optimal orientation. Other lesions that may impact eosinophil levels should be noted, e.g. *Helicobacter pylori*, coeliac disease, idiopathic inflammatory bowel disease (IBD), and microscopic colitis.

The ideal specimen will be oriented on edge with the surface clearly visualised on one side and the basement membrane or the *muscularis mucosae* on the other. Counting in poorly oriented areas may result in grossly inaccurate results. However, it is important to note that there will be times when the fields that have the greatest eosinophil density may not be the most appropriate for counting, e.g., areas adjacent to erosions, ulcerations, or neoplasia, or areas that have artefacts that can artificially affect the cell density, including over- or under-stained areas, crush artefact, or tissue folding. Fields predominantly void of tissue must be avoided to prevent falsely low counts. We also recommend against including multiple discontinuous fragments of tissue in a single field. An ideal field is one that does not overlap with any other counted field, is in a well-oriented area void of confounding histologic findings or artefacts, and that has the highest density of eosinophils. In time as one develops their own systematic method identifying such fields will become second nature. An example is included in **Figure 3.1.**

What to count?

Some authors have proposed strict criteria for the definition of a countable eosinophil, including the requirement to identify both lobes of the cell and at least a partial cytoplasmic membrane. Because histologic sections usually measure ~5 mμ in thickness, most eosinophils show only as partial portions of the cell, and may include only one lobe of the nucleus or none. Therefore, we recommend a more open definition of a countable eosinophil, a three-tiered definition of a countable eosinophil: (1) the rare picture-perfect intact eosinophil with red cytoplasmic eosinophilic granules and a bilobed nucleus; (2) a similar cell with only one lobe of the nucleus present; and (3) a cell-shaped sizable cluster of characteristic eosinophilic granules that appears to be membrane-bound but lacks an unequivocal nucleus. Scattered granules or smears, or wisps of granules should not be counted.

How to count?

Once proper fields are selected, the individual cells should be counted employing a systematic approach. A field can be examined using the "lawn mower" method sweeping back and forth, one side to the other, top to bottom, or dividing the field into segments of quadrants. Counts should be recorded as they are made, and one should attempt to be precise. Counts ending in 5 or 0 are a red flag for rounding and elicit the suspicion that a

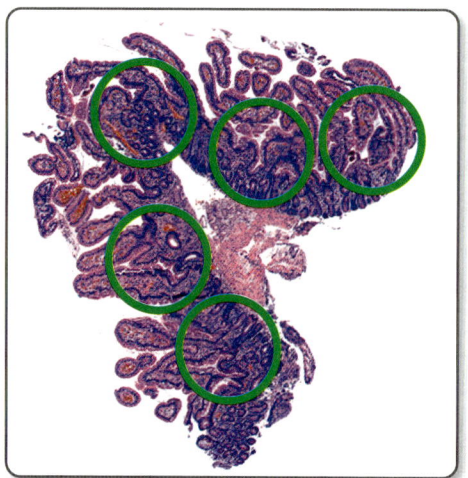

Figure 3.1 Gastric biopsy specimens with 5 non-overlapping high-power fields (HPF). Each HPF (green circles) represents an area of 0.237 mm², currently the most common area of the HPF in microscopes used in the US (40x lens with a 22-mm Ø ocular).

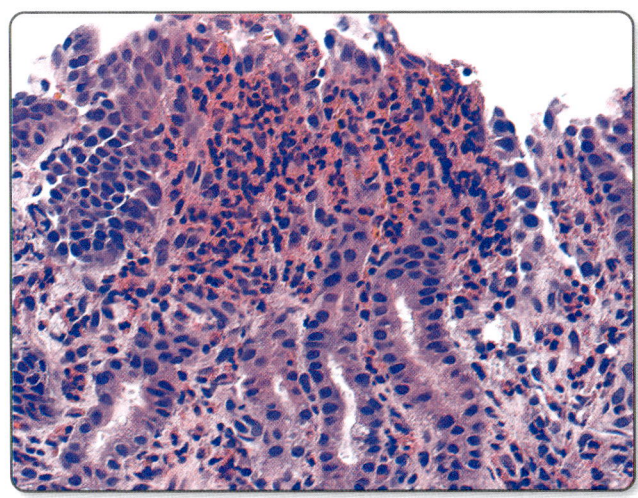

Figure 3.2 In this gastric biopsy, there is a large aggregate of eosinophils so close to one another to be essentially fused together. An accurate count in this area is impossible, and the observer should indicate that there is massive eosinophilic infiltration but that a definite number of eos/high-power field (HPF) cannot be provided.

reader makes estimated rather than counts. In cases of extremely high counts, numbers can be reported as, for example, ">200." If sheets of eosinophils are encountered that are not possible to numerate (**Figure 3.2**), a comment should be made that markedly increased eosinophils are present, but an accurate count cannot be provided.

We have observed that, regardless of a reader's preferred way of counting, the most reproducible results are achieved when a single preferred method is practised and consistently utilised. Some clinicians use counts to follow their patients' response to treatment. While interobserver variability is high amongst pathologists, a good degree of intraobserver consistency (that is, to agree with oneself) is attainable and important for assessing sequential procedures.

High-power field

The term "high-power field" is a nebulous term that represents a wide range of field areas depending on differences in equipment or values utilised. Colloquially, the HPF refers to a 40× objective on a microscope. However, the size of the field is not only determined by the objective magnification, but also the field number (FN) of the ocular piece. This results in HPFs ranging from 0.2 to 0.4 mm^2. The authors of this chapter have used microscopes with a 40× objective and a 22-mm ocular which results in the HPF area of 0.237 mm^2. This is the value we have used for all previous publications and the value that we input into digital viewers for HPF generation. As previously mentioned, we are aware of others that use various field areas, be it due to different equipment or different values inputted into digital viewers. To our knowledge, most investigators who study the quantification of cells use a field of areas between 0.2 and 0.3 mm^2. The remedy for this conundrum is rather than attempting to set a standardised field area, to standardise counts by converting them to eosinophils per mm^2. However, this step is unlikely to be widely adopted, in part because of the reluctance of many to embark even in simple calculations. For example, a count or 63 eosinophils in the HPF of 0.237 mm^2 would require a multiplication by 4.22 to achieve the count per square mm (266 eos/mm^2). For now, we recommend that pathologists should be aware of the size of their HPF in case such conversions become necessary in the future.

EOSINOPHILIC OESOPHAGITIS

Eosinophilic oesophagitis is a clinicopathologic condition characterised by mucosal eosinophilia of the oesophagus, oesophageal dysfunction, and associated symptoms. Before the mid-to-late 1990s, patients with complaints of dysphagia and intraepithelial eosinophils were usually diagnosed as having gastro-oesophageal reflux disease (GORD). It was not until scattered reports of patients with dysphagia, high levels of oesophageal eosinophils, allergic conditions, no obvious GORD symptoms began to emerge that EoO acquired its nosological status [17,18]. Initially received with skepticism by both clinicians and pathologists, over the following two decades evidence collected from exponentially increasing numbers of studies resulted in the establishment of in EoO as a distinct entity with published diagnostic criteria and therapeutic guidelines [19–21].

Epidemiology: Worldwide, EoO is estimated to have a prevalence of 50–100 per 100,000; it occurs in subjects of any age and is more prevalent in males than females that by a ratio (in the US) of approximately 3:1. There is evidence that its incidence is increasing worldwide, not only because it is increasingly recognised by both clinicians and pathologists, but likely because of yet unknown environmental risk factors [22–25].

Clinical manifestations: In adults, progressive dysphagia, with occasional solid food impaction, accompanied or not by gastro-oesophageal reflux, are characteristic symptoms. Regurgitation and failure to thrive are more common manifestations in infants and toddlers. Concurrent allergic conditions and asthma are common [26,27]. The classic endoscopic appearance of the oesophagus in EoO is characterised by furrows and rings (named "feline oesophagus"), as seen in **Figure 3.3** [28]. However, most patients have more subtle findings that somewhat limit the clinicians' ability to suspect EoO and transmit their suspicion to the pathologist [29]. As a result, many patients have to undergo multiple oesophagoscopies with biopsies before the correct diagnosis is made [6,30,31].

Histopathologic features: The oesophagus can mount only a limited set of injury patterns in response to different possible insults; even though we have identified parameters that are generally associated with EoO, none of them is, individually, either specific or

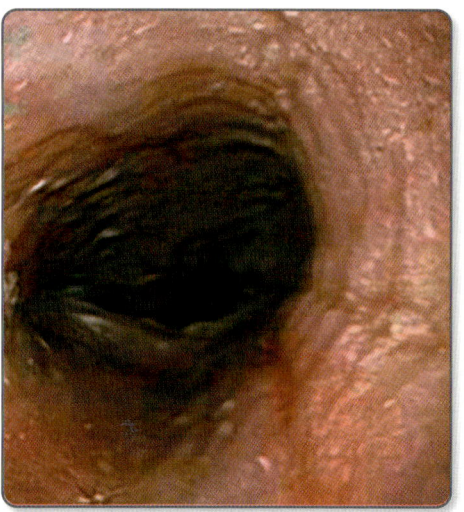

Figure 3.3 Endoscopic image from a patient with eosinophilic oesophagitis (EoO). The classic "feline oesophagus" is characterised by rings and longitudinal furrows that may run the entire length of the organ. Although quite specific, this appearance is not a sensitive marker of EoO, as many patients have only minimal endoscopic changes even in the presence of significant eosinophilic mucosal infiltrates.

diagnostic. Therefore, EoO is a clinicopathologic diagnosis that hinges upon a combination of clinical and histopathological findings. **Figure 3.4** illustrates the most characteristic features of EoO: (1) an intraepithelial infiltrate of at least 15 eosinophils per HPF; (2) dilated intercellular spaces; and (3) hyperplasia of the basal cell layer. The criterion of ≥15 eos/HPF was established by a consensus meeting in 2011 [19], and although it was made less stringent in later guidelines, it is still used in most specialised centres and in virtually all drug trials approved by the Federal Drug Administration [the Food and Drug Administration (FDA)]. In addition to the eosinophil density, pathologists involved in EoO studies are often asked to score oesophageal biopsies using the eosinophilic oesophagitis histologic scoring system (EoOHSS), a scoring system developed and validated by Collins et al [32]. The EoOHSS uses eosinophil density and seven additional features to create a grade and stage of disease severity. These features include basal cell hyperplasia (BCH), eosinophil abscess (EA), eosinophil surface layering (ESL), dilated intercellular spaces (DIS), surface epithelial alteration (SBA), dyskeratotic epithelial cells (DEC), and lamina propria fibrosis (LPF).

The distribution of eosinophils in an oesophagus affected by EoO may be very patchy [33,34]. Thus, to maximise the chance of adequate representations, an appropriate biopsy set must include at least two separate samples each from the proximal, mid, or distal oesophagus (>2 cm from the gastro-oesophageal junction). If the gastro-oesophageal junction is examined, eosinophils should be counted only in the squamous component;

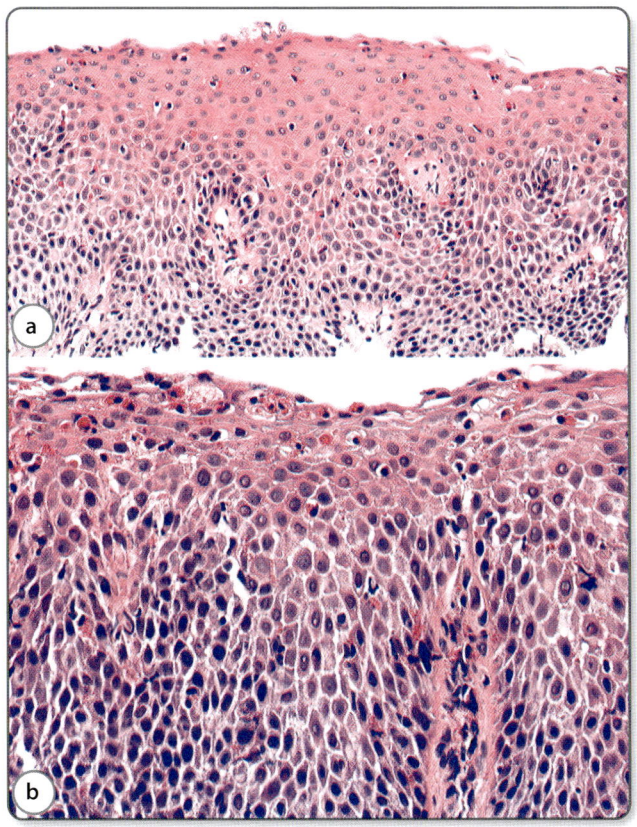

Figure 3.4 Panel (a) shows a low-power photomicrograph of an oesophageal biopsy from a patient with eosinophilic oesophagitis (EoO). There are scattered eosinophils, moderate basal cell hyperplasia, and dilatation of the intercellular spaces ("spongiosis") limited to the lower half of the mucosa. In panel (b) (from a patient with more severe changes), one can appreciate the eosinophils infiltrating the mucosal surface where they cause microscopic breaches (micro-erosions). Both spongiosis and basal cell hyperplasia extend to essentially the entire epithelium. The visible papilla shows fibrosis, a characteristic finding in advanced EoO.

however – particularly if the distal samples are the only ones available or the only ones with a significant density of eosinophils – the findings must be interpreted with care due to the overlapping features with GORD.

Reporting oesophageal biopsies submitted for the evaluation of EoO: If no HPFs with at least 15 eos/HPF can be identified in any of the submitted sample, the report should indicate the highest number counted and let clinicians draw their own conclusions. It would be imprudent and possibly misleading to state, e.g. that there are 13 eos/HPF and "no evidence of EoO."

If one or more HPFs with ≥15 eos/HPF are detected, the highest count should be provided, unless it is extremely high and an exact count is not practical to perform. In such case, it is acceptable to use a "greater than" expression such as >100 eos/HPF. Performing a full EoOHSS score can time-consuming and is best done only when requested by a study protocol. However, we suggest at least reporting in a comment the associated histologic features, as they can help in the diagnosis of EoO especially in the face of borderline counts. It is important to tailor the report to the clinical questions and the patient history provided, including the clinician's impressions. We strongly recommend avoiding generic semi-descriptive diagnoses such as "oesophageal mucosa with increased eosinophils;" these types of timid statements are rarely helpful clinically consequential.

The examples in **Table 3.1** are provided to show how we recommend reporting histologic findings in different clinical scenarios.

Table 3.1 Clinical Vignettes to show how we recommend reporting histologic findings in different clinical scenarios of oesophagitis					
Patient	**History**	**Endo/ Clinical impression**	**Histologic findings**	**Suggested diagnosis**
30-year-old male	Dysphagia Food impaction	White plaques History of EoO	Proximal: 70 eos/ HPF Mid: 90 eos/HPF Distal: 80 eos/HPF Basal hyperplasia, dilated intercellular space, lamina propria fibrosis, eosinophilic microabscesses	*Oesophageal mucosa with intraepithelial eosinophils consistent with eosinophilic oesophagitis; see comment* *Comment*: Sections of oesophageal mucosa show intraepithelial eosinophils numbering up to 90 in a HPF, basal cell hyperplasia, dilated intercellular spaces, lamina propria fibrosis, and eosinophilic microabscesses. The findings are consistent with the patient's reported history of eosinophilic oesophagitis
30-year-old male	Dysphagia Food impaction	White plaques Suspect EoO	Proximal: 70 eos/HPF Mid: 90 eos/HPF Distal: 80 eos/HPF Basal hyperplasia, dilated intercellular space, lamina propria fibrosis, eosinophilic microabscesses	*Oesophageal mucosa with increased intraepithelial eosinophils; see comment* *Comment*: Sections of oesophageal mucosa show intraepithelial eosinophils numbering up to 90 in a HPF, basal cell hyperplasia, dilated intercellular spaces, lamina propria fibrosis, and eosinophilic microabscesses. The findings are consistent with the reported suspicion of eosinophilic oesophagitis

Continues opposite

			Table 3.1 *Continued.*	
Patient	History	Endo/ Clinical impression	Histologic findings	Suggested diagnosis
19-year-old female	Dysphagia History of GORD	Normal oesophagus	Proximal: 11 eos/ HPF Mid: 10 eos/HPF Distal: 13 eos/HPF Basal hyperplasia, dilated intercellular space, lamina propria fibrosis	*Oesophageal mucosa with increased intraepithelial eosinophils; see comment* *Comment*: Sections of oesophageal mucosa show intraepithelial eosinophils numbering up to 90 in a HPF, basal cell hyperplasia, dilated intercellular spaces, and lamina propria fibrosis. This pattern of injury may be attributed to GORD; however, in light of the eosinophil density approaching the cutoff criteria and the presence of additional associated features, eosinophilc oesophagitis cannot be excluded histologically
40-year-old male	History of GORD	Normal oesophagus	Proximal: 70 eos/ HPF Mid: 90 eos/HPF Distal: 80 eos/HPF Basal hyperplasia, dilated intercellular space, lamina propria, fibrosis, eosinophilic microabscesses	*Oesophageal mucosa with increased intraepithelial eosinophils; see comment* *Comment*: Sections of oesophageal mucosa show intraepithelial eosinophils numbering up to 90 in a HPF, basal cell hyperplasia, dilated intercellular spaces, lamina propria fibrosis, and eosinophilic microabscesses. The findings are compatible with eosinophilic oesophagitis in the proper clinical setting
64-year-old female	Dysphagia	White plaques	Proximal: 41 eos/ HPF Mid: 52 eos/HPF Distal: 35 eos/HPF *Candida*, basal hyperplasia, dilated intercellular space, lamina propria, fibrosis, eosinophilic microabscesses, superficial eosinophil layering	*Oesophageal mucosa with increased intraepithelial eosinophils; see comment* *Comment*: Sections of oesophageal mucosa show fungal organisms consistent with *Candida*, intraepithelial eosinophils, basal cell hyperplasia, dilated intercellular spaces, lamina propria fibrosis, eosinophilic microabscesses, and superficial eosinophil layering. This pattern of injury may be related to the patient's fungal infection; however, in light of the presence of >15 eos/HPF eosinophilic oesophagitis cannot be excluded histologically

EoO, eosinophilic oesophagitis; GORD, gastro-oesophageal reflux disease; HPF, high-power field

EOSINOPHILIC GASTRITIS

The GI tract beyond the oesophagus is composed of glandular mucosa where eosinophils are a normal constituent of the lamina propria. The 1996 Updated Sydney System detailed many abnormalities of the stomach including intraepithelial eosinophils (as one of the types of "special gastritis") [35], but finding increased eosinophils within the lamina propria was not seen as a specific pathologic feature. Increased eosinophils in the gastric mucosa may be associated with a variety of conditions including infections (*Anisakis, Strongyloides stercoralis, Helicobacter* species, etc.), idiopathic IBD, various medications, allergic conditions, connective tissue and autoimmune disease, tumours, erosion and ulcers [36]. An interest in better defining EoG emerged only in the early 2000.

Epidemiology: In part because of the lack of established diagnostic criteria, clinical and pathological lack of awareness, the difficulty of maintaining EoG separate from other non-oesophageal EGIDs, and disease-coding inaccuracies, the true prevalence of EoG has not been determined. Data from national databases, however, suggest that the condition is rare, with fewer than 7 per 100,000 [22,37,38]. Several researchers have suggested, however, that these low figures may represent gross underestimates. For example, the IDEA database, a repository of approximately 2 million patients who underwent EGD with gastric biopsies in private endoscopy centres in the US, EoG was either diagnosed or mentioned as a viable candidate diagnosis in 1 every 700 patients (with a corresponding prevalence of 0.14%). EoG can occur in subjects of any age and, like other non-oesophageal EGIDs, is almost equally prevalent in males and females.

Clinical manifestations: The symptoms associated with EoG (dyspepsia, nausea, vomiting, and epigastric pain) are non-specific and overlap with many other gastric conditions. Therefore, except for specialised centres where patients are often referred after years of missed diagnoses [30], the index of suspicion amongst gastroenterologists is very low [5]. The endoscopic appearance of the gastric mucosa is often normal or minimally erythematous **(Figure 3.5)**. In the absence of histopathologic criteria for the diagnosis of

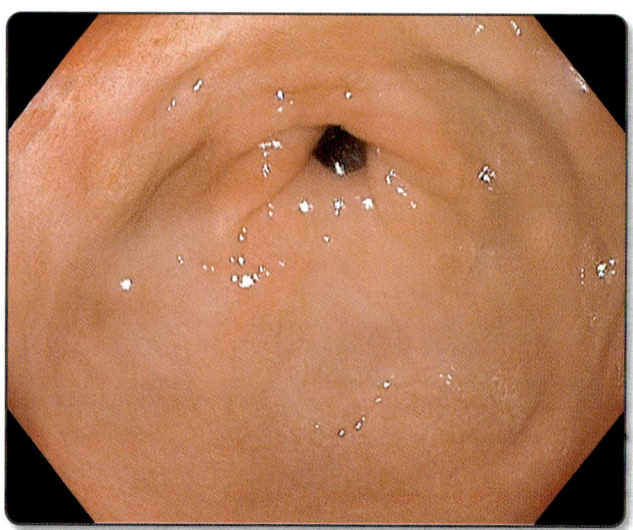

Figure 3.5 Only minimal erythema is seen endoscopically in this stomach from a patient with marked eosinophilic gastritis. The bland non-specific endoscopic appearance of eosinophilic gastrointestinal diseases (EGIDs) is at the root of their low level of suspicion amongst gastroenterologists.

EoG, pathologists, who underdiagnose EGIDs even when alerted by clinicians [6], tend to report eosinophilic infiltrates only when they are extremely prominent, and even then they prefer a descriptive comment to a diagnosis of EoG.

Histopathology features

The normal eosinophilic counts in the gastric mucosa: While most observers consider the presence of a few eosinophils in the lamina propria common, the Updated Sydney System incorrectly stated that intraepithelial eosinophils in gastric mucosa are always viewed as abnormal [35]. The limited information available regarding the normal range of gastric mucosal eosinophils is derived from often uncontrolled case series, isolated case reports, or brief sections in textbooks of GI pathology [39–41]. In the Kalixanda study, Talley et al found a mean eosinophil count of 11 eosinophils in five HPFs in biopsies from the cardia, body, and antrum of asymptomatic adult volunteers from Northern Sweden [42]. DeBrosse et al found peak eosinophil counts of eight eosinophils per HPF in antral and 11 in oxyntic mucosal biopsies from 19 children [41]. In a 2011 paper we enumerated eosinophils in the lamina propria of patients from a wide age range and geographic areas in the United States who had no known history of relevant GI disease and whose gastric biopsies were diagnosed as unremarkable [43]. The mean eosinophil count for 135 normal patients (age range 4–81 years) was four eosinophils per HPF (±4 SD), equivalent to 15 ± 17 SD eos/mm^2 (range 0–110). There were no significant differences between the counts in biopsies from the antrum and corpus, and no significant variation by either age or geographic location. Our findings were in essential agreement with those of both DeBrosse and Talley [41,42].

EoG: If a gastric biopsy specimen shows increased eosinophilic infiltrates, the pathologist should first attempt to exclude other possible causes of eosinophilia, which can often be found in the patient's history or in the features of the specimen under examination. Then, fields devoid of confounding factors (e.g. erosion, ulceration, neoplasm, and processing artefacts) can be chosen for counting. As previously mentioned, it is important to find a well-oriented area with surface epithelium on one side and the submucosal aspect of the tissue on the other. When examining the stomach, high magnification (200×) is usually required to detect optimal fields because eosinophils are often squeezed between glands and other lamina propria structures. This is especially true in the oxyntic mucosa where eosinophils can be nearly invisible at low power (**Figure 3.6**). Although no published consensus guidelines for the histopathologic diagnosis of EoG are available, many experts, including us, diagnose EoG when at least 5 HPFs with ≥30 eosinophils each are present in a set of gastric biopsies. The FDA has also allowed this criterion for several clinical eosinophilic gastritis pharmaceutical trials [44].

Many subjects with EoO have concurrent pathologic changes in the gastric mucosa in addition to increased eosinophils (**Figure 3.7**). Epithelial damage is almost always present, with foveolar hyperplasia that mimics reactive gastropathy. A variable degree of chronic inflammation, with prominent lymphocytic and plasma cell infiltrates is frequent. Long-standing cases may show advanced fibrosis, which in extreme cases separates the oxyntic mucosa in small nodules wrapped by fibrotic tissue, in an appearance that we have informally referred to as "gastric cirrhosis" (**Figure 3.8**).

Reporting oesophageal biopsies submitted for the evaluation of EoG: When requested to evaluate a gastric biopsy set for EoG in settings outside clinical studies, we suggest that pathologists count the eosinophils in the area with the greatest eosinophil density, and

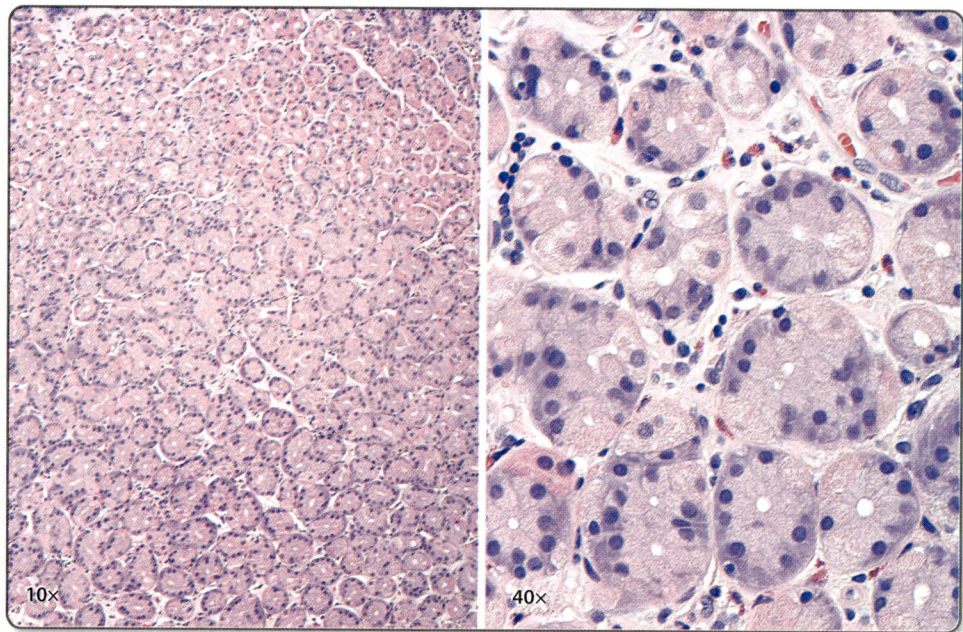

Figure 3.6 These photomicrographs illustrate the importance of suspecting that eosinophils may be found in the oxyntic mucosa. If only a brief low-power (10×, left panel) examination of the oxyntic mucosa were made, one could conclude that it was normal; however, a careful search for eosinophils at 40× (right panel) shows numerous cells between the oxyntic glands. Normally, no more than 2–5 is present per high-power field (HPF) in the oxyntic mucosa.

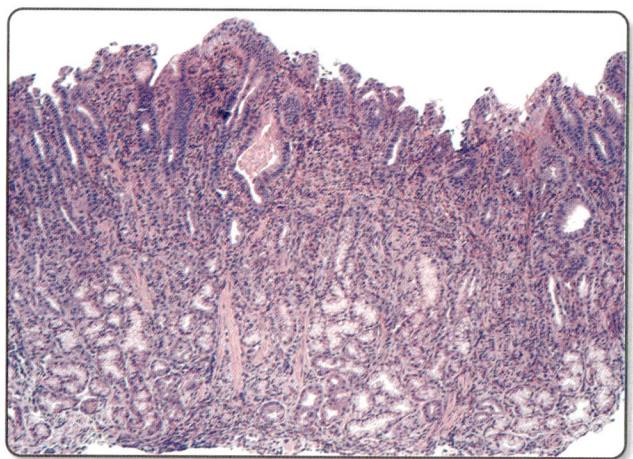

Figure 3.7 This biopsy from a subject with a very marked eosinophilic infiltration of the antral mucosa shows some of the other features of eosinophilic gastritis (EoG): marked chronic inflammation, epithelial damage, foveolar architectural irregularities, and prominent smooth muscle fibres, all features that could suggest reactive gastropathy.

report that number along with a comment that clarifies how diffuse the eosinophilic infiltration is. This is crucial for the diagnosis of EoO because a single focus of eosinophilia is much less likely to represent EoG than an uneven but diffuse infiltrate in several parts of the stomach. We are currently working on the evaluation of a single-field value that would alleviate the time-consuming practice of counting five fields and possibly making pathologists more likely to report gastric eosinophil counts [45]. The examples in **Table 3.2**

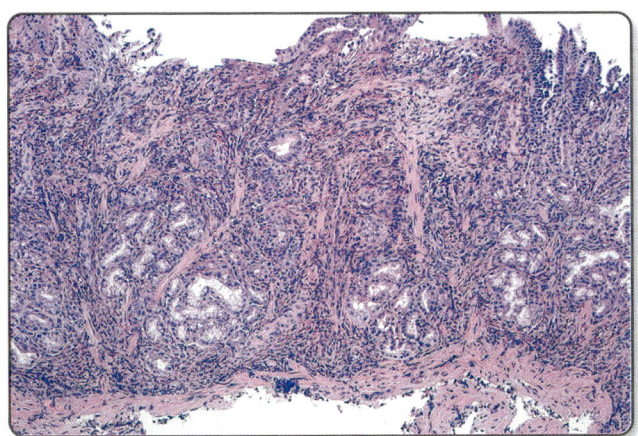

Figure 3.8 Marked fibrosis of the gastric mucosa is frequently found in patients with long-standing severe eosinophilic gastritis (EoG). In this case, sheets of eosinophils can be seen in and adjacent to the fibrous bands that engulf the remaining gastric glands and foveolae.

Table 3.2 Clinical vignettes to show how we recommend reporting histologic findings in different clinical scenarios of gastritis				
Patient	**History**	**Endo/Clinical impression**	**Histologic findings**	**Suggested diagnosis**
25-year-old female	Epigastric pain	Mild erythema	Increased gastric lamina propria eosinophils, numerous fields >30 with a peak count of 70	*Gastric mucosa with increased lamina propria eosinophils; see comment* *Comment*: Sections of gastric mucosa show increased lamina propria eosinophils (>30 eos/HPF in >5 fields; peak count of 70/HPF). These findings meet the criteria many experts use for the diagnosis of eosinophilic gastritis
25-year-old female	Dyspepsia, allergies, sister with history of eosinophilic gastroenteritis	Normal mucosa	Increased duodenal lamina propria eosinophils, numerous fields >100 with a peak count of >100	*Duodenal mucosa with increased lamina propria eosinophils; see comment* *Comment*: Sections of gastric mucosa show increased lamina propria eos (>100 eosinophils/HPF in >3 fields; peak count of >100/HPF). These findings are suggestive of eosinophilic duodenitis

Continues overleaf

Patient	History	Endo/Clinical impression	Histologic findings	Suggested diagnosis
25-year-old female	Dyspepsia, history of EoO	Mild erythema	Increased gastric and duodenal lamina propria eosinophils, numerous fields >30 with a peak count of 80	*Gastric and duodenal mucosa with increased lamina propria eosinophils; see comment* *Comment*: Sections of gastric mucosa show increased lamina propria eosinophils (>30 eos/HPF in >5 fields in the stomach and >3 fields in the duodenum; peak count of 80/HPF). The eosinophil density meets the criteria many experts use for the diagnosis of eosinophilic gastritis and duodenitis. Considering the patient's history of EoO the findings are consistent with eosinophilic gastritis and duodenitis with oesophageal involvement

Table 3.2 *Continued.*

EoO, eosinophilic oesophagitis; HPF, high-power field

are provided to show how we recommend reporting increased eosinophilia in different clinical scenarios.

Ideal biopsy sampling for the histopathologic diagnosis of EoG: Several studies have shown that four samples from the corpus and four from the antrum (delivered in two separate containers) provide excellent sampling that allows the detection of almost 100% of patients who have EoG [16,36,45,46].

EOSINOPHILIC DUODENITIS

Several studies have indicated that subgroups of patients with dyspepsia, post-prandial fullness or bloating, and other common and relatively vague digestive symptoms have increased numbers of duodenal eosinophils [9,11,42,47–49]. Although most of these studies have originated from a single centre in Australia, similar results have been obtained in later confirmatory studies and meta-analyses [50–52]. The main problem of applying these findings to real-life situations is the still undefined number of eosinophils in the duodenum of a normal subject. Although the reported numbers vary widely, we performed a systematic study on 370 patients with a histologically normal duodenum and no history of small intestinal disease and found mean counts of 8.2 eosinophils $\pm$ 6.3 SD, equivalent to ~35 $\pm$ 25 eos/mm^2 [53]. Based on this study, data from the literature, and our extensive experience on hundreds of duodenal biopsies collected from patients screened for drug studies, we concluded that 20 eos/HPF can be considered as a reasonable upper limit of normal.

Small intestinal eosinophilia can be associated with all the same local and systemic conditions that cause gastric eosinophilia (infections, idiopathic IBD, various medications, allergic conditions, connective tissue and autoimmune disease, tumours, and possibly erosion and ulcers). In this section, we will only discuss the condition that, albeit with some uncertainties, is currently referred to as eosinophilic duodenitis (EoD).

Epidemiology: Because it appears there is an even greater reluctance to make a histological diagnosis of EoD than one of EoG, the few data available show a minimal prevalence of this condition (<9/100,000 for gastroenteritis, so presumably much less for duodenitis) [22]; not surprisingly, no data exist on its incidence. In the IDEA database, the number of cases diagnosed as EoD was about one-tenth of those diagnosed as EoG.

Clinical manifestations: The same non-specific manifestations that characterise patients with EoG are encountered in those with EoD (dyspepsia, bloating, nausea and vomiting). Some patients with EoD have erosions and ulcers, and their manifestations include epigastric pain and, rarely, haematemesis. In the absence of lesions (erosions and ulcers), endoscopy shows either a normal or a mildly erythematous mucosa. Again, like in other EGIDs, neither clinical manifestations nor endoscopic findings lead gastroenterologists to suspect EoD. Only a carefully collected history of allergic conditions (e.g. asthma, atopic dermatitis) or peripheral eosinophilia may help to orient the astute clinician towards the possibility of EoD or, more generically, eosinophilic gastroenteritis. As in the case of EoG, most patients experience a long delay from the first symptoms to the diagnosis [6,30,31].

Histopathologic features: If a duodenal biopsy specimen shows markedly increased eosinophilic infiltrates, after excluding other possible causes of eosinophilia, the pathologist should attempt to count eosinophils in a few HPFs. We cannot overemphasise the importance of examining well-oriented areas with villi on one side and the muscularis mucosae on the other. However, in the duodenum, it can be more difficult to find adequate fields because the small intestine is more prone to poor orientation, and it can be difficult to fill the field with tissue due to its villous architecture. Eosinophils can be found in the villi as well as in the subjacent lamina propria, but it is important to not miss the deep part of the tissue between the bottom of the crypts and the muscularis mucosae. While in severe cases (those with very high counts) eosinophils are found everywhere (**Figure 3.9**), in mild to moderate cases the "sub-cryptal band" is where much of the infiltrates are found (**Figure 3.10**).

Although no published consensus guidelines for the histopathologic diagnosis of EoD are available, the FDA has agreed that for some pharmaceutical trials a criterion of "at least 30 eos/HPF in at least three HPFs" be used to categorise patients as having EoD [44]. In our experience, this threshold allows to establish a diagnosis of EoD in many borderline subjects which may not have the conditions. Therefore, we recommend using Collins's suggestion of 52 eos/HPF [54], perhaps rounding the number to 50.

When the numbers of eosinophils are very high, the villous architecture is altered and the mucosa may take an appearance suggestive of variable villous abnormality and, in some areas, be almost flat (**Figure 3.11**). However, once the eosinophils are detected – and the lack of significant intraepithelial lymphocytosis is confirmed – the differentiation from coeliac disease becomes obvious. Ulcers and fibrosis may be found in advanced cases.

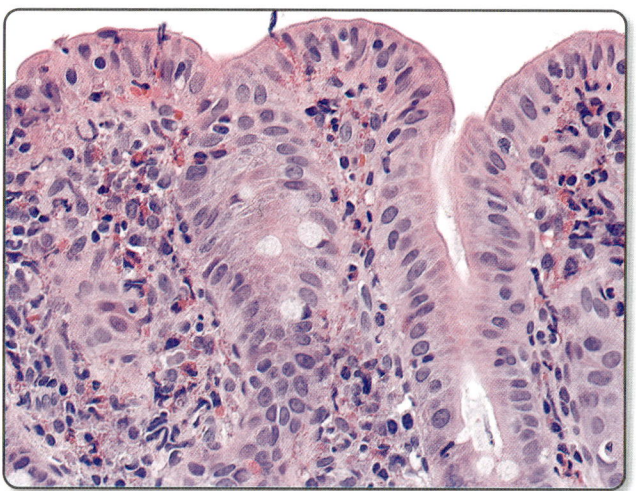

Figure 3.9 Marked eosinophilic infiltrates in the tips of duodenal villi in a subject with marked eosinophilic duodenitis (EoD). There is eosinophilic degranulation seeping into the surface epithelium.

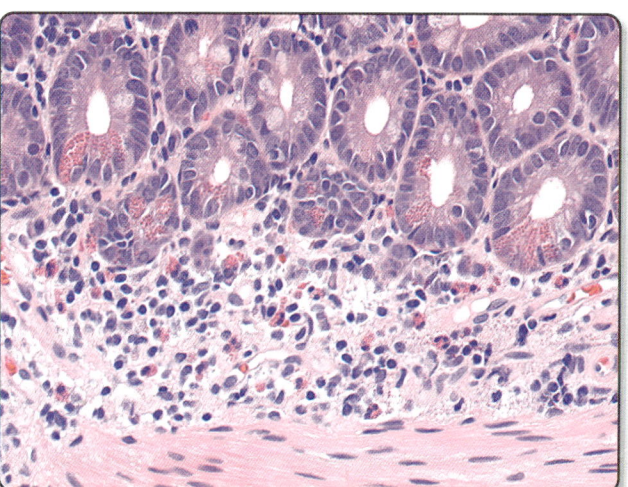

Figure 3.10 The area immediately below the lower tip of the duodenal crypts and above the muscularis mucosae is particularly rich in eosinophils, both in patients with normal counts and in those with eosinophilic duodenitis (EoD).

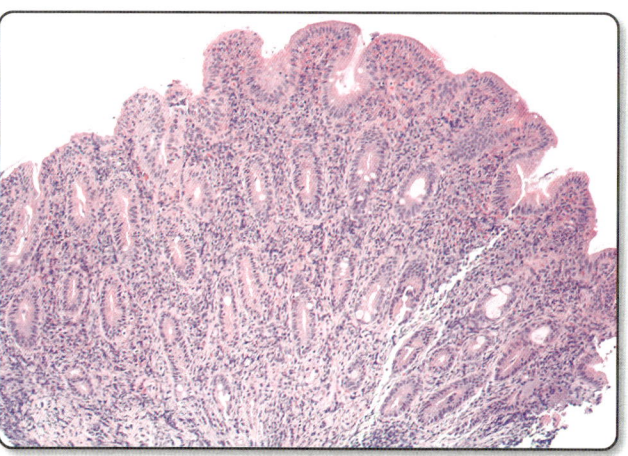

Figure 3.11 A low-power examination of the duodenal mucosa from patients with eosinophilic duodenitis (EoD) may give a first impression of complete or partial villous flattening, suggesting coeliac disease. Yet, the changes that affect the duodenal architecture in EoD are not accompanied by significant epithelial lymphocytosis; furthermore, a closer examination at higher power will reveal the eosinophilic infiltrates.

Reporting oesophageal biopsies submitted for the evaluation of EoD or eosinophilic gastroenteritis: A request to the pathologist to "rule out EoD" is extremely rare, and it almost never accompanies a duodenal biopsy taken during the patient's first EGD [5]. If a gastroenterologist has reasons to suspect EGID, will likely ask to rule out eosinophilic gastroenteritis. Because the only accessible portion of the small intestine is the duodenum (and the very proximal jejunum), a pathologist can only respond with a diagnosis of duodenitis. If the levels of eosinophils per HPF that the pathologist chooses to use (for example, either ≥30 eos/HPF in at least three HPFs, or >50 eos in at least one HPF) are detected, the counts should be reported and a diagnosis of "consistent with" or "suggestive of" EoD can be made. Lower numbers – those possibly associated with dyspepsia, but not yet defined or even proposed – could be reported. However, given the status of the relevant evidence, it would be imprudent to suggest that they could provide an explanation for the patient's reported dyspepsia, bloating, or other very non-specific symptoms. **Table 3.2** shows how we recommend reporting increased eosinophilia in different clinical scenarios.

Ideal biopsy sampling for the histopathologic diagnosis of EoD: Several studies have shown that four samples from any portion of the duodenum provide sufficient sampling to allow the detection of almost 100% of patients who have EoD [16,36,45,46].

EOSINOPHILIC COLITIS

Colonic eosinophilia, often referred to as eosinophilic colitis (EoC), remains a poorly understood condition. Until recently it was not even clear whether it represented a distinct disease or was a colonic manifestation of EGID or IBD. Classically, EoC was classified into allergic colitis of infancy and the most poorly characterised adolescent and adult allergic colitis. Both were diagnosed after exclusion of all other known causes of eosinophilia [55]. Allergic colitis in infancy (also known as the "dietary protein-induced proctocolitis of infancy syndrome") was considered to result from immune-mediated reactions to ingested proteins, such as cow's milk and soy proteins [56]. The pathogenesis of the adult form of the disease did not appear to be related to IgE-associated triggers and continues to remain elusive. However, a recent study established EoC transcriptomic profiles, identified mechanistic pathways, and integrated findings with parallel IBD and EGID data. These findings established EoC as a distinct disease compared with other EGIDs and IBD, thereby providing a basis for improving diagnosis and treatment [57].

Epidemiology: EoC is the least common of the EGIDs, with a reported prevalence of 1.6–2.1 per 100,000 in the US population [37,58]. In the IDEA database of 3.2 M US patients with colonic biopsies it was diagnosed histopathologically in <1 in 8,500 patients (or 0.012%).

Clinical manifestations: In one study, 38% of patients with colonic eosinophilia had no significant symptoms and the eosinophilia was discovered during a screening colonoscopy [7]. Amongst those who have manifestations prompting a colonoscopy, diarrhoea, abdominal pain, anaemia, rectal bleeding, and weight loss are the most common presentations. However, none of these manifestations are characteristic and they do not occur more frequently than in subjects with IBD, active colitis, or microscopic colitis. The endoscopic appearance is also non-contributory, with either a normal appearance (even in the presence of diffuse eosinophilic infiltrates), or erythema, erosions, and a pale granular mucosa. Thus, neither clinical manifestations nor endoscopic appearance are sufficiently characteristic to elicit the suspicion of colonic eosinophilia. This is reflected in the extremely rare requests from clinicians to ask for the investigation of possible EoC when submitting colonic biopsies for pathologic examination.

Histopathologic features

The normal eosinophilic counts in the colonic mucosa: The normal content of eosinophils in the adult colon and the criteria for the histopathologic diagnosis of EoC remain undefined. In a recent study, we counted the eosinophils in the right, transverse, and left colon of 159 adults with normal colonic histology. Using a database of 1.2 million patients with colonic biopsies, we extracted all adults with a diagnosis of colonic eosinophilia. We reviewed the slides from all cases and captured demographic, clinical, and pathologic data, including information about eosinophilia in other organs. We then compared the clinical manifestations of the study patients (those with no identifiable cause of eosinophilia) to those of patients with other types of colitis. The normal eosinophil counts (per HPF) were 55.7 ± 23.4 in the right (**Figure 3.12**), 41.0 ± 18.6 in the transverse, and 28.6 ± 17.2 in the left colon. Data from other sources are in the same range with our findings. The important message deriving from these studies is that there is no "normal number" of eosinophils in the colon: each segment of the organ has its own range of normal eosinophil density, with a considerable and progressive decrease from the right colon to the rectum.

Eosinophilic colitis: Most subjects with eosinophilic infiltrates in the colonic mucosa associated with primary EoC have a normal mucosal architecture and a normal or mildly increased mononuclear inflammatory component of the lamina propria [7,36,59]. This is an important feature that allows for an easy differentiation from the other more common causes of colonic eosinophilia, including IBD. Intramucosal parasites and their components (*S. stercoralis, T. trichura, Schistosoma* species eggs) tend to cause massive but localised eosinophilic responses that engulf the organism or its parts, which can often be detected by sequential sections of the biopsy specimens (**Figure 3.13**). As shown in **Figure 3.14**, the eosinophilic infiltrates can be extremely dense, obliterating the spaces between crypts, but generally without causing significant epithelial infiltration. In cases such as the one depicted

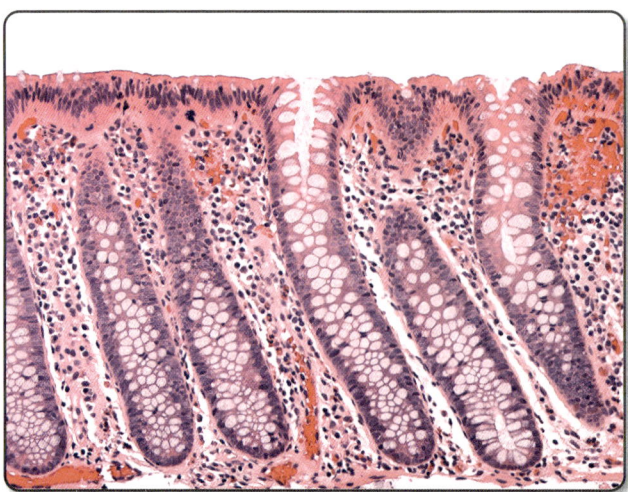

Figure 3.12 This section from the transverse colon from a normal control shows numerous eosinophils in the lamina propria. An inexperienced observer might suspect eosinophilia. However, the density of eosinophils is normal for the area of colon where the biopsy originated. Had it come from the distal sigmoid, it could be abnormally high.

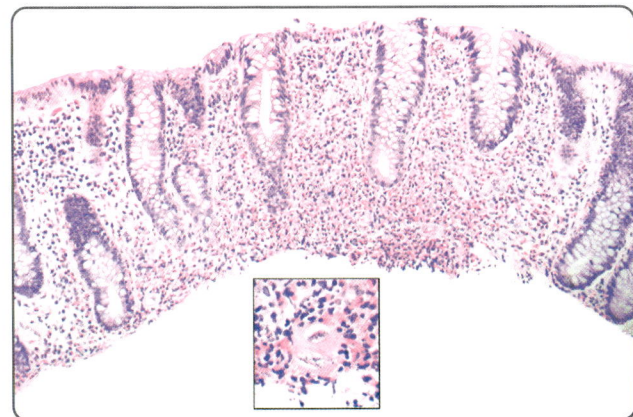

Figure 3.13 A massive focal infiltrate of eosinophils adjacent to an essentially normal colonic mucosa is most likely caused by a fragment of a parasitic helminth. Serial sections examined at high power (as shown in the inset) frequently reveal particles that sometimes can help to determine the organism responsible for the "eosinophilic abscess."

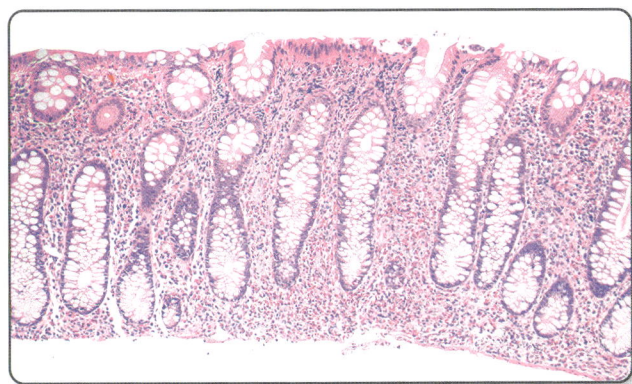

Figure 3.14 Severe and diffuse infiltrates in a background of a normal or almost normal glandular architecture are typical of idiopathic colonic eosinophilia (or eosinophilic colitis, EoC). Although such marked eosinophilic infiltrates are rarely present in patients with inflammatory bowel disease (IBD), the unaltered architecture is seen as a crucial histologic feature for the differentiation of EoC from IBD.

here, as it happened in most cases included in our study, the number of eosinophils is too large and, consequently, impossible to determine by visual counting.

Reporting colonic biopsies submitted for the evaluation of EoC: In spite of the disease-defining molecular findings in the study by Shoda et al [57], a diagnosis of EoC cannot be made in the absence of supporting clinical evidence, such as EGID in other organs, peripheral eosinophilia, documented the history of allergies or asthma. Since many patients with important eosinophilic infiltrates in the colon are asymptomatic, and molecular profiling is not yet clinically available, in most cases it may be preferable to report the eosinophil counts (when possible) and use the term "colonic eosinophilia" in the diagnostic line. EoC should be reserved to patients in which an EGID is documented. Clinical vignettes with similar histology but different manifestations are depicted in **Table 3.3**.

Ideal biopsy sampling for the histopathologic diagnosis of EoC: Considering the differences in the distribution of eosinophils throughout the colon, sampling should include at least two fragments from each of the following compartments: caecum; ascending colon; transverse colon; left colon; sigmoid; and rectum.

Table 3.3 Clinical vignettes to show how we recommend reporting histologic findings in different clinical scenarios of colitis

Patient	History	Endo/Clinical impression	Histologic findings	Suggested diagnosis
60-year-old male	Screening colonoscopy	Normal mucosa	Increased lamina propria eosinophils, numerous fields > 80 with a peak count of 120	*Colonic mucosa with increased lamina propria eosinophils; see comment* *Comment*: Sections of colonic mucosa show increased lamina propria eosinophils (>80 eos/HPF in multiple fields; peak count of 120/HPF). These findings may represent eosinophilic colitis in the proper clinical setting
60-year-old male	Diarrhoea	Normal mucosa	Increased lamina propria eosinophils, numerous fields > 60 with a peak count of 100	*Colonic mucosa with increased lamina propria eosinophils; see comment* *Comment*: Sections of colonic mucosa show increased lamina propria eosinophils (>80 eos/HPF in multiple fields; peak count of 120/HPF). In a patient with diarrhoea these findings are consistent with eosinophilic colitis

HPF, high-power field

MAST CELLS

An essential part of the immune system, mast cells play an important role in the pathogenesis of a variety of digestive diseases, including eosinophilic gastrointestinal disorders (EGID) and mastocytic enterocolitis. Surgical pathologists are seldom asked to comment on the distribution or density of mast cells in GI biopsy specimens, except for the rare patient suspected of having either systemic mastocytosis, mastocytic enterocolitis, or mast cell activation syndrome. However, in the last few years, requests to quantify small intestinal and colonic mast cells have increased considerably due to reports suggesting that a subset of patients with functional GI disease (functional dyspepsia and refractory irritable bowel syndrome) may have increased enteric mast cell density [60–64]. More recently, researchers and clinicians have turned their attention to the upper GI tract where increased mast cells have been associated with allergic conditions [26], EoO [65–67], gastritis [45], duodenitis [51,64]. **Figure 3.15** illustrates a case of EoO in which mast cell tryptase staining highlights a large population of mast cells, which are absent from the normal oesophagus. For now, only research protocols involve the requirement to evaluate the density of mucosal mast cells, and often count them, in several HPFs of EGID biopsies. It is not unlikely that pathologists will soon be faced with increasing requests to quantify mast cells in every compartment of the GI tract.

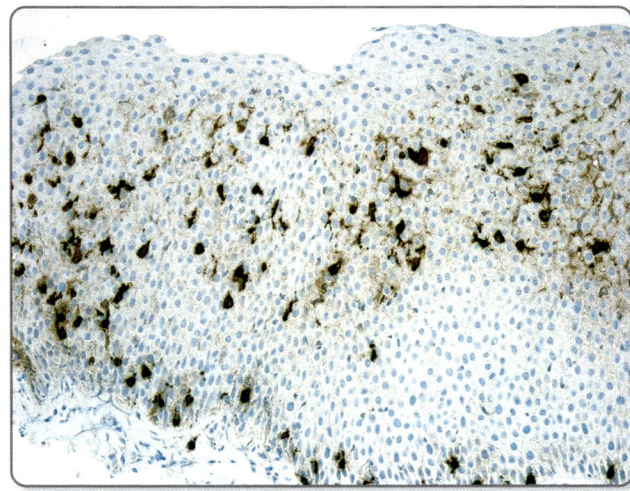

Figure 3.15 Oesophageal mucosa (stained with antimast cell tryptase) from a patient with eosinophilic oesophagitis (EoO). Mast cells are absent from the normal oesophageal epithelium. In EoO, their numbers may reach 30 or 40 per HPF and are beginning to be seen as a useful marker of response to therapy.

FUTURE DIRECTIONS

With the increasing availability of artificial intelligence computer-assisted diagnostics on whole slide images, we are now seeing programmes that can count a variety of cells and structures, including inflammatory cells, mitoses, Ki-67-stained proliferating cells, and evaluate the architectural integrity or disarray of the mucosa. Most pathologist will see this as a welcome addition to their toolbox, as these technologies show promising degrees of accuracy, sensitivity, and specificity. Eventually, tasks now perceived by many of our colleagues as mundane, tedious, and time-inefficient, will likely be performed quickly and effectively by non-complaining robots. For now, these tools are used primarily in research settings and, until they become more mainstream, pathologists will need to be comfortable quantifying eosinophils.

Key points for clinical practice

- It is important to differentiate between eosinophils and look-alikes such as neutrophils, Paneth cells and neuroendocrine cells.
- For eosinophil counting the optimal orientation of the specimen is on edge, with the surface clearly visualized on one side and the basement membrane or *muscularis mucosae* on the other.
- An ideal counting field has the highest density of eosinophils, does not overlap with any other counted field, and is in a well-oriented area void of confounding histologic findings or artifacts.
- Adequate sampling for eosinophilic oesophagitis requires at least two separate samples each from the proximal, mid, or distal esophagus (> 2 cm from the gastroesophageal junction).
- Eosinophilic oesophagitis is characterized by an intraepithelial infiltrate of at least 15 eosinophils per HPF, dilated intercellular spaces and hyperplasia of the basal cell layer.
- Adequate sampling for eosinophilic gastritis requires four samples from the corpus and four from the antrum, delivered in two separate containers.

- Eosinophilic gastritis can be diagnosed when at least 5 HPFs with ≥30 eosinophils each are present in a set of gastric biopsies; a single focus of eosinophilia is much less likely to represent EoG than an uneven but diffuse infiltrate in several parts of the stomach.
- Although no formally established criteria for a diagnosis of eosinophilic duodenitis have been published, a threshold of 50 eos/HPF in four biopsy samples is recommended; highest concentration of eosinophils is often found in sub-cryptal lamina propria.
- As the density of eosinophils differs considerably throughout the colon, biopsy ampling should include at least two fragments from cecum, transverse colon, left colon, sigmoid and rectum.
- Colonic eosinophilia is often found in inflammatory bowel disease, in association with intramucosal parasites and their components (*S. stercoralis, T. trichura, Schistosoma species.* eggs).
- A diagnosis of eosinophilic colitis cannot be made without supporting clinical evidence such as eosinophilic gastro-intestinal disease in other organs, peripheral eosinophilia, or a documented history of allergies or asthma.

REFERENCES

1. Gonsalves N. Eosinophilic Gastrointestinal Disorders. Clin Rev Allergy Immunol 2019; 57:272–285.
2. Reed C, Woosley JT, Dellon ES. Clinical characteristics, treatment outcomes, and resource utilization in children and adults with eosinophilic gastroenteritis. Dig Liver Dis 2015; 47:197–201.
3. Aceves SS, King E, Collins MH, et al. Alignment of parent- and child-reported outcomes and histology in eosinophilic esophagitis across multiple CEGIR sites. J Allergy Clin Immunol 2018; 142:130–138 e1.
4. Pesek RD, Reed CC, Collins MH, et al. Association Between Endoscopic and Histologic Findings in a Multicenter Retrospective Cohort of Patients with Non-esophageal Eosinophilic Gastrointestinal Disorders. Dig Dis Sci 2020; 65:2024–2035.
5. Genta RM, Dellon ES, Turner KO. Non-oesophageal eosinophilic gastrointestinal diseases are undersuspected clinically and underdiagnosed pathologically. Aliment Pharmacol Ther 2022; 56:240–250.
6. Saad AJ, Genta RM, Turner KO, et al. Do General Pathologists Assess Gastric and Duodenal Eosinophilia? Arch Pathol Lab Med 2022.
7. Turner KO, Sinkre RA, Neumann WL, Genta RM. Primary Colonic Eosinophilia and Eosinophilic Colitis in Adults. Am J Surg Pathol 2017; 41:225–233.
8. Chehade M. Eosinophilic gastrointestinal disorders: The journey to diagnosis remains arduous. Ann Allergy Asthma Immunol 2020; 124:229–230.
9. Ronkainen J, Aro P, Walker MM, et al. Duodenal eosinophilia is associated with functional dyspepsia and new onset gastro-oesophageal reflux disease. Aliment Pharmacol Ther 2019; 50:24–32.
10. Walker MM, Warwick A, Ung C, Talley NJ. The role of eosinophils and mast cells in intestinal functional disease. Curr Gastroenterol Rep 2011; 13:323–330.
11. Walker MM, Talley NJ. Functional gastrointestinal disorders and the potential role of eosinophils. Gastroenterol Clin North Am 2008; 37:383–395, vi.
12. Syeda MZ, Hong T, Zhang C, Ying S, Shen H. Eosinophils: A Friend or Foe in Human Health and Diseases. Kidney Dis (Basel) 2023; 9:26–38.
13. Fettrelet T, Gigon L, Karaulov A, Yousefi S, Simon HU. The Enigma of Eosinophil Degranulation. Int J Mol Sci 2021; 22:7091.
14. Klion AD, Ackerman SJ, Bochner BS. Contributions of Eosinophils to Human Health and Disease. Annu Rev Pathol 2020; 15:179–209.

15. Redd WD, Dellon ES. Eosinophilic Gastrointestinal Diseases Beyond the Esophagus: An Evolving Field and Nomenclature. Gastroenterol Hepatol (N Y) 2022; 18:522–528.

16. Turner KO, Collins MH, Walker MM, Genta RM. Quantification of Mucosal Eosinophils for the Histopathologic Diagnosis of Eosinophilic Gastritis and Duodenitis: A Primer for Practicing Pathologists. Am J Surg Pathol 2022; 46:557–566.

17. Straumann A, Spichtin HP, Bernoulli R, Loosli J, Vogtlin J. Idiopathic eosinophilic esophagitis: a frequently overlooked disease with typical clinical aspects and discrete endoscopic findings. Schweiz Med Wochenschr 1994; 124:1419–1429.

18. Straumann A, Bauer M, Fischer B, Blaser K, Simon HU. Idiopathic eosinophilic esophagitis is associated with a T(H)2-type allergic inflammatory response. J Allergy Clin Immunol 2001; 108:954–961.

19. Liacouras CA, Furuta GT, Hirano I, et al. Eosinophilic esophagitis: updated consensus recommendations for children and adults. J Allergy Clin Immunol 2011; 128:3–20 e6; quiz 21–22.

20. Aceves SS, Dellon ES, Greenhawt M, et al. Clinical guidance for the use of dupilumab in eosinophilic esophagitis: A yardstick. Ann Allergy Asthma Immunol 2022.

21. Dellon ES, Khoury P, Muir AB, et al. A Clinical Severity Index for Eosinophilic Esophagitis: Development, Consensus, and Future Directions. Gastroenterology 2022; 163:59–76.

22. Jensen ET, Martin CF, Kappelman MD, Dellon ES. Prevalence of Eosinophilic Gastritis, Gastroenteritis, and Colitis: Estimates From a National Administrative Database. J Pediatr Gastroenterol Nutr 2016; 62:36–42.

23. Henderson CJ, Ngeow J, Collins MH, et al. Increased prevalence of eosinophilic gastrointestinal disorders in pediatric PTEN hamartoma tumor syndromes. J Pediatr Gastroenterol Nutr 2014; 58:553–560.

24. Pesek RD, Reed CC, Muir AB, et al. Increasing Rates of Diagnosis, Substantial Co-Occurrence, and Variable Treatment Patterns of Eosinophilic Gastritis, Gastroenteritis, and Colitis Based on 10-Year Data Across a Multicenter Consortium. Am J Gastroenterol 2019; 114:984–994.

25. Rothenberg ME, Hottinger SKB, Gonsalves N, et al. Impressions and aspirations from the FDA GREAT VI Workshop on Eosinophilic Gastrointestinal Disorders Beyond Eosinophilic Esophagitis and Perspectives for Progress in the Field. J Allergy Clin Immunol 2022; 149:844–853.

26. Spergel JM, Aceves SS, Kliewer K, et al. New developments in patients with eosinophilic gastrointestinal diseases presented at the CEGIR/TIGERS Symposium at the 2018 American Academy of Allergy, Asthma & Immunology Meeting. J Allergy Clin Immunol 2018; 142:48–53.

27. Dunn JLM, Rothenberg ME. 2021 year in review: Spotlight on eosinophils. J Allergy Clin Immunol 2022; 149:517–524.

28. Aceves SS, Alexander JA, Baron TH, et al. Endoscopic approach to eosinophilic esophagitis: American Society for Gastrointestinal Endoscopy Consensus Conference. Gastrointest Endosc 2022; 96:576–592 e1.

29. Schoepfer AM, Hirano I, Coslovsky M, et al. Variation in Endoscopic Activity Assessment and Endoscopy Score Validation in Adults With Eosinophilic Esophagitis. Clin Gastroenterol Hepatol 2019; 17:1477–1488 e10.

30. Chehade M, Kamboj AP, Atkins D, Gehman LT. Diagnostic Delay in Patients with Eosinophilic Gastritis and/or Duodenitis: A Population-Based Study. J Allergy Clin Immunol Pract 2021; 9:2050–2059 e20.

31. Lenti MV, Savarino E, Mauro A, et al. Diagnostic delay and misdiagnosis in eosinophilic oesophagitis. Dig Liver Dis 2021; 53:1632–1639.

32. Collins MH, Martin LJ, Alexander ES, et al. Newly developed and validated eosinophilic esophagitis histology scoring system and evidence that it outperforms peak eosinophil count for disease diagnosis and monitoring. Dis Esophagus 2017; 30:1–8.

33. Jamali E, Kazeminezhad B, Ahadi M, Moradi A, Khabbazi H. Quantity and Distribution of Eosinophils in Esophageal Specimens of Adults: An Iranian Population-Based Study. Iran J Pathol 2022; 17136–142.

34. Min S, Shoda T, Wen T, Rothenberg ME. Diagnostic merits of the Eosinophilic Esophagitis Diagnostic Panel from a single esophageal biopsy. J Allergy Clin Immunol 2022; 149:782–787 e1.

35.   Dixon MF, Genta RM, Yardley JH, Correa P. Classification and grading of gastritis. The updated Sydney System. International Workshop on the Histopathology of Gastritis, Houston 1994. Am J Surg Pathol 1996; 20:1161–1181.

36.   Hurrell JM, Genta RM, Melton SD. Histopathologic diagnosis of eosinophilic conditions in the gastrointestinal tract. Adv Anat Pathol 2011; 18:335–348.

37.   Mansoor E, Saleh MA, Cooper GS. Prevalence of Eosinophilic Gastroenteritis and Colitis in a Population-Based Study, From 2012 to 2017. Clin Gastroenterol Hepatol 2017; 15:1733–1741.

38.   Zhang M, Li Y. Eosinophilic gastroenteritis: A state-of-the-art review. J Gastroenterol Hepatol 2017; 32:64–72.

39.   Chaudhary R, Shrivastava RK, Mukhopadhyay HG, Diwan RN, Das AK. Eosinophilic gastritis--an unusual cause of gastric outlet obstruction. Indian J Gastroenterol 2001; 20:110.

40.   Ayyub M, Almenawi L, Mogharbel MH. Eosinophilic gastritis; an unusual and overlooked cause of chronic abdominal pain. J Ayub Med Coll Abbottabad 2007; 19:127–130.

41.   DeBrosse CW, Case JW, Putnam PE, Collins MH, Rothenberg ME. Quantity and distribution of eosinophils in the gastrointestinal tract of children. Pediatr Dev Pathol 2006; 9:210–218.

42.   Talley NJ, Walker MM, Aro P, et al. Non-ulcer dyspepsia and duodenal eosinophilia: an adult endoscopic population-based case-control study. Clin Gastroenterol Hepatol 2007; 5:1175–1183.

43.   Lwin T, Melton SD, Genta RM. Eosinophilic gastritis: histopathological characterization and quantification of the normal gastric eosinophil content. Mod Pathol 2011; 24:556–563.

44.   Dellon ES, Peterson KA, Murray JA, et al. Anti-Siglec-8 Antibody for Eosinophilic Gastritis and Duodenitis. N Engl J Med 2020; 383:1624–1634.

45.   Reed CC, Genta RM, Youngblood BA, Wechsler JB, Dellon ES. Mast Cell and Eosinophil Counts in Gastric and Duodenal Biopsy Specimens From Patients With and Without Eosinophilic Gastroenteritis. Clin Gastroenterol Hepatol 2021; 19:2102–2111.

46.   Dellon ES, Gonsalves N, Rothenberg ME, et al. Determination of Biopsy Yield That Optimally Detects Eosinophilic Gastritis and/or Duodenitis in a Randomized Trial of Lirentelimab. Clin Gastroenterol Hepatol 2022; 20:535–545 e15.

47.   Walker MM, Potter MD, Talley NJ. Tangible pathologies in functional dyspepsia. Best Pract Res Clin Gastroenterol 2019; 40–41:101650.

48.   Halland M, Talley NJ, Jones M,et al. Duodenal Pathology in Patients with Rumination Syndrome: Duodenal Eosinophilia and Increased Intraepithelial Lymphocytes. Dig Dis Sci 2019; 64:832–837.

49.   Walker MM, Salehian SS, Murray CE, et al. Implications of eosinophilia in the normal duodenal biopsy - an association with allergy and functional dyspepsia. Aliment Pharmacol Ther 2010; 31:1229–1236.

50.   Barreyro FJ, Caronia MV, Elizondo K, et al. Clinical Implications of Low-grade Duodenal Eosinophilia in Functional Dyspepsia: A Prospective Real-life Study. J Clin Gastroenterol 2023; 57:362–369.

51.   Shah A, Fairlie T, Brown G, et al. Duodenal Eosinophils and Mast Cells in Functional Dyspepsia: A Systematic Review and Meta-Analysis of Case-Control Studies. Clin Gastroenterol Hepatol 2022; 20:2229–2242, e29.

52.   Jarbrink-Sehgal ME, Sparkman J, Damron A, et al. Functional Dyspepsia and Duodenal Eosinophil Count and Degranulation: A Multiethnic US Veteran Cohort Study. Dig Dis Sci 2021; 66:3482–3489.

53.   Genta RM, Sonnenberg A, Turner K. Quantification of the duodenal eosinophil content in adults: a necessary step for an evidence-based diagnosis of duodenal eosinophilia. Aliment Pharmacol Ther 2018; 47:1143–1150.

54.   Collins MH, Capocelli K, Yang GY. Eosinophilic Gastrointestinal Disorders Pathology. Front Med (Lausanne) 2017; 4:261.

55.   Rothenberg ME. Eosinophilic gastrointestinal disorders (EGID). J Allergy Clin Immunol 2004; 113:11–28; quiz 29.

56.   Odze RD, Bines J, Leichtner AM, Goldman H, Antonioli DA. Allergic proctocolitis in infants: a prospective clinicopathologic biopsy study. Hum Pathol 1993; 24:668–674.

57.   Shoda T, Collins MH, Rochman M, et al. Evaluating Eosinophilic Colitis as a Unique Disease Using Colonic Molecular Profiles: A Multi-Site Study. Gastroenterology 2022; 162:1635–1649.

58.   DiTommaso LA, Rosenberg CE, Eby MD, et al. Prevalence of eosinophilic colitis and the diagnoses associated with colonic eosinophilia. J Allergy Clin Immunol 2019; 143:1928–1930, e3.

59. Paramo-Zunzunegui J, Ortega-Fernandez I, Benito-Barbero S, Rubio-Lopez L. Eosinophilic colitis: an infrequent disease with difficult diagnose. BMJ Case Rep 2020; 13:e235804.
60. Burns G, Carroll G, Mathe A, et al. Evidence for Local and Systemic Immune Activation in Functional Dyspepsia and the Irritable Bowel Syndrome: A Systematic Review. Am J Gastroenterol 2019; 114:429–436.
61. Jakate S, Demeo M, John R, Tobin M, Keshavarzian A. Mastocytic enterocolitis: increased mucosal mast cells in chronic intractable diarrhea. Arch Pathol Lab Med 2006; 130:362–367.
62. Sethi A, Jain D, Roland BC, et al. Performing colonic mast cell counts in patients with chronic diarrhea of unknown etiology has limited diagnostic use. Arch Pathol Lab Med 2015; 139:225–232.
63. Talley NJ, Alexander JL, Walker MM, et al. Ileocolonic Histopathological and Microbial Alterations in the Irritable Bowel Syndrome: A Nested Community Case-Control Study. Clin Transl Gastroenterol 2020; 12:e00296.
64. Walker MM, Talley NJ, Prabhakar M, et al. Duodenal mastocytosis, eosinophilia and intraepithelial lymphocytosis as possible disease markers in the irritable bowel syndrome and functional dyspepsia. Aliment Pharmacol Ther 2009; 29:765–773.
65. Abonia JP, Blanchard C, Butz BB, et al. Involvement of mast cells in eosinophilic esophagitis. J Allergy Clin Immunol 2010; 126:140–149.
66. Aceves SS, Chen D, Newbury RO, et al. Mast cells infiltrate the esophageal smooth muscle in patients with eosinophilic esophagitis, express TGF-beta1, and increase esophageal smooth muscle contraction. J Allergy Clin Immunol 2010; 126:1198–1204, e4.
67. Ben-Baruch Morgenstern N, Ballaban AY, Wen T, et al. Single-cell RNA sequencing of mast cells in eosinophilic esophagitis reveals heterogeneity, local proliferation, and activation that persists in remission. J Allergy Clin Immunol 2022; 149:2062–2077.

Chapter 4

Mesonephric-like adenocarcinoma of the gynaecologic tract

Ridin Balakrishnan, Ricardo R Lastra

INTRODUCTION

Mesonephric remnants are relics of the embryonic mesonephric (Wolffian) ducts and can occur anywhere along the path where mesonephric duct regress in biologic females. They are generally found in the mesosalpinx or the lateral aspect of the cervix but can rarely be present in the lateral wall of the vagina and uterine corpus. Mesonephric carcinomas are rare tumours that arise from these mesonephric remnants in the uterine cervix [1]. Within the last few years, tumours with mesonephric-like morphology and immunohistochemical profile have been described in sites in which mesonephric remnants are not usually expected, particularly the uterine corpus and the ovaries. In the seminal paper by McFarland et al in 2015, the authors reported a series of uterine and ovarian adenocarcinomas with distinct morphological and immunophenotypic profile, resembling mesonephric carcinomas [2]. The ovarian cases demonstrated foci of endometriosis in the same ovary. In all uterine cases, none involved the myometrium without predominant involvement of the endometrium. Notably, the authors did not identify any benign mesonephric remnants in association with the uterine tumours or in the cervix [2]. Given the uncertainty of the origin of these tumours at that time (i.e. did these represent mesonephric carcinomas arising in unusual location or variations of Müllerian-derived carcinomas), the authors recommended that they are termed "mesonephric-like" adenocarcinomas until their histogenesis was firmly established.

Although recent molecular data supports the notion that these tumours are, indeed, of Müllerian origin, mesonephric-like adenocarcinoma (MLA) retained their initial descriptive name because of the morphological, immunophenotypic, and molecular overlap with classic mesonephric carcinomas [1,3,4]. The morphologic spectrum and scarcity of mesonephric carcinomas and MLA tend to cause substantial problems in their recognition and diagnosis. However, the aggressive nature of these deceptively low-grade appearing lesions has since been well established, with the majority presenting at advanced stage and with distant metastases [4]. Hence, the importance of their recognition

Ridin Balakrishnan MD, Department of Pathology, LSU Health Center, New Orleans, Louisiana
E-mail: ridin.balakrishnan@gmail.com

Ricardo R Lastra MD, Department of Pathology, University of Chicago Medicine, Chicago, Illinois
E-mail: ricardo.lastra@bsd.uchicago.edu

and proper diagnosis has become evident, resulting in its inclusion as a new entity in the latest 2020 WHO Classification of Female Genital Tumors [5].

EPIDEMIOLOGY

Mesonephric-like adenocarcinomas are rare tumours with an incidence of approximately 1% amongst all endometrial carcinomas [6,7]. In one comprehensive study, the mean age of diagnosis of endometrial MLA was 60 years (median: 61 years, range from 28 to 91 years) with the most common presenting symptom being vaginal bleeding, followed by post-menopausal bleeding and abnormal uterine bleeding [4]. Patients with MLA of the ovary most commonly present with pelvic pain, post-menopausal/abnormal uterine bleeding and/or abdominal distension and bloating [4].

PATHOGENESIS

The cell of origin in MLA has been a subject of debate for several years. In all uterine cases, including those in the seminal description by McFarland et al, tumours arose from the endometrium rather than the myometrium; in addition, a majority of the ovarian MLA were associated with endometriosis [2]. Direct transition between ovarian MLA and concomitant endometriosis has been reported [8]. An extensive literature review of MLA by Deolet et al in 2021 showed that some of the tumours were associated with underlying Müllerian-derived processes, including adenomyosis, endometriosis, atypical hyperplasia of the endometrium, serous borderline tumours, serous cystadenoma, borderline endometrioid adenofibroma, low-grade endometrioid endometrial carcinoma, and low-grade serous ovarian carcinoma [9]. These point favourably to the notion that MLAs do not arise from mesonephric remnants, but perhaps rather from Müllerian structures differentiating along a mesonephric pathway [2]. Attempts to differentiate mesonephric carcinomas and MLA based on proteomic analysis have shown no difference, and various studies have shown clonality between the background Müllerian-derived lesions and concomitant MLA present within the same case (see Molecular Findings) [10–13].

GROSS FINDINGS

In the original series, when gross findings were available, the ovarian MLA ranged from 4 to 32 cm, with a predominantly solid and cystic, yellow-tan or gray-white cut surface [2]. In other studies, ovarian MLA ranged from 7 to 15 cm with solid and cystic gross appearance. Papillary excrescences, fleshy and gelatinous cut-surfaces have also been described **(Figure 4.1)** [9,11]. Gross findings of uterine MLA are not specifically mentioned in the literature.

HISTOLOGIC FEATURES

There is significant overlap in morphology between MLA and conventional mesonephric carcinomas. A variety of growth patterns are typically present, including glandular, tubular, solid, slit-like, sex-cord like, trabecular, retiform, sieve-like, glomeruloid, spindle-cell, and papillary [2,14]. The classic architecture is usually a tubular growth pattern containing

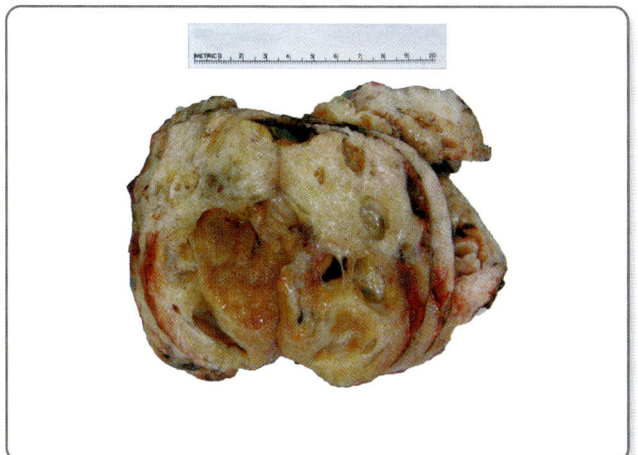

Figure 4.1 Ovarian MLA demonstrating a yellow-tan, solid and cystic mass with focal papillary excrescences involving the lining of the cystic spaces.

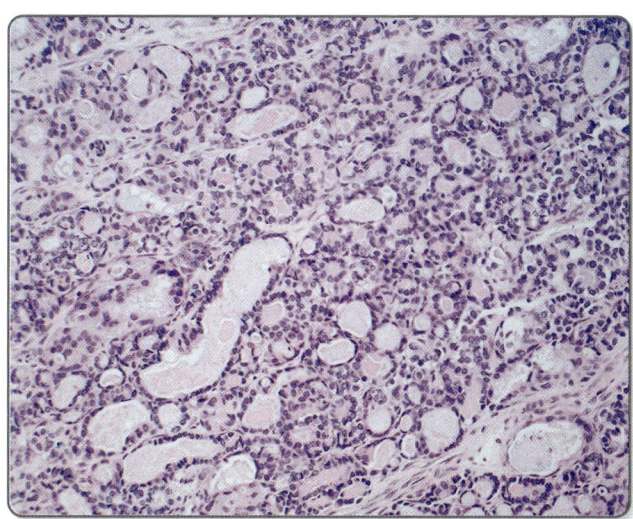

Figure 4.2 Tubular growth pattern with intraluminal eosinophilic colloid-like material (H&E, 200×).

eosinophilic colloid-like material in the lumen **(Figure 4.2)**, although this can be focal or absent. The neoplastic cells typically show moderate nuclear atypia **(Figure 4.3)** with nuclear overlapping, nuclear clearing, nuclear membrane angulations, nuclear grooves, and small nucleoli, often reminiscent of the classic nuclear features seen in papillary thyroid carcinoma **(Figure 4.4)** [2]. The cytoplasm is generally scant and in some solid areas, a spindled morphology can be seen [2]. No mucinous, ciliated, or squamous differentiation or metaplasia should be present, and no identifiable mesonephric remnants should be identified; if either of these features is present, the possibility of an unusual endometrioid carcinoma or a true mesonephric carcinoma, respectively, should be strongly considered **(Figure 4.5)** [15]. The morphologic spectrum of MLA is further highlighted in **Figure 4.6**. There are no reported differences in morphologies between ovarian and endometrial MLA [3].

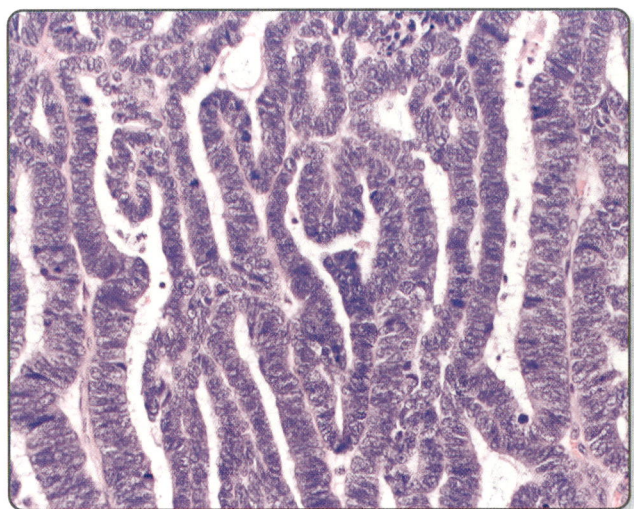

Figure 4.3 Moderate nuclear atypia with nuclear overlapping and conspicuous mitotic activity (H&E, 400×).

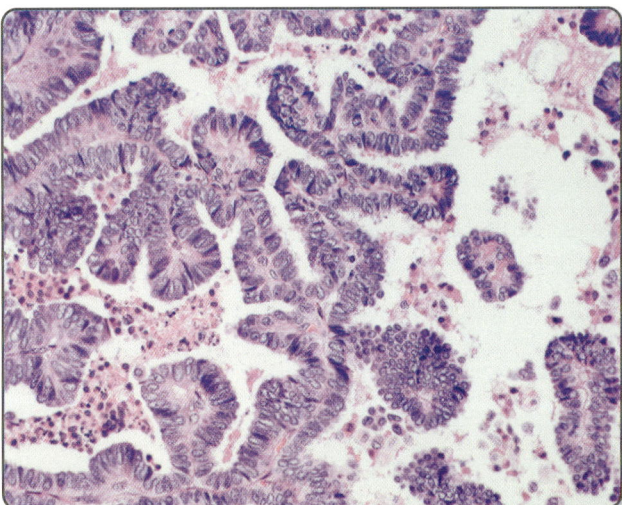

Figure 4.4 MLA demonstrating nuclear clearing, nuclear overlapping, nuclear grooves, and small nucleoli, reminiscent of the nuclear features of papillary thyroid carcinoma (H&E, 400×).

IMMUNOHISTOCHEMISTRY

The typical immunohistochemical profile for MLA is as follows **(Figure 4.7)** [15].

- *PAX-8*: Positive; nuclear
- *GATA-3 and TTF-1*: Variably positive; nuclear
- *CD10*: Luminal staining
- *Calretinin*: Focal staining; nuclear and cytoplasmic
- *Oestrogen receptors (OR/ER) and progesterone receptors (PR)*: Negative

It must be noted that focal/weak positivity for ER can be seen, as shown in multiple studies, which does not preclude a diagnosis of MLA, with PR being a more reliably

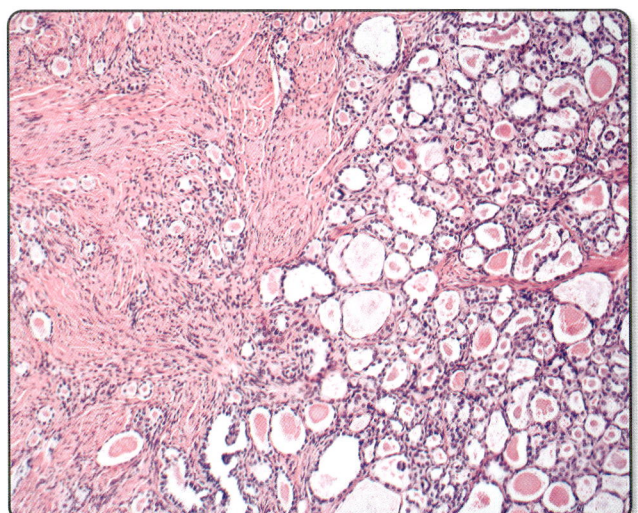

Figure 4.5 The presence of mesonephric hyperplasia (top left) adjacent to a carcinoma with mesonephric features (right) provides strong evidence for a diagnosis of cervical mesonephric carcinoma over MLA (H&E, 200×).

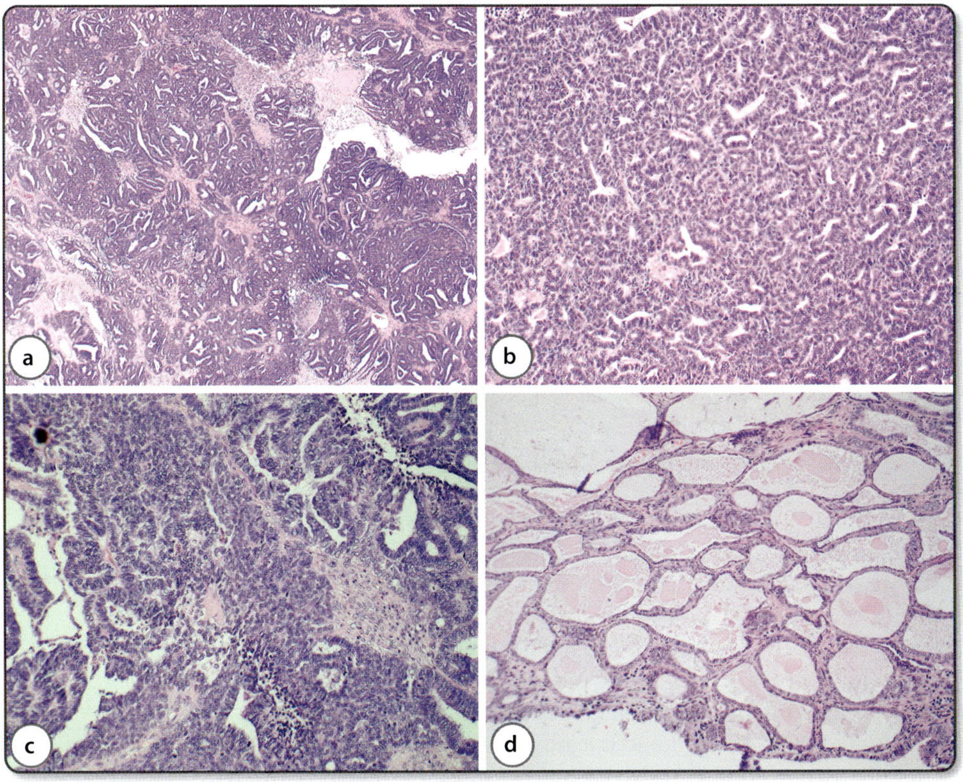

Figure 4.6 Histologic spectrum of MLA: (a) Glandular morphology with slit-like spaces and papillary architecture (H&E, 100×); (b) closely packed tubules (H&E, 200×); (c) focal solid growth (H&E, 200×); (d) cystic and dilated glands with attenuated lining (H&E, 200×).

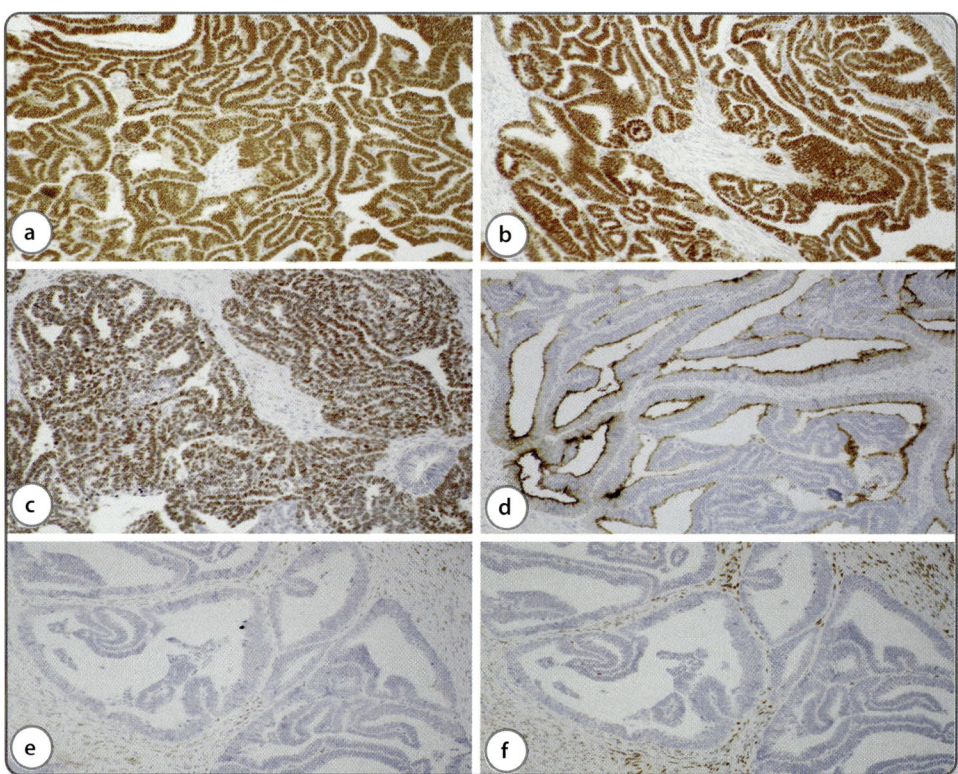

Figure 4.7 Typical immunohistochemical profile of MLA: (a) PAX-8 nuclear positivity (200×); (b) GATA-3 nuclear positivity (200×); (c) TTF-1 nuclear positivity (200×); (d) luminal positivity with CD10 (200×); (e) negative staining for ER (200×); (f) negative staining for PR (200×).

negative marker [4,6,16–19]. In fact, the absence of diffuse ER and PR expression in tumours that are initially considered to be low-grade endometrioid carcinomas is extremely unusual; this discrepancy should hint to the possibility of the tumour representing MLA, and additional immunohistochemical staining would be warranted. Interestingly, GATA-3 and TTF-1 often show an inverse staining pattern which can be useful in small biopsies where GATA-3 is negative **(Figure 4.8)** [19]. Because CD10 invariably stains surrounding endometrial stroma and calretinin can be non-specific, these stains are often difficult to interpret. MLAs show wild-type *p53* expression and patchy *p16* positivity, as well as negative staining for WT-1. Recent studies have demonstrated that they are typically mismatch-repair protein proficient, with retained expression of *MLH1, PMS2, MSH2* and *MSH6*, and the loss of expression of any of these markers should put in doubt a diagnosis of MLA [15].

Although TTF-1 is considered the most specific marker for MLA, GATA-3 is the best overall stain when combining both sensitivity and specificity, followed by TTF-1, CD10, and calretinin. Greater TTF-1 positivity in MLA when compared to mesonephric carcinoma may be secondary to the fact that the two are biologically distinct. Focal GATA-3 positivity may be seen in a subset of mesonephric carcinomas, limiting its utility in distinguishing MLA from true mesonephric carcinomas [10].

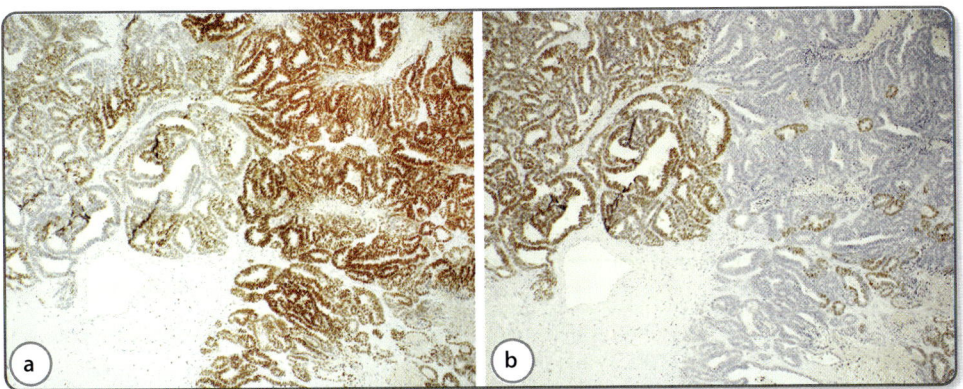

Figure 4.8 Characteristic inverse staining pattern of MLA with GATA-3 and TTF-1: (a) GATA-3 demonstrating strong expression in the right half of the image with weak expression on the left; (b) TTF-1 demonstrates strong expression in the left half with decreased to absent expression in the right half.

MOLECULAR FINDINGS

Mesonephric-like adenocarcinomas are characterised by molecular findings which overlap between endometrioid carcinomas and mesonephric carcinomas. As such, they often demonstrate recurrent *KRAS* mutations (often seen in mesonephric carcinomas), as well as *PIK3CA* and *ARID1A* mutations (commonly seen in endometrioid carcinomas) but lack the characteristic *PTEN* mutations seen in endometrioid carcinomas [3,20]. Gains of chromosomes 1q, 10, and 12 have also been described as a recurrent feature [3].

There are a few caveats to keep in mind when using molecular findings to aid in the diagnosis. Copy number changes are not specific to MLA and can be seen in a subset of endometrioid carcinomas [21]. *KRAS* and *ARID1A* mutations are common in both mesonephric and endometrioid carcinomas and are not useful in determining the Müllerian origin of MLA [3,21]. *PIK3CA* mutations are also commonly seen in endometrioid carcinomas and MLA, but not in mesonephric carcinomas [21], raising the possibility that MLA could possess dual endometrioid and mesonephric differentiation or, more likely, derive from Müllerian epithelium but exhibit predominantly mesonephric differentiation [3].

Interestingly, one study demonstrated the presence of 1q gain in all ovarian tumours but only in one uterine tumour, while gains of chromosomes 10 and 12 were only observed in uterine MLAs [3]. In the same study, all ovarian MLA had G12D *KRAS* mutations and all uterine MLA harboured G12V *KRAS* mutations [3]. While the biologic significance of this distinction is not known, the G12D mutation has been linked to adverse clinical behaviour in some gastrointestinal carcinomas [22,23].

Lastly, MLAs have not been shown to have mutations in *TP53*, are microsatellite stable (MSS), and have not been shown to harbour *POLE* mutations. As such, when endometrial based, they belong to the "No specific molecular profile (NSMP)" group of endometrial tumours [21]. It is speculated that a proportion of patients with poor survivals seen in this TCGA (The Cancer Genome Atlas) group may be explained by their tumours being unrecognised MLA [15].

DIFFERENTIAL DIAGNOSIS

The diagnosis of MLA is challenging, particularly because these are newly described and unusual tumours with diverse histology. As a result, they are often misdiagnosed, generally as low-grade endometrioid carcinomas. Even though MLAs commonly have tubular and glandular growth patterns, they are characterised by extensive architectural heterogeneity. Cytological findings such as nuclear grooves and vesicular chromatin are usually not observed in endometrioid carcinomas, which are characterised by columnar cells with pseudostratified nuclei. On the other hand, the presence of metaplastic changes, including mucinous and squamous metaplasia, is not expected in MLA and would favour a diagnosis of endometrioid carcinoma. Similarly, the presence of atypical hyperplasia/endometrial intraepithelial neoplasia (AH/EIN) favours an endometrioid carcinoma, but there are described instances in which these precursor lesions are found co-existing with *bona fide* MLA [4]. MLAs are characterised by the expression of GATA-3 and/or TTF-1, not normally seen in endometrioid carcinomas. Additionally, low-grade endometrioid carcinomas are classically ER and PR positive; when dealing with an architecturally low-grade appearing tumour reminiscent of an endometrioid carcinoma demonstrating absence of ER and PR expression, MLA must be strongly considered as an alternative diagnosis. Conversely, while MLA may occasionally demonstrate focal staining for ER, the presence of strong and diffuse ER and PR expression generally argues against a diagnosis of MLA. Lastly, as mentioned above, MLAs are generally mismatch-repair protein proficient; loss of expression of any of the four mismatch-repair proteins would be unusual for this diagnosis, and endometrioid carcinoma should be considered instead.

When confronted with a tumour demonstrating mesonephric-like features, the possibility of cervical mesonephric carcinomas with uterine corpus involvement must always be considered and excluded. Radiologic correlation and determination of the location of the bulk of the tumour can help to determine site of origin, and aid in this distinction; the identification of background mesonephric hyperplasia of the cervix in association to the cervical component of the tumour should be taken as a strong indication of a true primary cervical mesonephric carcinoma with secondary uterine corpus involvement. MLAs of the uterine corpus typically arise in the endometrium, while mesonephric carcinomas, on the other hand, potentially arise in the lateral walls of the myometrium where mesonephric remnants are expected to exist [15]. Immunohistochemical overlap exists between these two entities, with both usually staining negative for ER and PR. GATA-3, calretinin, and CD10 can be positive in both. However, MLAs tend to have more TTF-1 staining in comparison to mesonephric carcinomas [19]. Additional molecular testing can be performed if needed to aid in this distinction, and although MLA and mesonephric carcinomas share *KRAS* mutations, the presence of concurrent *PIK3CA* mutations favours the diagnosis of the former within this differential.

While less likely to be included in the differential diagnosis, the diagnostic differences between MLA and the other Müllerian-derived carcinomas (namely high-grade serous carcinoma and clear-cell carcinoma) are worth mentioning. High-grade nuclear atypia, particularly in the context of a papillary growth pattern, should raise the possibility of serous carcinoma. While MLAs act in an aggressive manner, the cytologic atypia characteristic of serous carcinomas is not seen in MLAs, which in fact usually demonstrate only mild-to-moderate nuclear atypia. Evidently, serous carcinomas demonstrate aberrant *p53* staining patterns and often show block positivity with *p16*, features rarely ever seen in MLA. Since ER and PR may be negative in serous carcinomas, these are less helpful in this differential.

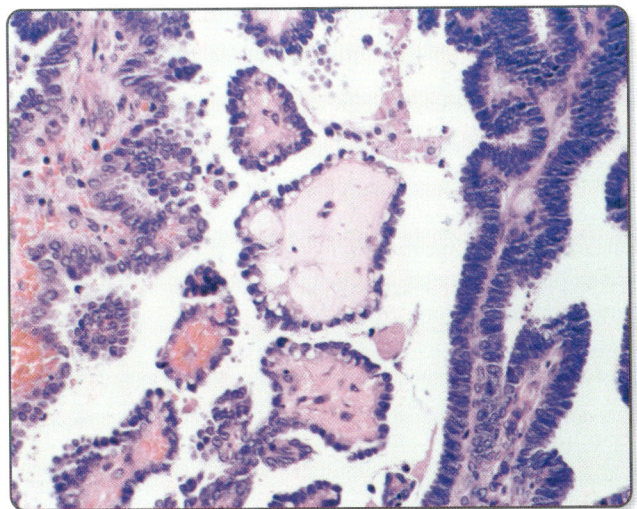

Figure 4.9 Stromal hyalinisation, hobnailing, and focal cytoplasmic clearing in MLA, mimicking the morphology of clear cell carcinoma (H&E, 400×).

Clear-cell carcinomas, which may also demonstrate a multitude of architectural growth patterns, are also generally negative for ER and PR, as are MLAs. However, the cytoplasmic clearing, hobnailing, and prominent nucleoli, classically seen in clear-cell carcinomas, are not characteristics of MLA. In addition, the classic stromal hyalinisation often seen in clear-cell carcinomas is also lacking in MLA. However, there can be areas that mimic these features in MLA (**Figure 4.9**). Immunohistochemical stains used to help diagnose clear-cell carcinoma, such as Napsin-A and hepatocyte nuclear factor-1-beta (HNF-1β) can be focally positive in MLA and are thus of limited utility [24]. GATA-3 and TTF-1 are typically negative in clear-cell carcinomas, which as is the case with endometrioid carcinomas, can also be DNA mismatch-repair protein deficient.

Owing to the frequent positivity with TTF-1 and characteristic nuclear features, an additional diagnosis to keep in the differential, mainly when dealing with an ovarian lesion, is metastatic papillary thyroid carcinoma (PTC) or malignant struma ovarii with a papillary thyroid carcinoma component [25]. This is even more challenging when the MLA is associated with a teratoma [9]. The use of additional thyroid-specific markers, such as thyroglobulin, is usually sufficient to establish the correct diagnosis.

Female adnexal tumour of probable Wolffian origin (FATWO) may also enter in the differential diagnosis. While FATWO and MLA both have varied architectural patterns, the former does not show the papillary thyroid carcinoma-like nuclear features, and more frequently demonstrate a sieve-like architecture [25]. Unlike MLA, and in addition to being positive for inhibin, FATWOs are more likely to also be positive for ER and are usually negative for PAX-8, TTF-1 and GATA-3 [26].

A scenario where immunohistochemical staining can cause a dilemma is when MLA metastasises to the lungs. Positive TTF-1 with negative hormone receptors can make it hard to delineate metastatic MLA from a lung adenocarcinoma [15]. In these cases, the clinical history is crucial in avoiding a misdiagnosis. As such, if there is a known history of a gynaecologic malignancy, or if there are clinico-radiologic features concerning for a potential endometrial or ovarian lesion (including abnormal vaginal bleeding and/or the presence of a pelvic mass), doing a PAX-8 is invaluable [15]. Morphological clues such as pseudo-endometrioid glands and small tubules with eosinophilic secretions provide clues for MLA. GATA-3, CD10, and calretinin can be used for confirmation, if deemed necessary.

PROGNOSIS

Even though MLAs generally have low-grade histologic features, they have been shown to act in an aggressive manner. In comparison to other endometrial adenocarcinomas, uterine MLA have a worse overall survival compared to International Federation of Gynaecology and Obstetrics (FIGO) grade 1 and 2 endometrial endometrioid carcinomas, similar overall survival to FIGO grade 3 endometrial endometrioid carcinomas, and slightly better overall survival than serous carcinomas and carcinosarcomas [4]. Metastasis to the lungs and recurrences are common [4,6,7,14,20]. Even low-stage tumours tend to metastasise frequently and characteristics such as large tumour size (>4 cm), advanced FIGO stages (III to IV), ill-defined tumour borders, tumour necrosis, increased mitotic activity (>10 mitotic figures per 10 high-power fields) and lymphovascular invasion are significantly associated with an increased risk of dissemination [20].

Based on the data available in the literature, ovarian MLAs tend to have a worse prognosis than clear cell and endometrioid ovarian carcinomas [27].

TREATMENT

Unfortunately, as of now, there is not an established optimal regimen of treatment with respect to chemotherapy or radiation for MLA. Historically, cases have undergone hysterectomy with bilateral salpingo-oophorectomy. Pelvic and para-aortic lymph node dissections are occasionally performed. Various combinations of adjuvant therapy (carboplatin with paclitaxel), radiation, and radiation with chemotherapy have been attempted. However, there are currently no tumour-specific treatments for MLA.

A recent study by Arslanian et al has demonstrated a case with a potentially actionable *PIK3CA H1047Q* mutation [28]. Although mutations in the *PIK3CA* gene have been reported in *KRAS* mutated MLAs, this variant is a new finding. Variants in this hotspot have shown response to a combination of ER antagonist and alpha-specific PI3K inhibitors in ER-positive breast carcinoma, demonstrating improved progression free and overall survival [29,30]. While the therapeutic prospective has not been elucidated specifically in MLA, future studies in ER-expressing MLA may shed light on the potential of this treatment option.

CONCLUSION

Given the significant prognostic implication of this diagnosis, proper recognition of MLA is crucial for adequate patient management. As mentioned in this review, the most common misdiagnosis when dealing with MLA is that of a low-grade endometrioid carcinoma. Since low-grade and low-stage endometrioid carcinomas are generally followed with observation only, this misdiagnosis could result in withholding of necessary adjuvant therapy in misdiagnosed MLAs, with negative impact on patient's outcomes. Features such as heterogeneous architectural patterns, with a predominant tubular and glandular architecture, intratubular eosinophilic secretions, papillary thyroid carcinoma-like nuclear features, and the absence of squamous or mucinous differentiation, are all important clues in avoiding this diagnostic pitfall. A low index of suspicion is necessary to request confirmatory immunohistochemical stains in order to adequately diagnose these uncommon but clinically relevant carcinomas, including PAX-8, GATA-3, TTF-1, ER and PR as first-line markers [19]. In challenging cases, CD10, calretinin, and mismatch-repair protein immunohistochemistry might be helpful. Molecular alterations in *KRAS*, *PIK3CA*, and/or *ARID1A*, in the absence of *PTEN* aberrations, would also support this diagnosis, but are seldom required.

Finally, MLAs are tumours with deceptively low-grade morphology that should be considered high-grade carcinomas. The tendency to metastasise and recur makes it imperative to recognise and differentiate it from its close mimics. While treatment options and therapeutic modalities are inadequate as of today, further research must be undertaken to understand the biology and pathogenesis of this tumour.

Key points for clinical practice

- Mesonephric-like adenocarcinoma (MLA) of the female genital tract is a recently recognised carcinoma of the gynaecologic tract, occurring in the uterine corpus and ovaries.
- It is considered to be a Müllerian-derived adenocarcinoma differentiating along mesonephric lines.
- These tumours show overlapping morphological, immunohistochemical, and molecular features with mesonephric carcinomas of the cervix and endometrial endometrioid carcinomas, leading to complexities in identification and diagnosis.
- MLAs have a significantly more aggressive clinical behaviour, particularly when endometrial based, compared to low-grade endometrioid carcinomas. Metastasis to the lungs and recurrences are common.
- Morphological features such as heterogeneous architectural patterns, with a predominant tubular and glandular architecture, intratubular eosinophilic secretions, and papillary thyroid carcinoma-like nuclear features, and the absence of squamous or mucinous differentiation, are all important clues for diagnosis.
- Confirmatory immunohistochemical stains include PAX-8, GATA-3, TTF-1, ER, and PR.
- Although not necessary, molecular alterations in *KRAS*, *PIK3CA*, and/or *ARID1A*, in the absence of *PTEN* aberrations, can support diagnosis.

REFERENCES

1. McCluggage WG. Progress in the pathological arena of gynecological cancers. Int J Gynecol Obstet 2021; 155:107–114.
2. McFarland M, Quick CM, McCluggage WG. Hormone receptor-negative, thyroid transcription factor 1-positive uterine and ovarian adenocarcinomas: report of a series of mesonephric-like adenocarcinomas. Histopathology 2016; 68:1013–1020.
3. Mirkovic J, McFarland M, Garcia E, et al. Targeted Genomic Profiling Reveals Recurrent KRAS Mutations in Mesonephric-like Adenocarcinomas of the Female Genital Tract. Am J Surg Pathol 2018; 42:227–233.
4. Pors J, Segura S, Chiu DS, et al. Clinicopathologic Characteristics of Mesonephric Adenocarcinomas and Mesonephric-like Adenocarcinomas in the Gynecologic Tract: A Multi-institutional Study. Am J Surg Pathol 2021; 45:498–506.

5.   Quick CM, Malpica A, Hoang LN. Mesonephric-like adenocarcinoma. In: WHO Classification of Tumours Editorial Board (Ed). WHO classification of tumours: Female Genital Tumours, 5th Edition. WHO, France: the International Agency for Research on Cancer Publications, 2020.

6.   Kolin DL, Costigan DC, Dong F, Nucci MR, Howitt BE. A Combined Morphologic and Molecular Approach to Retrospectively Identify KRAS-Mutated Mesonephric-like Adenocarcinomas of the Endometrium. Am J Surg Pathol 2019; 43:389–398.

7.   Horn LC, Höhn AK, Krücken I, et al. Mesonephric-like adenocarcinomas of the uterine corpus: report of a case series and review of the literature indicating poor prognosis for this subtype of endometrial adenocarcinoma. J Cancer Res Clin Oncol 2020; 146:971–983.

8.   Chang CS, Carney ME, Killeen JL. Two Cases of Mesonephric-like Carcinoma Arising From Endometriosis: Case Report and Review of the Literature. Int J Gynecol Pathol 2023; 42:101–107.

9.   Deolet E, Arora I, Van Dorpe J, et al. Extrauterine Mesonephric-like Neoplasms: Expanding the Morphologic Spectrum. Am J Surg Pathol 2022; 46:124–133.

10.   Gibbard E, Cochrane DR, Pors J, et al. Whole-proteome analysis of mesonephric-derived cancers describes new potential biomarkers. Hum Pathol 2021; 108:1–11.

11.   Chapel DB, Joseph NM, Krausz T, Lastra RR. An Ovarian Adenocarcinoma With Combined Low-grade Serous and Mesonephric Morphologies Suggests a Müllerian Origin for Some Mesonephric Carcinomas: Int J Gynecol Pathol 2018; 37:448–459.

12.   McCluggage WG, Vosmikova H, Laco J. Ovarian Combined Low-grade Serous and Mesonephric-like Adenocarcinoma: Further Evidence for A Müllerian Origin of Mesonephric-like Adenocarcinoma. Int J Gynecol Pathol 2020; 39:84–92.

13.   Yano M, Shintani D, Katoh T, et al. Coexistence of endometrial mesonephric-like adenocarcinoma and endometrioid carcinoma suggests a Müllerian duct lineage: a case report. Diagn Pathol 2019; 14:54.

14.   Euscher ED, Bassett R, Duose DY, et al. Mesonephric-like Carcinoma of the Endometrium: A Subset of Endometrial Carcinoma With an Aggressive Behavior. Am J Surg Pathol 2020; 44:429–443.

15.   Deolet E, Van Dorpe J, Van de Vijver K. Mesonephric-Like Adenocarcinoma of the Endometrium: Diagnostic Advances to Spot This Wolf in Sheep's Clothing. A Review of the Literature. J Clin Med 2021; 10:698.

16.   Ando H, Watanabe Y, Ogawa M, et al. Mesonephric adenocarcinoma of the uterine corpus with intracystic growth completely confined to the myometrium: a case report and literature review. Diagn Pathol 2017; 12:63.

17.   Kenny SL, McBride HA, Jamison J, McCluggage WG. Mesonephric Adenocarcinomas of the Uterine Cervix and Corpus: HPV-negative Neoplasms That Are Commonly PAX8, CA125, and HMGA2 Positive and That May Be Immunoreactive with TTF1 and Hepatocyte Nuclear Factor 1-β. Am J Surg Pathol 2012; 36:799–807.

18.   Patel V, Kipp B, Schoolmeester JK. Corded and hyalinized mesonephric-like adenocarcinoma of the uterine corpus: report of a case mimicking endometrioid carcinoma. Hum Pathol 2019; 86:243–248.

19.   Pors J, Cheng A, Leo JM, et al. A Comparison of GATA3, TTF1, CD10, and Calretinin in Identifying Mesonephric and Mesonephric-like Carcinomas of the Gynecologic Tract. Am J Surg Pathol 2018; 42:1596–1606.

20.   Na K, Kim HS. Clinicopathologic and Molecular Characteristics of Mesonephric Adenocarcinoma Arising From the Uterine Body. Am J Surg Pathol 2019; 43:14.

21.   The Cancer Genome Atlas Research Network, Levine DA. Integrated genomic characterization of endometrial carcinoma. Nature 2013; 497:67–73.

22.   Modest DP, Ricard I, Heinemann V, et al. Outcome according to KRAS-, NRAS- and BRAF-mutation as well as KRAS mutation variants: pooled analysis of five randomized trials in metastatic colorectal cancer by the AIO colorectal cancer study group. Ann Oncol 2016; 27:1746–1753.

23.   Bournet B, Muscari F, Buscail C, et al. KRAS G12D Mutation Subtype Is A Prognostic Factor for Advanced Pancreatic Adenocarcinoma. Clin Transl Gastroenterol 2016; 7:e157.

24.   Kajiwara H, Hirasara T, Kawashima M, et al. Three cases of mesonephric-like adenocarcinoma in the female genital organs. Obstet Gynecol Rep 2020; 4:1–7.

25.   McCluggage WG. Mesonephric-like Adenocarcinoma of the Female Genital Tract: From Morphologic Observations to a Well-characterized Carcinoma With Aggressive Clinical Behavior. Adv Anat Pathol 2022; 29:208–216.

26.   Goyal A, Masand RP, Roma AA. Value of PAX-8 and SF-1 Immunohistochemistry in the Distinction Between Female Adnexal Tumor of Probable Wolffian Origin and its Mimics: Int J Gynecol Pathol 2016; 35:167–175.

27.   Davis M, Rauh-Hain JA, Andrade C, et al. Comparison of clinical outcomes of patients with clear cell and endometrioid ovarian cancer associated with endometriosis to papillary serous carcinoma of the ovary. Gynecol Oncol 2014; 132:760–766.

28.   Arslanian E, Singh K, James Sung C, Quddus MR. Somatic mutation analysis of Mesonephric-Like adenocarcinoma and associated putative precursor Lesions: Insight into pathogenesis and potential molecular treatment targets. Gynecol Oncol Rep 2022; 42:101049.

29.   André F, Ciruelos EM, Juric D, et al. Alpelisib plus fulvestrant for PIK3CA-mutated, hormone receptor-positive, human epidermal growth factor receptor-2–negative advanced breast cancer: final overall survival results from SOLAR-1. Ann Oncol 2021; 32:208–217.

30.   Juric D, Janku F, Rodón J, et al. Alpelisib Plus Fulvestrant in PIK3CA-Altered and PIK3CA-Wild-Type Estrogen Receptor–Positive Advanced Breast Cancer: A Phase 1b Clinical Trial. JAMA Oncol 2019; 5:e184475.

Chapter 5

Soft-tissue tumours with an epithelioid morphology – diagnostic challenges

Kyle D Perry, Anamarija M Perry

INTRODUCTION

Soft-tissue tumours with an epithelioid morphology can be an exceptionally difficult area for pathologists. While a pleomorphic or spindled appearance can be a strong indicator that a tumour is likely mesenchymal in nature, an epithelioid tumour is much less specific. Before considering an epithelioid mesenchymal tumour, a pathologist should consider other cellular lines of differentiation, including haematolymphoid neoplasms (e.g. anaplastic large cell lymphoma, Hodgkin lymphoma), germ-cell tumours (e.g. yolk sac tumours), metastatic or primary melanoma, and primary or metastatic carcinoma.

Immunohistochemistry can be helpful in excluding many of these entities. Anaplastic large cell lymphoma and Hodgkin lymphoma will typically be positive for CD30. SALL4 will often be positive in germ-cell tumour. Melanomas typically stain for S100 and SOX10. Carcinomas are usually positive for pancytokeratin. However, the specificity of these stains is not absolute, as epithelioid mesenchymal tumours can have overlapping staining profiles. Pancytokeratin staining can be seen in many tumours with epithelioid morphology, including epithelioid sarcoma (ES), epithelioid haemangioma, epithelioid haemangioendothelioma (EHE), and epithelioid angiosarcoma (EA). Additionally, schwannomas with epithelioid features or clear-cell sarcoma will typically show strong staining with S100 or SOX10. While historically used to identify a tumour as mesenchymal in nature, vimentin has been virtually abandoned in soft-tissue pathology as it is unable to confirm or exclude a tumour as mesenchymal in nature.

Given the limitations of ancillary studies, it is important to consider the clinical context of the mass when formulating and executing a differential diagnosis. In patients who have had a previous history of malignancy, excluding recurrence or metastasis should be a top priority for the pathologist. This can sometimes be difficult as tumours can sometimes lose their original staining characteristics (e.g. metaplastic carcinoma losing AE1/AE3 staining or "dedifferentiated melanoma" losing staining for SOX10). If the mass is arising in or

Kyle D Perry MD, Pathology and Laboratory Medicine, Henry Ford Health System, Detroit, MI, US
Email: kperry4@hfhs.org (for correspondence)

Anamarija M Perry MD, Department of Pathology, University of Michigan, Ann Arbor, MI, US
E-mail: anaperry@med.umich.edu

adjacent to a parenchymal organ, attention should be paid to whether the tumour appears to be arising from the respective epithelium or if there is a background in-situ neoplastic component. When considering a metastasis from a germ-cell tumour in a male patient, a pathologist should encourage imaging and clinical examination for assessment for a testicular mass. However, it should also be noted that patients can sometimes have primary malignancies which will undergo spontaneous regression, such as the case of a patient with a "burned out testicular germ-cell tumour."

The purpose of this chapter is to highlight some epithelioid mesenchymal tumours which can be encountered in practice. As numerous soft-tissue neoplasms can exhibit an "epithelioid variant", this discussion is by no means exhaustive. Entities addressed in this chapter include ES, clear-cell sarcoma, alveolar soft-part sarcoma, sclerosing epithelioid fibrosarcoma (SEF), ossifying fibromyxoid tumour (OFMT) of soft tissue, EA, and epithelioid haemangioendothelioma.

EPITHELIOID SARCOMA

Epithelioid sarcoma is a rare malignant soft-tissue tumour composed of multinodular aggregates of epithelioid cells surrounded by stromal mesenchymal spindle cells. Two types of ES are recognised: (1) the usual type, as originally described by Enzinger in 1970 [1], and (2) a proximal type ES described by Guillou et al in 1997 [2]. The clinicopathologic features of these tumours have been reviewed on several occasions [3–6]. Nevertheless, they still present a formidable diagnostic pitfall to the unsuspecting pathologist and clinician.

Clinical presentation and gross features

The usual-type ES is a tumour of young adults and is two times more common in men than women. It is found mostly in the dermis and subcutis of the distal parts of the upper extremities, often involving the hands and fingers. It usually presents as a slow-growing solitary mass, but it may also occur in the form of multiple nodules. The tumour has a firm consistency, but may show surface ulcerations. On sectioning, these nodules typically show a central area of softening due to necrosis. Local metastases are typically found in lymph nodes. Distal haematogenous metastases may be found in the lungs or other organs.

Proximal-type ES presents as larger deep-seated masses, which are, by definition, located more proximally than the usual-type ES. Thus, they can be found in the axilla or inguinal region, flank and even in the pelvic region. Clinically, these tumours are more aggressive than the distal, usual-type ES [3,4].

Microscopic features

Microscopically, the usual-type ES consists of confluent nodules composed of relatively uniform, polygonal epithelioid cells that have well-developed eosinophilic cytoplasm (**Figure 5.1**). The nuclei of these cells are deceivingly uniform and bland at low power, which sometimes results in ES being misdiagnosed as a non-neoplastic granulomatous process. Infiltrates of lymphocytes can also further masquerade an ES as an inflammatory process. At the periphery of these tumours, epithelioid cells merge with the spindle cells of fibroblastic and even desmoplastic stroma. Foci of necrosis, haemorrhage, or haemosiderin deposits are common. The proximal-type ES shows greater cytologic atypia than usual-type ES and its cells may have rhabdoid features (**Figure 5.2**). Several morphologic variants of ES have been described, including myxoid, angiomatoid, and fibroma-like.

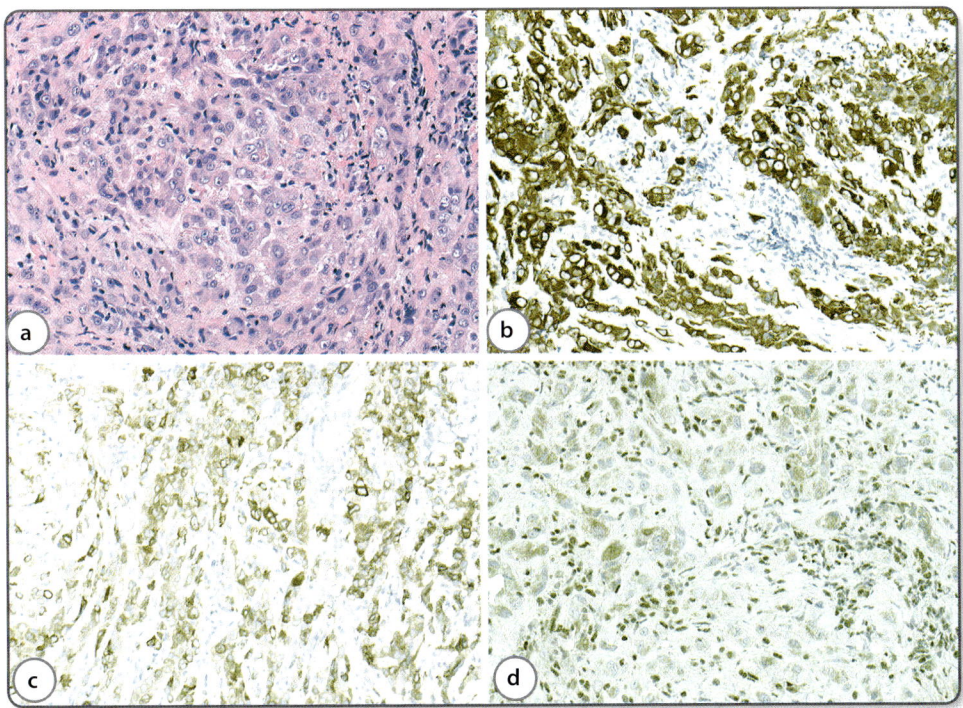

Figure 5.1 Epithelioid sarcoma, usual type. Tumour is composed of polygonal epithelioid cells with relatively bland vesicular nuclei and abundant eosinophilic cytoplasm (a). They are positive for cytokeratin AE1/AE3 (b), CK5/6 (c), and show loss of INI-1 (d).

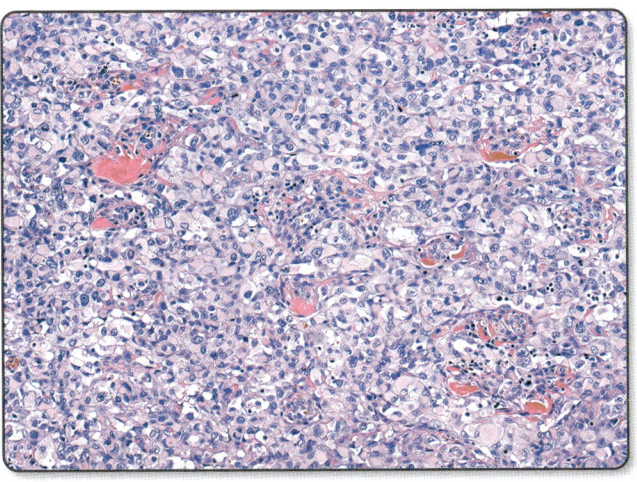

Figure 5.2 Epithelioid sarcoma, proximal variant. Sheets of tumour cells with rhabdoid features.

Immunohistochemical studies are essential for the proper diagnosis. Typically, >90% of all tumours react positively with antibodies to pancytokeratin and ERG and are negative for INI-1. CD34 is positive in about one-half of all tumours. Cytokeratin 5/6 is positive in about 30% of cases **(Figure 5.1)** [7].

Differential diagnosis

The differential diagnosis of ES includes non-neoplastic granulomatous diseases, non-keratinising squamous-cell carcinoma, and vascular tumours (both benign and malignant) and immunohistochemical stains could be useful in this respect. Granulomatous inflammation is positive for CD163 and negative for AE1/AE3. Squamous-cell carcinomas will generally retain INI-1 staining. Pseudomyogenic haemangioendothelioma (sometimes called "ES-like haemangioendothelioma") is a tumour which can mimic ES both clinically and histologically. Vascular tumours (including pseudomyogenic haemangioendothelioma) will be positive for CD31 and retain INI-1 staining [7].

CLEAR-CELL SARCOMA OF SOFT TISSUE

Clear-cell sarcoma of soft tissue (CCSST) is a rare malignant tumour composed of glycogen-rich clear cells. Originally described by Enzinger [8] as clear-cell sarcoma of tendons and aponeuroses, it was also termed "malignant melanoma of soft parts" [9]. This link to melanoma was promoted further by immunohistochemical studies, which showed that these two tumours share the same immunophenotype [10]. However, subsequent genetic studies revealed that most CCSSTs are associated with a t(12;22)(q13-14;q12) translocation, which is not found in malignant melanomas. CCSST also shares some features with clear-cell sarcoma of the gastrointestinal tract. There are, however, differences between these tumour types, and the gastrointestinal tumour is therefore called clear-cell sarcoma-like gastrointestinal tumour [11].

Clinical presentation and gross features

Clear-cell sarcoma of soft tissues are mostly diagnosed in young adults, 20–40 years of age [10]. The median age at the time of diagnosis is 39 years. 5- and 10-year survival is 50% and 38%, respectively [12]. CCSSTs are slow-growing tumours most commonly arising from tendon sheaths and aponeuroses. The majority of these tumours are located in the soft tissue of the lower limbs, particularly around the ankles. CCSSTs infiltrate the normal connective tissue and cannot be shelled out. Tumours arising in the upper extremities and chest wall are rare.

Microscopic features

Microscopically, CCSSTs are composed of invasive epithelioid to spindled cells enclosed by a densely fibrotic stroma. Tumour cells have vesicular nuclei and prominent nucleoli, and abundant clear or eosinophilic cytoplasm. Multinucleated tumour giant cells and melanin pigment in the cytoplasm of some cells can be seen (**Figure 5.3**).

Immunohistochemically, these cells react with antibodies to S100, SOX10, HMB-45, and Melan A and thus resemble melanoma (**Figure 5.3b, inset**) [8].

Genetics

Genetically, CCSSTs differ from melanomas and exhibit an *EWSR1-ATF1* fusion transcript, which is not found in melanomas. Interestingly *EWSR1-ATF1* is not specific for this tumour, as this fusion has been identified in completely unrelated entities such as angiomatoid fibrous histiocytoma, hyalinising clear-cell carcinoma of the salivary gland and primary pulmonary myxoid sarcoma [13].

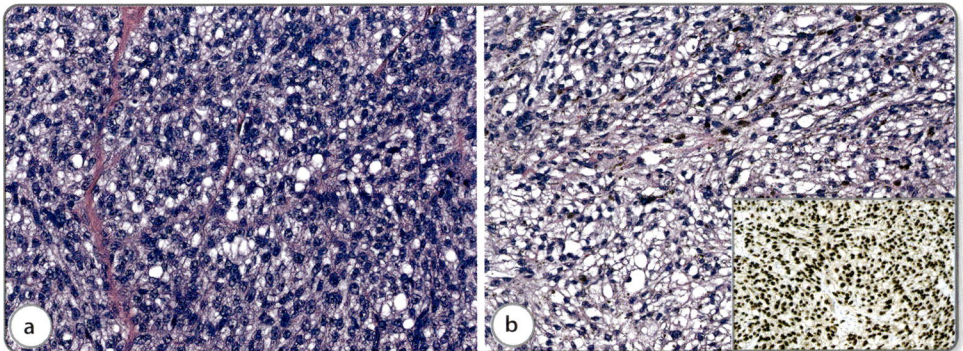

Figure 5.3 Clear-cell sarcoma is composed of epithelioid (a) or spindled cells (b), with vesicular nuclei, conspicuous nucleoli, and abundant eosinophilic cytoplasm. Scattered melanin pigment can be seen (b). Tumour cells are positive for SOX10 (b-inset).

Differential diagnosis

Differential diagnosis includes melanoma, and other soft-tissue sarcomas that might have epithelioid and spindle cells, such as synovial sarcoma or perhaps malignant peripheral nerve sheath tumour. The presence of strong S100, HMB45 and Melan-A staining, supported by molecular biology data demonstrating an *EWSR-ATF1* fusion transcript, makes it easy to distinguish CCSST from these histological mimickers.

ALVEOLAR SOFT-PART SARCOMA

Alveolar soft-part sarcoma (ASPS) is an uncommon soft-tissue neoplasm accounting for <1% of soft-tissue sarcomas [7].

Clinical presentation and gross features

Alveolar soft-part sarcoma is predominantly a tumour of adolescents and young adults, most commonly occurring in patients 15–35 years of age. It is more common in females and quite rare in patients younger than 5 and older than 50 years old. It usually occurs in the lower extremities (particularly the anterior thighs and buttocks), while in infants and children the head and neck are the most common sites. Patients present with a slow growing, painless mass that can be easily overlooked. Metastatic disease (frequently to the brain and lungs) is frequently a first presenting symptom in patients with ASPS [7,14]. The prognosis of patients with ASPS is generally unfavourable. Metastatic disease can occur early in the disease course or many years after the initial diagnosis. In one study, patients with localised and metastatic disease had an overall 5-year survival of 87% and 20%, respectively [15]. Only approximately 15% of patients survive 20 years after the initial diagnosis. The prognosis seems to be better in children, as they present with smaller and more resectable tumours. The primary mode of treatment is surgical resection. Chemotherapy and radiotherapy might be beneficial in some cases [16]. Furthermore, some patients benefit from tyrosine kinase inhibitor sunitinib, as well as other related drugs (e.g. crizotinib) [7,17,18].

Grossly, ASPS is typically a poorly circumscribed friable mass that is tan-yellow on sectioning with areas of haemorrhage and necrosis.

Microscopic features

Histologically, ASPS is composed of nests or aggregates of cells separated by thin fibrovascular septa. Characteristically, these nests will show degeneration and loss of cell cohesiveness, resulting in pseudoalveolar pattern, after which this tumour was named. Importantly, some cases (especially in infants and children) show more solid sheets of malignant cells, with less obvious nesting and lack of pseudoalveolae, which can be challenging to diagnose (**Figure 5.4**). The tumour cells are large or polygonal and have eosinophilic and granular cytoplasm, often with prominent nucleoli. Occasionally, they may show clear cytoplasm (**Figure 5.5**). Nuclear pleomorphism, including multinucleation, has been described. Mitoses are usually rare [7].

By immunohistochemistry, the neoplastic cells are positive for TFE3 (nuclear), cathepsin K, and desmin (variable). They are negative for S100, smooth muscle actin (SMA), SOX10,

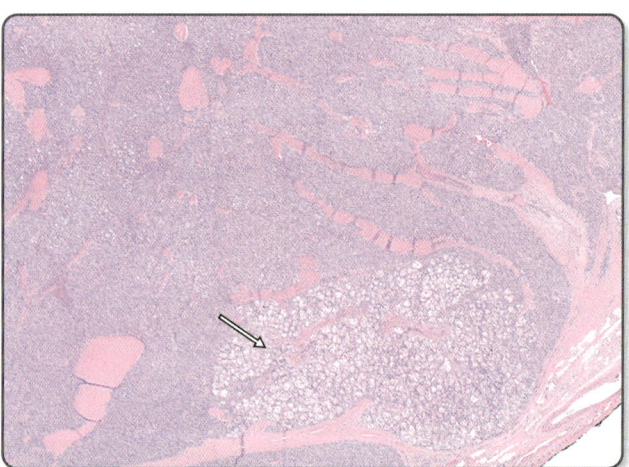

Figure 5.4 Alveolar soft-part sarcoma. Majority of tumour shows solid sheets of cells with focal area of pseudoalveolar pattern (arrow).

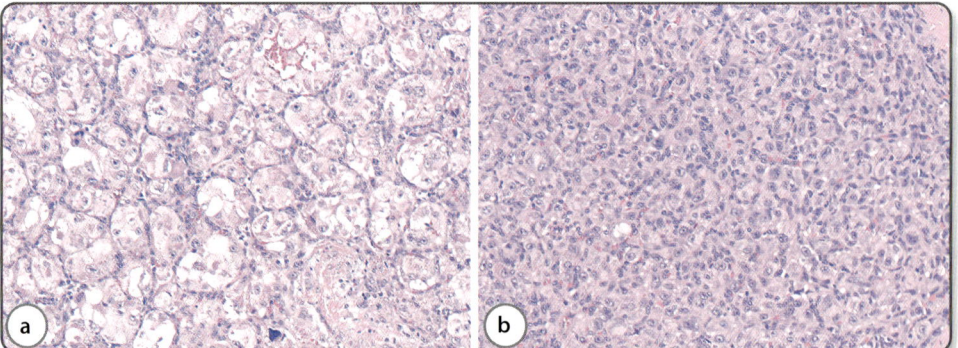

Figure 5.5 Alveolar soft-part sarcoma. Tumour cells show nesting and pseudoalveolar pattern (a) or sheets of cells with no obvious nesting pattern (b). The cells are large with vesicular nuclei, small nucleoli, and abundant eosinophilic granular cytoplasm.

cytokeratins, myogenin, MyoD1. A PAS stain highlights diastase-resistant intracytoplasmic crystals [7,19].

Genetics

Alveolar soft-part sarcoma shows a characteristic chromosomal alteration, der(17)t(X;17) (p11.2;q25), leading to *ASPSCR1-TFE3* gene fusion [20].

Differential diagnosis

While the classic morphology of alveolar soft-part sarcoma is a strong tipoff to its diagnosis, the alveolar features are often only found in a limited area of the tumour. Often, in a needle core biopsy, the pathologist might only encounter a sheet-like arrangement of eosinophilic epithelioid mesenchymal cells. When encountered in anatomic sites such as the proximal lower extremity or buttock, the differential diagnosis would include entities such as a (cellular) extraskeletal myxoid chondrosarcoma, proximal variant of ES, metastatic renal cell carcinoma, or a granular cell tumour. Extraskeletal myxoid chondrosarcoma usually exhibits epithelioid-like cells in a myxoid matrix; however, they can occasionally be almost completely composed of epithelioid cells. These tumours typically exhibit fusion transcripts involving the *NR4A3* gene (usually *EWSR1-NR4A3*). The proximal variant of ES can have rhabdoid-like cells with enlarged vesicular nuclei and prominent nucleoli. These tumours generally show complete loss of nuclear expression of the SMARCB1 (INI-1) protein. Granular cell tumour shows robust staining with S100 and SOX10 stains. Renal-cell carcinoma exhibits a particular proclivity to metastasise to unusual sites, including soft tissue. As some variants of renal-cell carcinoma can show translocations involving the *TFE* gene (including Xp11 translocation renal-cell carcinoma which can also show an *ASPSCR1-TFE3* fusion transcript), a pathologist should be generous in correlating with radiology findings and utilising PAX8 (often positive in renal-cell carcinoma) to exclude the possibilty of a renal primary [21].

SCLEROSING EPITHELIOID FIBROSARCOMA

Sclerosing epithelioid fibrosarcoma is an agressive variant of fibrosarcoma which can be diagnostically problematic for a pathologist [7,22].

Clinical presentation and gross features

Sclerosing epithelioid fibrosarcoma mostly commonly presents as a mass in deep soft tissue of the lower extremities. Other frequent locations include the upper extremities, trunk, and head and neck region. The median age of diagnosis is 45 years, but these tumours have been reported over a broad age range. There is no gender predilection. SEF is an aggressive neoplasm, characterised by late local recurrences and distal metastasis and requires long-term follow-up. A relatively small series showed that after 5 years of follow-up, approximately 50% or people deveoped local recurrence and 40% developed metastatic disease, most commonly to the lungs [7,23].

Grossly, SEF appears as well-circumsribed and lobulated lesions, with myxoid change or calcifications occasionally present.

Microscopic features

Histologically, SEF is typically infiltrative and extends into the surrounding soft tissue. The tumour cells have round to ovoid nuclei, vesicular nuclei, inconspicuous or small nucleoli and scant pale cytoplasm. They are arranged into nests of cords and embedded into densely hyalinised stroma (**Figure 5.6**) [7]. Many SEFs have a component of tumour which morphologically resembles low-grade fibromyxoid sarcoma (LGFMS). LGFMS features include spindled cells with varying amounts of hyalinised and myxoid stroma, arcuate vessels, and hyalinised collagen rosettes. These tumours are often referred to as hybrid sclerosing epithelioid fibrosarcoma-low-grade fibromyxoid sarcoma (hybrid SEF-LGFMS). The survival rates of SEF and SEF-LGFMS have been found to be similar [24].

By immunohistochemistry, the neoplastic cells are positive for MUC4 (**Figure 5.6**), the most useful stain for supporting the diagnosis of this tumour [25]. EMA is positive in about half of all cases, while cytokeratins, S100, SMA, desmin, and CD34 stains are negative.

Genetics

Both SEF and SEF-LGFMS tumours exhibit relatively consistent translocations involving the *CREB3L2* and *CREB3L1* genes. Pure SEFs tend to show *EWSR1-CREB3L2* or *EWSR1-CREB3L1* fusions. SEF-LGFMS more often exhibit *FUS-CREB3L2* fusion transcripts. This tendency is not absolute, however, and SEF with *FUS* gene translocations have been reported [7].

Differential diagnosis

The differential diagnosis of SEF is broad. SEF can be positive for EMA which can simulate a metastatic carcinoma. Unlike carcinoma, SEF is typically negative for pancytokeratin markers. Lymphoma and melanoma can also be seen in the background of dense sclerosis. However, these tumours have remarkably different immunoprofiles (positive for CD45 and S100/SOX10, respectively). Sclerosing rhabdomyosarcoma can have a very similar morphology. Unlike SEF, this variant of rhabdomyosarcoma will be positive for desmin (often dot like) and stain for MyoD1. SEF can be mistaken for OFMT of soft tissue. Additionally, both tumours can be positive for MUC4 which can also create confusion.

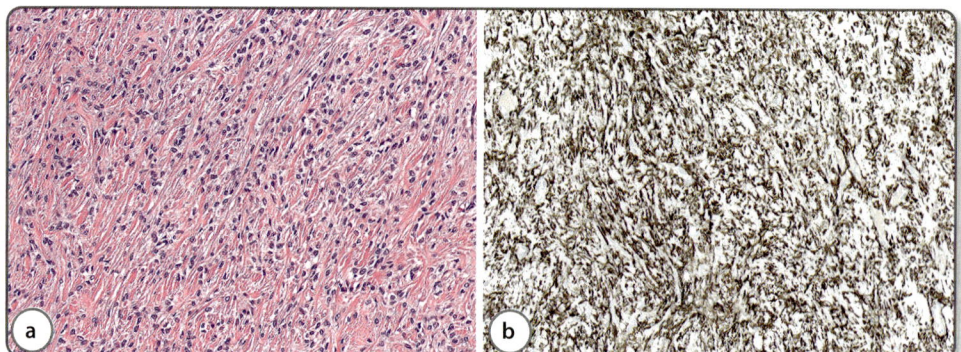

Figure 5.6 Sclerosing epithelioid fibrosarcoma. Sheets of small cells with round to ovoid nuclei, inconspicuous nucleoli, and scant pale cytoplasm are embedded into densely hyalinised stroma (a). Tumour cells are positive for MUC4 (b).

Unlike SEF, OFMT does not exhibit translocations involving the *EWSR1* and *FUS* genes. Finally, it should be understood that the category of "sclerosing epithelioid fibrosarcoma" is somewhat dynamic. Recently recurrent *YAP1* and *KMT2A* gene rearrangements have been identified in a subset of "MUC4-negative sclerosing epithelioid fibrosarcomas" [26].

OSSIFYING FIBROMYXOID TUMOUR OF SOFT TISSUE

Ossifying fibromyxoid tumour of soft tissue is a relatively rare neoplasm which is of an uncertain line of differentiation. This tumour can be diagnostically problematic as it shows a diversity of histologies spanning from benign to malignant appearing lesions. The clinical behaviour of these tumours is difficult to predict but roughly correlates with the histologic appearance, with local recurrences and distant metastases being much more frequent in OFTs with malignant histology [7,27].

Clinical presentation and gross features

Ossifying fibromyxoid tumour primarily occurs in adults (median age at diagnosis of 50 years) and is more common in males. It typically arises in the extremities (around 70% of all cases) as a subcutaneous and well-defined mass. It can occasionally occur in other sites such as the head and neck, trunk, mediastinum and retorperitoneum. As mentioned above, OFMTs with bland (typical) histology rarely locally recur (around 10% of cases) and only exceptionally metastasise. Malignant appearing OFMTs will locally recur and metastasise in over 50% of cases [7].

Grossly, OFMT is typically a well-circumscribed and often lobulated mass with a thick-fibrous pseudocapsule. On sectioning, the mass is tan white and can contain focal areas of calcifications, giving it a gritty appearance.

Microscopic features

Histologically, OFMT is surrounded by a pseudocapsule and is composed of nests and cords of round to ovoid or spindled cells embedded in a variably myxoid or fibrous stroma. The cells have vesicular nuclei, small to inconspicuous nucleoli and a small amount of eosinophilic cytoplasm. In the majority of cases (approximately 75%), periphery of the tumour contains at least partial areas of bone which can sometimes be quite abundant (**Figure 5.7**). Although most OFMTs have a monomorphic bland morphology, some tumours have atypical of frankly malignant features. Folpe and Weiss proposed a histologic classification system of OFMT that combines nuclear features, cellularity and mitotic activity. Tumours with low cellularity, low nuclear grade and <2 mitoses/50 high-power fields (HPF) are classified as typical OFMT. In contrast, tumours with high cellularity, high nuclear grade (defined as irregular nuclear contours, macronucleoli and/or coarse chromatin) and >2 mitoses/HPF are malignant. Atypical OFMTs not meeting the criteria for typical or malignant are designated as atypical [7,27].

Tumour cells express S100 in approximately 70% of cases with variable intensity of staining. Other stains that were found to be positive include cytokeratins, desmin, CD56, CD57, neuron-specific enolase (NSE), glial fibrillary acidic protein (GFAP), and SMA. In approximately 70% of cases there is a partial loss of expression of the SMARCB1/INI1 tumour suppressor gene that results in a mosaic pattern of nuclear expression [7,28]. A minority of OFMTs have also been found to express MUC4 [29].

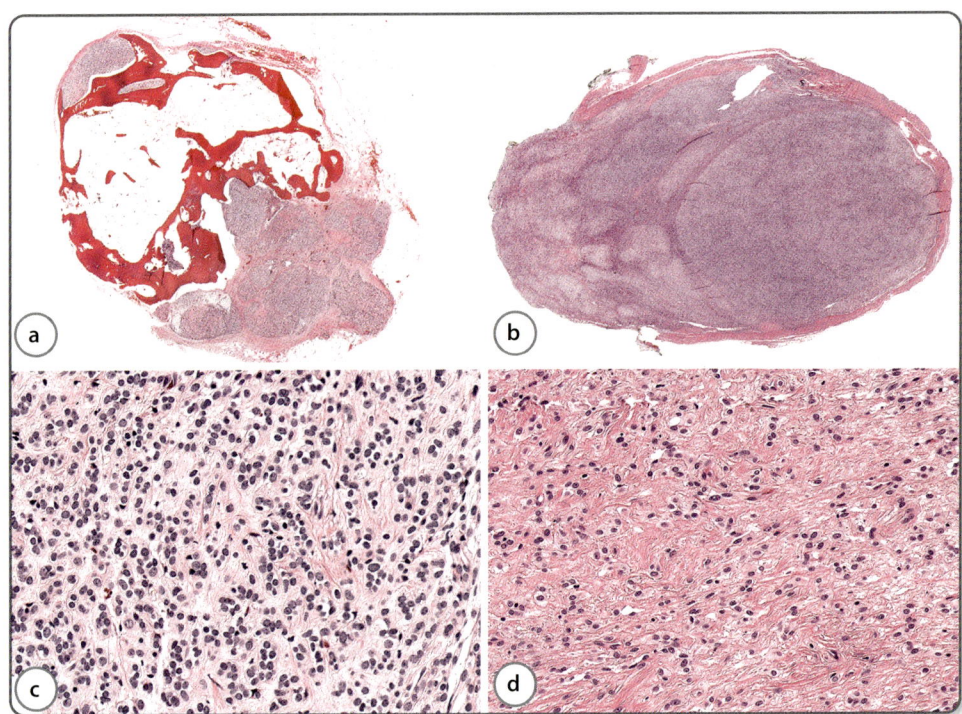

Figure 5.7 Ossifying fibromyxoid tumour of soft tissue. The tumour contains abundant area of mature bone (a); prominent pseudocapsule is seen (b). Tumour is composed of nests and cords of round to ovoid cells embedded in a loose fibrous stroma (c). In some areas, stroma is more abundant (d).

Genetics

The most frequently encountered genetic abnormalities in OFMT involve rearrangements of the *PHF1* gene (up to 80% of cases) [30,31]. The most frequent fusion gene is *PHF1-EP400*; however, numerous other fusions have been identified in this tumour, including *KDM2A-WWTR1*, *EPC-PHF1*, *PHF1-TFE3*, *ZC3H7B-BCOR*, *MEAF6-PHF1*, and *CREBBP-BCOR* [31–33]. A small percentage of OFMT have been reported to exhibit a *PHF1-TFE3* gene fusion. At present, from the limited amount of cases in the literature, tumours with this fusion transcript are less likely to have associated calcifications and are disproportionately found to have malignant histologic features [31]. Additionally, a recent report of a novel *MEAF6-SUZ12* fusion was recently described in a case of OFMT [34]. This tumour showed some unusual histologic features such as a multilobular growth pattern and a more haphazard distribution of ossification than typically associated with OFMTs. It should be emphasised that utilisation of genetic and molecular diagnostics should be interpreted in the context of the morphologic findings as many of the fusion transcripts of OFMT can be found in other mesenchymal tumours such as endometrial stromal sarcoma [33].

Differential diagnosis

When encountered in classical histological form, the diagnosis of OFMT can be a relatively straightforward affair. However, when the tumour is viewed in the context of limited sampling (i.e. needle core biopsy) or variant morphology, the diagnosis can be more problematic. If no calcification is identified, then cutaneous adnexal (e.g. chondroid syringoma) or myoepithelial neoplasms can be considered, but should have more robust staining with epithelial markers and SOX10. If OFMT has a spindled component (and is positive for *MUC4*), then a pathologist could potentially mistake it for a LGFMS or SEF. Both LGFMS and SEF typically exhibit translocations that involve the *CREB3L1* or *CREB3L2* gene. OFMTs can sometimes mimic other matrix producing mesenchymal tumours such as paraosteal osteosarcoma; however, such bone tumours have not been described as sharing the characteristic molecular fusion transcripts seen in OFMT [35].

EPITHELIOID ANGIOSARCOMA

Epithelioid angiosarcoma is a rare variant of angiosarcoma composed predominantly of endothelial cells that have epithelioid features, often expressing both epithelial and vascular immunohistochemical markers [36–39].

Clinical presentation and gross features

Epithelioid angiosarcoma occurs most often in older adults with a peak incidence in the seventh decade of life. The majority of cases have been identified in the deep soft tissue of extremities and are commonly intramuscular. EA may also be less commonly found in the dermis and internal organs. Tumours tend to metastasise early to lungs and other organs and are lethal in a relatively short period after the diagnosis.

Microscopic features

Epithelioid sarcoma is composed of large, mildly to moderately pleomorphic, round or polygonal epithelioid cells, that have well developed eosinophilic cytoplasm and vesicular nuclei containing prominent nucleoli. Tumour cells are usually arranged into sheets and solid nests, which may resemble malignant epithelial tumours or melanomas. Nevertheless, most tumours also contain areas composed of anastomosing vascular spaces indicative of their rudimentary vasoformative potential (**Figure 5.8**). Sheeted areas contain

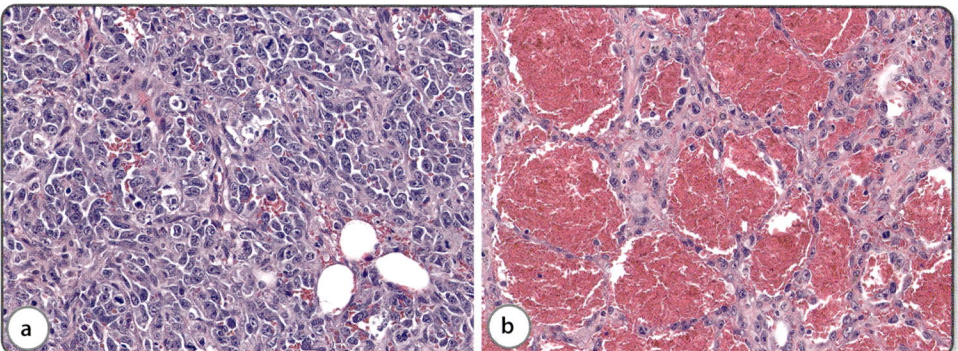

Figure 5.8 Epithelioid angiosarcoma. Majority of the tumour is composed of large pleomorphic cells with irregular nuclei, prominent nucleoli, and eosinophilic cytoplasm (a). Tumour also shows areas composed of anastomosing vascular spaces lined by malignant cells (b).

scant stroma which can be highlighted with the reticulin stain. In other areas, stroma may be more prominent, loosely myxomatous or desmoplastic. Mitoses and areas of necrosis are usually prominent, indicative of rapid growth of this neoplasm.

Immunohistochemistry is useful to show the hybrid nature of tumour cells which express both epithelial and mesenchymal markers. As with all types of angiosarcoma, AE is positive for vimentin, CD31, factor VII, and Fli-1. CD34 positivity ranges from 40% to 100%. Antibodies to pancytokeratin stain react with most tumour cells, although one should note that cytokeratin positivity can be found in about one-third of all angiosarcomas [38].

Differential diagnosis

Differential diagnosis includes carcinomas, and vascular tumours that are not as malignant as the EA, such as epithelioid haemangioma and haemangioendothelioma. The differential diagnosis with ES was mentioned before. EHE is a less malignant tumour than AE, and thus these two neoplasms need to be distinguished one from another. Both of them are composed of cells that have epithelioid features and are often sheeted. However, EHEs show lower mitotic activity (<2 per 10 HPF), and secondary signs of high malignancy such as necrosis and haemorrhage are not prominent. Their nuclei are usually less hyperchromatic and without prominent nucleoli. Many individual cells display intracytoplasmic lumina, occasionally containing red blood cells. Immunohistochemically, these cells are positive for CD31, CD34 and ERG. EAs, however, lack the *WWTR1-CAMTA1* (WW domain containing transcription regulator 1 and calmodulin-binding transcription activator 1) fusion transcript associated with epithelioid haemangioendothelioma.

EPITHELIOID HAEMANGIOENDOTHELIOMA

Epithelioid haemangioendothelioma is another vascular tumour with epithelioid morphology which can be diagnostically problematic for pathologist. While not typically as clinically aggressive as EA, these tumours are still considered malignant and correct diagnosis is important.

Clinical presentation and gross features

These tumours usually present in adults and are often found within or around a vessel in the superficial or soft tissue. Other sites include pleura, lungs, bone, and liver. They can be present as a single mass or have a multicentric presentation. The mass can often be painful [40].

Microscopic features

Microscopically, EHEs typically have a much less vasoformative architecture than other vascular neoplasms. Instead, the tumour is usually composed of individual, cords or small nests of epithelioid cells in the background of myxohyalinised stroma (**Figure 5.9**). Often, the tumour can be centred in a vascular space that extends through the vessel wall into the adjacent soft tissue. The cells typically have eosinophilic cytoplasm with vesicular nuclei. Intracellular cytoplasmic vacuolisation, sometimes containing an erythrocyte can be seen. Although EHEs are not "graded" by Fédération Nationale des Centres de Lutte Contre

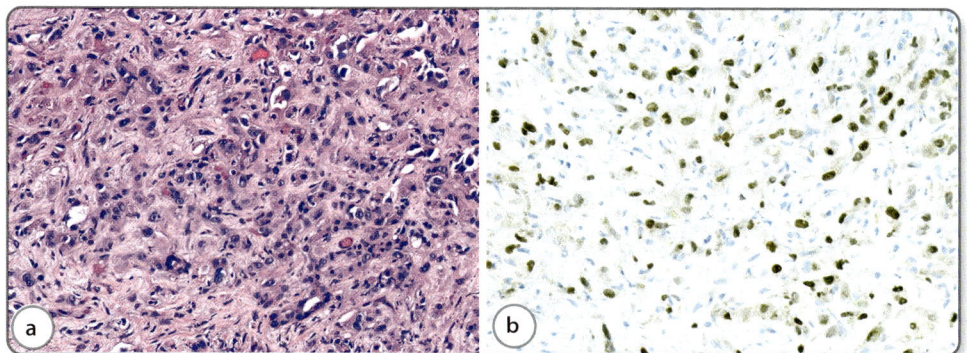

Figure 5.9 Epithelioid haemangioendothelioma is composed of small nests and cords of epithelioid cells with round nuclei, vesicular chromatin and eosinophilic cytoplasm. (a) Tumour cells are positive for CAMTA1 (b).

le Cancer (FNCLCC) criteria, risk stratification systems have been published which can help to determine clinical behaviour of this tumour. One of the most commonly used was published by Deyrup and colleagues, in which a two-tiered system was proposed. High-risk tumours had >3 mitoses/50 HPF or ≥3 cm in the greatest dimension. The low-risk group had tumours <3 cm in dimension and had ≤3 mitoses/50 HPF. In the high-risk group, the 5-year disease-specific survival was 59% and 32% of patients experienced metastasis. In the low-risk group, there was no tumour-specific mortality and only 15% of patients experienced metastasis [41].

Epithelioid haemangioendothelioma is consistently positive for vascular markers such as CD31 and ERG. CD34 is considered to be less sensitive (81% of cases) [42]. *WWTR1-CAMTA1* fusion transcripts have been identified in most EHEs which have been particularly helpful in increasing the accuracy and consistency of diagnosis. This fusion can be identified by molecular sequencing. Alternatively, the *CAMTA1* immunohistochemical stain can also infer this fusion by highlighting nuclear expression of the CAMTA1 protein **(Figure 5.9)** [43].

Differential diagnosis

The diagnosis of EHE primarily rests on excluding it from other epithelioid vascular tumours such as epithelioid haemangioma or EA. In brief, EAs typically exhibit much more pleomorphism and have more prominent areas of vasoformative architecture. Epithelioid haemangiomas typically retain a vaguely lobular distribution and also exhibit areas of a more vasoformative appearance. This distinction, however, can sometimes be difficult and the use of *CAMTA1* immunostain has been immensely helpful in distinguishing these entities (positive in EHE and negative in EA and epithelioid haemangioma).

As EHE can be positive for cytokeratin, one must be careful not to mistake this for a metastatic carcinoma, particularly when the tumour arises in common anatomic sites of metastasis such as the lungs or the liver. This confusion can be further compounded as EHEs can also rarely express synaptophysin [42]. Liberal use of vascular markers with subsequent *CAMTA1* immunohistochemistry can help to prevent a misdiagnosis.

Key points for clinical practice

- Numerous soft-tissue neoplasms can exhibit epithelioid morphology and can be very challenging for pathologists.
- These neoplasms are generally overall rare and need to be distinguished from more common tumours with epithelioid morphology, such as carcinoma, melanoma, lymphoma, or germ-cell tumours
- Liberal use of immunohistochemical stains to exclude non-mesenchymal entities is encouraged. However, care should be taken since mesenchymal tumours with epithelioid morphology can have overlapping staining profiles, and can, for example, stain for cytokeratins or melanoma markers.
- Among soft-tissue tumours with epithelioid morphology, different entities can have overlapping morphologic features. Immunohistochemical stains and/or molecular sequencing studies are frequently needed to resolve the differential diagnosis.

REFERENCES

1. Enzinger FM. Epithelioid sarcoma. A sarcoma simulating a granuloma or a carcinoma. Cancer 1970; 26:1029–1041.
2. Guillou L, Wadden C, Coindre JM, Krausz T, Fletcher CD. "Proximal-type" epithelioid sarcoma, a distinctive aggressive neoplasm showing rhabdoid features. Clinicopathologic, immunohistochemical, and ultrastructural study of a series. Am J Surg Pathol 1997; 21:130–146.
3. Fisher C. Epithelioid sarcoma of Enzinger. Adv Anat Pathol 2006; 13:114–121.
4. Deyrup AT. Epithelioid Lesions. Surg Pathol Clin 2011; 4:865–885.
5. Armah HB, Parwani AV. Epithelioid sarcoma. Arch Pathol Lab Med 2009; 133:814–819.
6. Needs T, Fillman EP. Epithelioid Sarcoma. In: StatPearls [Internet]. Treasure Island (FL): StatPearls Publishing, 2023.
7. Weiss SW, Goldblum JR, Folpe A. Enzinger and Weiss Soft Tissue Tumors, 7th edition. Philadelphia, PA: Elsevier, 2020.
8. Enzinger FM. Clear-Cell Sarcoma of Tendons and Aponeuroses. An Analysis of 21 Cases. Cancer 1965; 18:1163–1174.
9. Chung EB, Enzinger FM. Malignant melanoma of soft parts. A reassessment of clear cell sarcoma. Am J Surg Pathol 1983; 7:405–413.
10. Zamora EA, Cassaro S. Soft Tissue Clear Cell Sarcoma. In: StatPearls [Internet]. Treasure Island (FL): StatPearls Publishing, 2023.
11. Segawa K, Sugita S, Aoyama T, et al. Detection of specific gene rearrangements by fluorescence in situ hybridization in 16 cases of clear cell sarcoma of soft tissue and 6 cases of clear cell sarcoma-like gastrointestinal tumor. Diagn Pathol 2018; 13:73.
12. Gonzaga MI, Grant L, Curtin C, et al. The epidemiology and survivorship of clear cell sarcoma: a National Cancer Database (NCDB) review. J Cancer Res Clin Oncol 2018; 144:1711–1716.
13. Perry KD, Montecalvo J, Perry AM. Sarcomas of the mediastinum with epithelioid morphology. Mediastinum 2021; 5:4.
14. Ordonez NG. Alveolar soft part sarcoma: a review and update. Adv Anat Pathol 1999; 6:125–139.
15. Portera CA, Jr, Ho V, Patel SR, et al. Alveolar soft part sarcoma: clinical course and patterns of metastasis in 70 patients treated at a single institution. Cancer 2001; 91:585–591.
16. Orbach D, Brennan B, Casanova M, et al. Paediatric and adolescent alveolar soft part sarcoma: A joint series from European cooperative groups. Pediatr Blood Cancer 2013; 60:1826–1832.
17. Ghose A, Tariq Z, Veltri S. Treatment of multidrug resistant advanced alveolar soft part sarcoma with sunitinib. Am J Ther 2012; 19:e56–e58.

18. Schoffski P, Wozniak A, Stacchiotti S, et al. Activity and safety of crizotinib in patients with advanced clear-cell sarcoma with MET alterations: European Organization for Research and Treatment of Cancer phase II trial 90101 'CREATE'. Ann Oncol 2017; 28:3000–3008.

19. Rekhi B, Ingle A, Agarwal M, et al. Alveolar soft part sarcoma 'revisited': clinicopathological review of 47 cases from a tertiary cancer referral centre, including immunohistochemical expression of TFE3 in 22 cases and 21 other tumours. Pathology 2012; 44:11–17.

20. Ladanyi M, Lui MY, Antonescu CR, et al. The der(17)t(X;17)(p11;q25) of human alveolar soft part sarcoma fuses the TFE3 transcription factor gene to ASPL, a novel gene at 17q25. Oncogene 2001; 20:48–57.

21. Argani P, Zhong M, Reuter VE, et al. TFE3-Fusion Variant Analysis Defines Specific Clinicopathologic Associations Among Xp11 Translocation Cancers. Am J Surg Pathol 2016; 40:723–737.

22. Murshed KA, Al-Bozom I, Ammar A. Sclerosing epithelioid fibrosarcoma: in-depth review of a genetically heterogeneous tumor. APMIS 2021; 129:455–460.

23. Meis-Kindblom JM, Kindblom LG, Enzinger FM. Sclerosing epithelioid fibrosarcoma. A variant of fibrosarcoma simulating carcinoma. Am J Surg Pathol 1995; 19:979–993.

24. Argani P, Lewin JR, Edmonds P, et al. Primary renal sclerosing epithelioid fibrosarcoma: report of 2 cases with EWSR1-CREB3L1 gene fusion. Am J Surg Pathol 2015; 39:365–373.

25. Doyle LA, Moller E, Dal Cin P, et al. MUC4 is a highly sensitive and specific marker for low-grade fibromyxoid sarcoma. Am J Surg Pathol 2011; 35:733–741.

26. Kao YC, Lee JC, Zhang L, et al. Recurrent YAP1 and KMT2A Gene Rearrangements in a Subset of MUC4-negative Sclerosing Epithelioid Fibrosarcoma. Am J Surg Pathol 2020; 44:368–377.

27. Folpe AL, Weiss SW. Ossifying fibromyxoid tumor of soft parts: a clinicopathologic study of 70 cases with emphasis on atypical and malignant variants. Am J Surg Pathol 2003; 27:421–431.

28. Graham RP, Dry S, Li X, et al. Ossifying fibromyxoid tumor of soft parts: a clinicopathologic, proteomic, and genomic study. Am J Surg Pathol 2011; 35:1615–1625.

29. Miettinen M, Finnell V, Fetsch JF. Ossifying fibromyxoid tumor of soft parts—a clinicopathologic and immunohistochemical study of 104 cases with long-term follow-up and a critical review of the literature. Am J Surg Pathol 2008; 32:996–1005.

30. Graham RP, Weiss SW, Sukov WR, et al. PHF1 rearrangements in ossifying fibromyxoid tumors of soft parts: A fluorescence in situ hybridization study of 41 cases with emphasis on the malignant variant. Am J Surg Pathol 2013; 37:1751–1755.

31. Suurmeijer AJH, Song W, Sung YS, et al. Novel recurrent PHF1-TFE3 fusions in ossifying fibromyxoid tumors. Genes Chromosomes Cancer 2019; 58:643–649.

32. Kao YC, Sung YS, Zhang L, et al. Expanding the molecular signature of ossifying fibromyxoid tumors with two novel gene fusions: CREBBP-BCORL1 and KDM2A-WWTR1. Genes Chromosomes Cancer 2017; 56:42–50.

33. Antonescu CR, Sung YS, Chen CL, et al. Novel ZC3H7B-BCOR, MEAF6-PHF1, and EPC1-PHF1 fusions in ossifying fibromyxoid tumors--molecular characterization shows genetic overlap with endometrial stromal sarcoma. Genes Chromosomes Cancer 2014; 53:183–193.

34. Killian K, Leckey BD, Naous R, et al. Novel MEAF6-SUZ12 fusion in ossifying fibromyxoid tumor with unusual features. Genes Chromosomes Cancer 2021; 60:631–634.

35. Ogose A, Otsuka H, Morita T, Kobayashi H, Hirata Y. Ossifying fibromyxoid tumor resembling parosteal osteosarcoma. Skeletal Radiol 1998; 27:578–580.

36. Fletcher CD, Beham A, Bekir S, Clarke AM, Marley NJ. Epithelioid angiosarcoma of deep soft tissue: a distinctive tumor readily mistaken for an epithelial neoplasm. Am J Surg Pathol 1991; 15:915–924.

37. Meis-Kindblom JM, Kindblom LG. Angiosarcoma of soft tissue: a study of 80 cases. Am J Surg Pathol 1998; 22:683–697.

38. Hart J, Mandavilli S. Epithelioid angiosarcoma: a brief diagnostic review and differential diagnosis. Arch Pathol Lab Med 2011; 135:268–272.

39. Bacchi CE, Silva TR, Zambrano E, et al. Epithelioid angiosarcoma of the skin: a study of 18 cases with emphasis on its clinicopathologic spectrum and unusual morphologic features. Am J Surg Pathol 2010; 34:1334–1343.

40.   Mentzel T, Beham A, Calonje E, Katenkamp D, Fletcher CD. Epithelioid hemangioendothelioma of skin and soft tissues: clinicopathologic and immunohistochemical study of 30 cases. Am J Surg Pathol 1997; 21:363–374.

41.   Deyrup AT, Tighiouart M, Montag AG, Weiss SW. Epithelioid hemangioendothelioma of soft tissue: a proposal for risk stratification based on 49 cases. Am J Surg Pathol 2008; 32:924–927.

42.   Flucke U, Vogels RJ, de Saint Aubain Somerhausen N, et al. Epithelioid Hemangioendothelioma: clinicopathologic, immunhistochemical, and molecular genetic analysis of 39 cases. Diagn Pathol 2014; 9:131.

43.   Doyle LA, Fletcher CD, Hornick JL. Nuclear Expression of CAMTA1 Distinguishes Epithelioid Hemangioendothelioma From Histologic Mimics. Am J Surg Pathol 2016; 40:94–102.

Chapter 6

Molecular biology of gliomas

Peter P Molnar

INTRODUCTION

Five thousand years have elapsed since the first documentation of cancer [1]. Still, we have not found a comprehensive explanation for the basic questions: What makes cancer cells grow uncontrollably and, in about half of the cases, kill their host? Beginning with Virchow's concept of cellular pathology [2], the search for answers has focussed on morphological aberrations of neoplastic cells. Abnormal nuclear morphology (hyperchromasia, chromatin clumping, or clearing) of neoplastic cells as well as cytoplasmic changes have been recognised for over a century. Regarding glial tumours, Bailey's and Cushing's seminal work characterised the microscopic features of glial tumour cells but also attempted to find similarities between these features and those of their putative precursor cells [3]. Their findings fundamentally influenced all research endeavours to understand cerebral neoplasia. It is now widely accepted that morphology per se is insufficient to explain brain tumour heterogeneity and biological potential.

Classifications using visual impressions and information dominated, but their inadequacies became unequivocal by the early years of the 21st century [4]. It is fascinating to dissect the "splitting" and "lumping" strives of traditional histopathological categories applied to diverse groups of tumours [5]. The underlying aim has always been finding proper names reflecting the clinical prognosis of various neoplastic entities.

The names suggested for glial tumours put together groups of similar tumours, but the behaviour of individual tumours may be different. Thus, oncologists often faced a daunting dilemma when trying to predict the outcome of an individual neoplasm. Interobserver differences, which result from subjectivity, represented a major hurdle [4]. Intratumoural cytological and histological heterogeneity severely heightened these difficulties. Let alone confusing names, the clinical dependence on precise tumour grades complicated all these conundrums further. The problem was mostly rooted in the lack of understanding of the crucial steps of tumorigenesis. The launch of international collaborative studies partially clarified the notion that the clinical/biological behaviour of brain tumours varies considerably according to the age of the patient, histological type and location of the tumours, and their grade.

Peter P Molnar MD PhD DSc, Professor Emeritus of Pathology and Neuropathology, University of Debrecen, Clinical Centre, Department of Pathology, Debrecen, Hungary, Consultant Neuropathologist, Department of Pathology, BAZ County Hospital, Szentpeteri kapu, Hungary
Email: ppmolnar@gmail.com; molnarp@med.unideb.hu

THE EARLY ERA OF MOLECULAR ONCOLOGY

The introduction of immunohistochemistry (IHC) was a crucial step towards a scientific analysis of abnormal cellular growth [6]. This technique supplied insight into spatial protein distribution in neoplastic cells and their microenvironment. Since the early 1990s, IHC studies generated an immense amount of data that broadened the standard microscopic studies and began to shed light on cancer biology at molecular level. As an example, the detection of GFAP in tumour cells provided final proof of their glial origin. IHC markers like Ki-67 (also known as Mib-1, the monoclonal antibody most often used in IHC staining), became essential in various tumour grading schemes. Diagnostic, prognostic, and predictive markers were defined, resulting in radical changes in histopathology reports. The concurrent rapid evolution of sequencing technology furthermore confirmed the association between tumour histotypes and gene abnormalities, confirming that cancer is a disease of genes.

Changes in brain tumour diagnostics and classification perfectly mirror the conceptual evolution outlined above. Groundbreaking research in the early 1990s resulted in a revolutionary switch from the purely morphological interpretation of CNS tumours to attempts to understand the underlying molecular mechanisms. In the 1993 WHO classification [7] grading of tumours was nonetheless based solely on morphological criteria and remained somewhat subjective. Despite utilising ultrastructural features, terms such as spongioblasts, astroblasts, and medulloblastoma lingered. An important update was the heavy emphasis on IHC markers. The classification included characteristic genetic alterations (e.g. *TP53* mutations, *EGFR* amplification, and chromosomal abnormalities), which were crucial for the understanding of astrocytic tumorigenesis and progression. However, these data were insufficiently comprehensive to override morphological characteristics as determinants for tumour classification.

A refined and broadening list of molecular and genetic events kept popping up and became ever more critical in the following classifications of CNS neoplasia. In the 2000 WHO classification of CNS tumours [8] IARC introduced a new approach to tumour classification including genetic classification criteria. This approach was explicit in the 2001 WHO volume on haemopoietic neoplasia, which demonstrated for leukaemias and lymphomas that cytogenetic and molecular genetic characteristics offered reliable criteria for classification [9]. This concept was applied subsequently in further analyses of the biology of brain tumours. Genetic alterations operative in the evolution of glioblastoma (GB) were often the focus of research. Early on, *TP53* mutations, amplification, mutation of *EGFR*, loss of p16 expression, overexpression/amplification of *CDK*s, or loss of *Rb* function gained attention [10]. The notion of differentiating primary and secondary glioblastomas gained acceptance. These concepts were included in the 2007 edition of the WHO classification of CNS tumours [11], which clarified the relationship between various tumour types and numerous genetic alterations. IHC remained an essential tool in glioma classification [12].

In parallel, computational analysis of genomic data and understanding of cell signalling and stem-cell characteristics established that histologically similar tumours may behave differently due to unique (combinations of) genetic abnormalities, as elaborated in a crucial 2007 paper describing molecular aspects of astrocytic tumour development [13]. An integrative analysis of alterations in DNA copy number, gene expression, and DNA methylation in glioblastomas was published in 2008 [14].

Further study of the data established that these molecular/genetic changes occur in a defined order along the progression of low-grade tumours towards high-grade tumours. Mutations of the *TP53* gene appeared to be an early event that preceded loss or modification of *PTEN* and amplification of *EGFR* [10,15], the latter two events characterising higher-grade tumours. In oligodendrogliomas, allelic loss of 1p and 19q occurred in many WHO grade 2 tumours, whereas loss of 9p21 was confined mainly to WHO grade 3 tumours. A groundbreaking event was the finding of mutations of the isocitrate dehydrogenase genes (*IDH1* or *IDH2*) [16,17]. Importantly, codeletion of 1p19q was not observed in IDH wild-type tumours. The discovery of involvement of these molecular pathways in gliomagenesis suggested new approaches towards targeted therapy. However, this was not readily confirmed in clinical trials [18].

In 2016, an Updated 4th WHO classification of CNS tumours was published which was based upon a combination of specific molecular alterations and traditional histological methods [19]. It was called Updated 4th WHO Classification rather than 5th Edition in view of the profound impact of new molecular genetic data on tumour classification, which justified an official update before full revision of the classification. Integrating phenotypic and genotypic parameters improved tumour type designation and added greater objectivity to the diagnostic process. Since its introduction, classifying cerebral neoplasms has incorporated clinical, morphologic, immunophenotypic, and genetic information.

The updated edition presented the "*layered (integrated) diagnosis*" as a new format of histopathology reports, which proved helpful for clinicians in interpreting molecular pathological findings [20]. The consortium responsible for the classification aimed at defining "more biologically homogeneous and narrowly defined diagnostic entities." Morphological and molecular/genetic features became essential for defining gliomas with different phenotypes and grades, resulting in *IDH*-wildtype (IDHwt) and *IDH*-mutant (IDHmut) glioblastoma, *H3 K27M*-mutant diffuse midline glioma, *RELA* fusion-positive ependymoma, *WNT*-activated and *SHH*-activated medulloblastoma, *C19MC*-altered embryonal tumour with multilayered rosettes. Oligodendrogliomas were defined as IDH-1-mutant, ATRX-wildtype, 1p19q co-deleted tumours, while astrocytomas comprised IDH-mutant, ATRX-mutant, 1p/19q-intact neoplasms. Thus, the somewhat subjective and controversial "oligoastrocytoma" diagnosis was omitted.

An essential sequel of these definitions was that the molecular fingerprint could overrule the morphological phenotype. As an example, a tumour resembling an oligodendroglioma by light microscopy but with *IDH, ATRX* and *TP53* mutations and *intact* 1p and 19q had to be reported as *IDH-1* mutant, 1p19q intact astrocytoma. Application of these criteria to gliomas with a more circumscribed growth pattern and *BRAF* or *TSC1/TSC2* mutations, but lacking *IDH* gene family alterations (pilocytic astrocytoma, pleomorphic xanthoastrocytoma, subependymal giant cell astrocytoma), allowed the pathologist to separate these tumours from diffuse astrocytomas. This approach resembled the naming conventions for haematopoietic/lymphoid neoplasms. The proposal suggested that the histopathological name comes first, followed by the list of genetic characteristics as adjectives, as for example in diffuse midline glioma, *H3K27M*–mutant.

According to the revised 4th edition of the WHO classification [19], a lesion might be diagnosed as *IDH*-wildtype when IHC for mutant R132H IDH1 protein was negative and *IDH1* codon 132 and *IDH2* codon 172 gene were wildtype. This scenario was considered identical to wildtype *IDH1* codon 132 and *IDH2* codon 172 gene only. The WHO experts recognised that diagnostic categories requiring genotyping might create testing and reporting challenges, due to variable availability of a full array of genotyping or surrogate assays in different countries while nonetheless a diagnosis must still be formulated in each case. As a solution, it was proposed to add the designation NOS (i.e. not otherwise specified) to a morphological diagnosis when molecular diagnostic testing could not be performed [21].

CURRENT VIEWS ON THE MOLECULAR BIOLOGY OF GLIOMAS

Propelled by advances in DNA and RNA sequencing, DNA fluorescence in situ hybridisation, RNA expression profiling, and broadening "*omics*" analysis, detailed molecular characterisation of various brain tumour types continued after the publication of WHO 2016. A consortium to Inform Molecular and Practical Approaches to CNS Tumour Taxonomy" (cIMPACT-NOW) published seven consecutive updates leading to the 5th Edition of the WHO classification of CNS tumours published in 2021 [22–24]. The substantial changes are rooted in advanced molecular diagnostics based on histological findings supported by ancillary tissue-based tests. Methylome profiling has shown unprecedented efficacy in characterising some tumours with unusual morphological features and seems to prevail as the recommended tool to identify some rare tumour types and subtypes.

The data gathered to that point showed unquestionably that the subcellular events which drive tumorigenesis and progression encompass a host of mechanisms, including chromosomal abnormalities (translocations, deletions, and complex rearrangements), loss-of-function/gain-of-function mutations, gene amplifications, gene fusions, gene rearrangements, and small duplications of genes, and gene overexpression. These findings had significant impact on the discussions that led to the 5th Edition of the WHO classification of CNS tumours [24]. It was felt that identifying the chain of molecular steps in the development of any particular tumour type could facilitate finding therapeutically targetable alterations for these neoplasms. Therefore, critical emphasis was on separating tumour types by detailed description of the involved molecular pathway. In WHO CNS-5, tumour "types" and "subtypes" were replaced by the terms "entities" and "variants." The segregation of *paediatric* from *adult* tumour types was based on the substantially different pathways responsible for their development and progression. The new classification also adapted the "Not Elsewhere Classified (NEC)" designation, to be used in the layered diagnosis when the results of the relevant molecular analyses failed to categorise the tumour in one of the recognised categories.

In newly recognised tumour names, molecular mechanisms were frequently incorporated; examples are diffuse astrocytoma, MYB- or MYBL1-altered, CNS tumour with *BCOR* internal tandem duplication, and diffuse hemispheric glioma, *H3* G34-mutant. Other names such as atypical teratoid/rhabdoid tumour (AT/RT) did not include molecular terms, but the entities they referred to required a molecular characteristic to allow for final diagnosis. "Essential" (= must have) and "desirable" (= nice to have) diagnostic criteria were formulated for each tumour type, and both requirements often relied on molecular/genetic features, many of which required DNA-methylation analysis. The use of an integrated diagnosis was introduced as an absolute requirement, optimally combining a specific histological term with a specific molecular genetic mechanism.

Conceptual changes in the grading schemes are also based on molecular data. A major revision in the approach to grading was the shift to *within-tumour-type grading* rather than grading across different tumour types. Earlier, tumours with radically different histogenesis (i.e. astrocytoma and meningioma) but with the same histological grade were assumed to have similar biological behaviour. In reality, tumours with the same grade could have very different outcome. The explanation was found in underlying differences in molecular profile. Two astrocytomas, both showing relatively bland histology, may show very different behaviour. One, an *IDH*-mutant astrocytoma, will indeed have a favourable outcome while the other, *IDH* wildtype astrocytoma with a *CDKN2A/B* homozygous deletion, *TERT* promoter mutation, *EGFR* amplification, and/or +7/−10 copy number changes will show clinical outcome typical of a grade 4 astrocytoma (i.e. glioblastoma). This clinically useless and biologically false concept was avoided by *grading within tumour type,* which brought cerebral tumour grading in conformity with WHO grading of non-CNS tumour types. Another essential modification (which had already been included in the updated 4th edition) was that a (molecular) grade 4 (Arabic numerals now replaced Roman numerals for grading) might be assigned to a neoplasm that would histologically qualify as a lower-grade tumour.

Traditionally, CNS-tumour grading intended to predict clinical behaviour of neoplasms before treatment. However, the presently available therapeutic interventions drastically changed the outcome of some otherwise highly malignant entities, e.g. *WNT-activated medulloblastomas.* Patients who suffer from such a tumour may live much longer, which might justify assigning a lower grade. However, changing a grade based upon the response to treatment might result in erroneous clinical judgement and therefore the traditional (pre-treatment) grading approach was retained.

Radiological imaging studies have continued to provide valuable information, but this was considered to be beyond the scope of this chapter. Recent reviews are available for imaging details [25,26].

MOLECULAR FEATURES OF CANCER IN GENERAL

It would be pointless to separate molecular aspects of glial neoplasia from the mechanisms governing cancer growth and development, as lucidly elaborated by Weinberg and Hanahan in their "Hallmarks of cancer" concept in 2000 [27] and expanded in 2011 with the introduction of "*enabling features*" [28]. A recent publication by Hanahan [29] summarises our present understanding of these components, as shown in **Figure 6.1**. Recent publications confirm that the hallmarks, including the *enabling features*, also apply to glial tumours [30–42]. The following paragraphs will detail how these "hallmarks" apply to neuro-oncology.

Particular attention will be paid to isocitrate dehydrogenase (*IDH*) gene mutations, as these occur in several brain tumour types. *IDH* mutations have gained particular significance in understanding molecular brain tumour biology, and this will be discussed under the hallmark headings.

Sustaining proliferative signalling

Cancer cells have the capacity to grow autonomously due to disturbances in cell cycle regulation, with active support from their microenvironment. In glial tumours, various and frequent alterations of the *PI3K–AKT–mTOR* and *RAS-RAF-MAPK* molecular pathways,

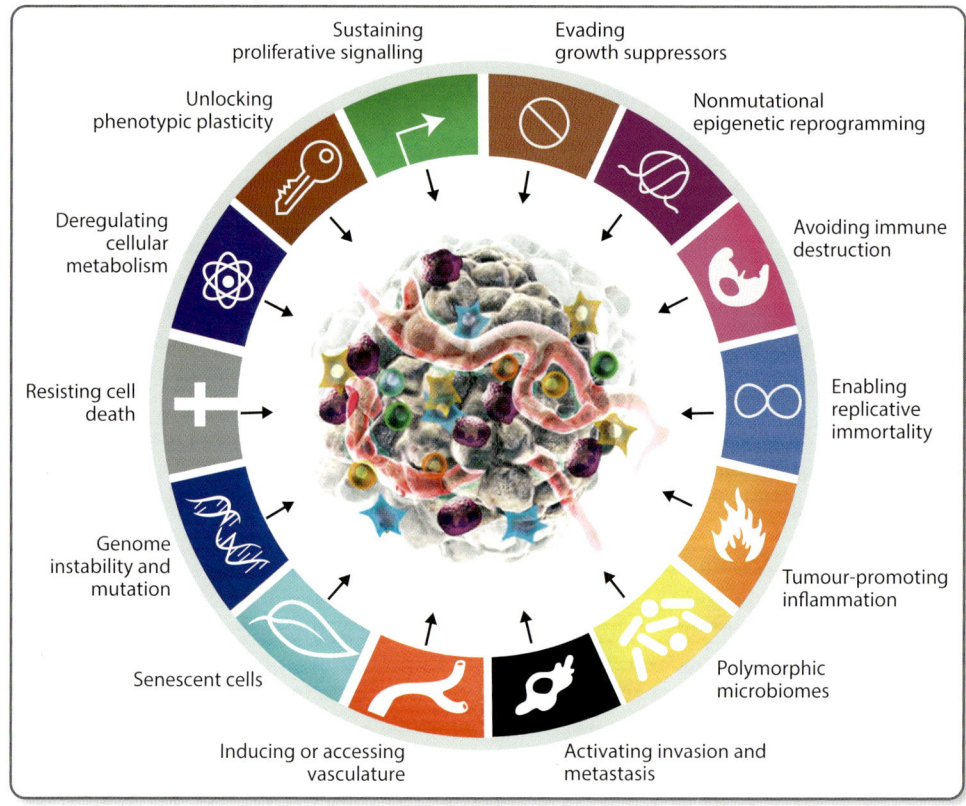

Figure 6.1 The canonical and prospective new additions to the 'Hallmarks of Cancer'.

Source: Reprinted with permissiom from the American Association of Cancer Research.

which regulate the cell cycle, exemplify this hallmark's manifestation. Oncogenes provide self-sufficiency in growth signals, and co-expression of *PDGF* and *PDGFR* represent this scenario in glioblastoma. *IDH* is essential for cellular homeostasis and energy provision and its mutations occur in a majority of high-grade gliomas.

Evading growth suppressors

In transformed cells, the standard control of cell cycling is disrupted, and this can result in growth-stimulating molecules. In various gliomas, *CDK4* amplification is regularly observed, loss of *RB1*, activation of *TP53* via deletion of *CDKN2A* gene and deficiency of the CDK4 suppressor p16^{INK4a} are frequent, and all these alterations result in functional inactivation of *Rb*. Schwannomas and meningiomas often arise due to mutations affecting the tumour suppressor *NF1* or *NF2* genes, resulting in sporadic and familial tumours. Mutated *PTCH*, an inhibitor of Hedgehog signalling, is involved in medulloblastomas.

Non-mutational epigenetic re-programming

Epigenetic signatures maintain cell-specific transcriptional profiles, and many gene-regulation networks control them. The genome-wide erasure and re-establishment of epigenetic marks, including methylation status, is a well-established process during tumorigenesis and progression. Regulation of the higher-order organisation of DNA (e.g. looping of enhancer elements onto gene promoters) is often aberrant in brain tumours. Histone *H3* variants have paramount significance in paediatric gliomas and other cerebral neoplasms. Epigenetic factors crucially affect the glial tumour cell lineage or differentiation state. In addition, epigenetic elements determine whether Notch receptors behave as tumour suppressors or function as oncogenes. *IDH* mutations play a significant role as they inhibit various components of the epigenetic machinery, including histone- and DNA-demethylases.

Avoiding immune destruction

Cancer cells may activate various mechanisms that neutralise dominantly cell-mediated defence mechanisms of the host. Selective outgrowth of antigen-negative variants may occur, and tumour cells may reduce the expression of histocompatibility antigens or induce immunosuppression by secreting transforming growth factor-beta (TGF-β) or programmed death ligand 1 (PD-L1) ligands. The GB microenvironment is rich in immunomodulatory factors, including TGF-β, interleukin-10 (IL-10) and prostaglandin E-2 (PGE2). In GB patients, systemic immunosuppression affects primary and secondary lymphoid organs, and *IDH* mutations are critical players in this process, although the responsible mechanisms are largely unknown.

Enabling replicative immortality

In malignant cells, hotspot mutations in the promoter region of the *TERT* (transcriptase) gene reactivate the telomerase complex, enabling cellular immortalisation through infinite maintenance of telomere length. These mutations occur in over 80% of *IDH*wt glioblastomas.

Tumour-promoting inflammation

Various inflammatory cells produce factors that enhance growth, survival, angiogenesis and reactive oxygen species that can cause additional mutations in cancer cells. Gliomas with unmutated (wild-type) *IDH* prompt more robust immune responses, increasing tumour aggressiveness and reducing survival. CD4+/CD8+ T cells and T regulatory cells (Tregs) express high levels of CTLA-4 and PD-1 and accumulate in glial tumours. High levels of CTLA-4, PD-1 and PD-L1 in glioma cells correlate with WHO high grade and short survival. The number of infiltrating immunosuppressive myeloid cells, immunosuppressive macrophages, exhausted T cells, and Tregs creates a tumour-supportive tumour micro-environment (TME, inflammatory micro-milieu). *IDH* mutations effectively regulate the nature of the inflammatory microenvironment.

Polymorphic microbiomes

Recent studies have shown that tumour-related microbiomes are associated with a variety of cancer types, and this has now also been reported in gliomas. It is quite surprising that bacterial DNA is detectable in glioblastomas without direct connection with the external environment. It is relatively easy to understand how colonic bacteria interact with the organism, alter host cell characteristics, and participate in carcinogenesis. Metabolic products of bacteria may alter the tumour microenvironment and thus influence tumorigenesis.

Activating invasion and metastasis

Cells of a neoplasm may destroy host tissue and colonise distant sites via modified interactions with components of their microenvironment. Although glioma metastases are extremely rare, most glial tumours tend to invade pre-existing parenchyma of the CNS early and extensively, rendering them incurable by surgery. *IDH* mutations enhance GB cell mobility (invasiveness) via modulating the PI3K/AKT/mTOR pathway.

Inducing or accessing vasculature

Tumour cells acquire the ability to enhance neovascularisation and thus fulfil the increased oxygen and nutrient needs for expansion. The recurrent activation of the *MAPK–RAS–PI3K* pathway shows the relevance of this hallmark in brain tumours; its activation is often due to binding of vascular endothelial growth factor (VEGF) to vascular endothelial growth factor receptor (VEGFR), resulting in active new vessel formation. Another angiogenesis promoter is angiopoietin 2. The latter destabilises tumour vessels and thus promotes angiogenesis. Notch receptors are overexpressed in gliomas, and the Notch pathway promotes angiogenesis. Neo-angiogenesis in the form of microvascular proliferation (MVP) is a diagnostic and grade-determining event in GB. These blood vessels develop under unique gene expression profiles. Such vascular abnormalities are associated with high expression of angiogenic factors, including VEGF, TGF-β2, and pleiotrophin (PTN).

Senescent cells

The biology of neoplastic growth is fundamentally influenced by interactions between tumour cells and the unique micromilieu they induce *in loco*. Senescent cells are significant players in these interactions. The latter are typically in mitotic arrest and have altered transcriptional, metabolic, and secretory phenotypes. The growth of glioma stem cells (GSCs) contributes to glioma malignancy, and senescent cells often acquire stem cell characteristics. Animal experiments and patient studies confirmed the detrimental function of persistent senescent cells in glial tumours.

Genome instability and mutation

The p53 protein (encoded by the *TP53* gene) is a cellular gatekeeper for growth and division, and its dysfunction is crucial in gliomagenesis. *TP53* mutations were among the early genetic abnormalities discovered in glioma genesis. Abnormal p53 proteins allow unchecked growth, provide glioma cells with a growth advantage, and lead to genomic instability secondary to a lack of proper DNA repair checkpoints. *ATRX* deficiency plays a role in genomic instability in several glial tumours. DNA replication errors are common in various cancers and usually are repaired by the mismatch repair complex. If this function is lost, microsatellite instability often creates mutated alleles. *IDH* mutations are critical players in genomic instability.

Resisting cell death

Neoplastic cells overwrite signals that otherwise would force them to disintegrate via apoptosis, pyroptosis, or other molecular mechanisms of cell death. Loss of *PTEN* as primary regulator, which is common in diffuse gliomas, along with activated *RTK* signalling, results in increased activity of the *PI3K/AKT1* pathway, leading to inhibition of apoptosis and increased survival.

Deregulating cellular metabolism

Utilising the "Warburg effect," defined as an increase in the rate of glucose uptake and preferential production of lactate, energy and essential components of proteins, DNA, and lipids are provided for the continuous proliferation of cancerous cells. Glycolysis is part of glioma energy production. GSCs can switch metabolism between glycolysis and oxidative phosphorylation, proving that the metabolism of glioma cells varies according to the cell's microenvironment. However, only <50% of acetyl-CoA production originates from glucose metabolism. Meanwhile, fatty-acid oxidation enzymes are conspicuously active within glioma tissues. Wild-type and mutated *IDH* are pivotal in metabolic reprogramming in glial tumours.

Unlocking phenotypic plasticity

Cellular plasticity involves the repression of genes associated with a given cell type along with activation of genes that determine the characteristics of another cell type. Unlocking phenotypic plasticity therefore changes cellular identity through dedifferentiation or transdifferentiation. In gliomas, mutant *IDH* or cell-permeable 2HG has been associated with repression of expression of lineage-specific differentiation genes which blocks differentiation. To elucidate the still largely unknown mechanisms involved, GSCs and cell lineages in various glioma subtypes should be characterised.

D-2-HYDROXYGLUTARATE IS AN ONCOMETABOLITE PLAYING A CRUCIAL EARLY STEP IN GLIOMA GENESIS

Dissection of these uniformly shared features that initiate/drive tumorigenesis and progression provides detailed insight. At the same time, in-depth analysis of the individual hallmarks instinctively propels integrative, holistic endeavours since cancer hallmarks form a highly intertwined network. In the following paragraphs, we will discuss how one particular molecule fulfils a role in several hallmarks.

A crucial step in understanding the molecular basis of glial tumours was the observation that in a high percentage of glial tumours the genes encoding the isocitrate dehydrogenase enzymes, *IDH1* and *IDH2*, are mutated [16]. The literature on *IDH* mutations has proliferated "faster than the most aggressive type of glioblastoma". Hence, the reader is referred to two excellent recent reviews and isolated references for each statement will not be used [43–45].

Isocitrate dehydrogenase enzymes are present in various cancers at various levels. *IDH1* is downregulated in early skin cancer, upregulated in non-small cell lung carcinoma (NSCLC), and in 65% of GBM cases [42]. *IDH1* mutations primarily involving the hotspot arginine at codon R132 were first recognised. Eventually, *IDH1* mutations were also reported in other codons (R132H, R132S, R132C, and R132G) and R172 for *IDH2*. The IDH1 protein is cytoplasmic or localises in peroxisomes and the endoplasmic reticulum. The enzyme catalyses oxidative decarboxylation of isocitrate to alpha-ketoglutarate (α-KG). Alpha-KG-dependent dioxygenases (α-KGDDs) comprise a heterogeneous group of enzymes responsible for DNA/histone demethylation, ubiquitination, and hydroxylation (**see Figure 6.2**). These proteins also regulate epigenetic changes, control protein stability, and significantly affect signalling pathways like HIF-1. α-KG regulates cell migration by modulating the *PI3K/AKT/mTOR* axis. A high concentration of 2-HG also promotes

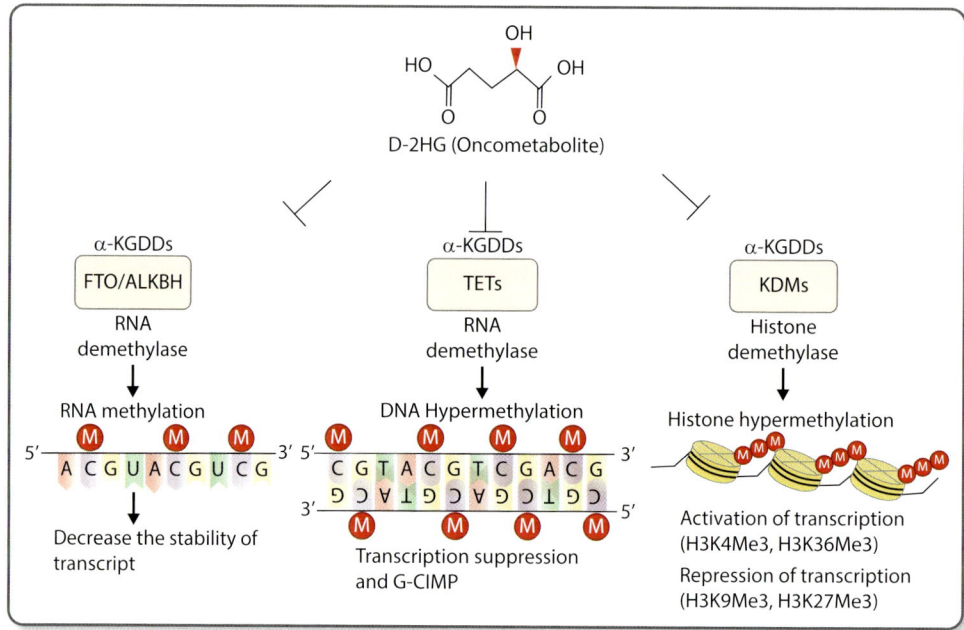

Figure 6.2 Epigenetic alterations of D-2HG. D-2HG alters the methylation status of DNA, RNA, and histone to regulate gene expression, and RNA stability via inhibition of various types of α-KDGG. D-2HG, D-2hydroxyglutarate.

α-KDGG, alpha ketoglutarate dependent dioxygenase.

Source: Redrawn with permission Chou FJ, et al. (2021) [44]

angiogenesis via inhibiting prolyl-hydroxylases and stabilisation of the hypoxia-inducible factor-1 alpha (HIF-1α). HIF-1α is a heterodimeric transcription factor that controls genes promoting cell adaptation to hypoxia via enhancing transcription, e.g. VEGF [46].

The mutant IDH1 enzyme reduces α-KG to D2-hydroxyglutarate (D2-HG). The reaction is NADPH dependent, resulting in decreased NADPH and α-KG levels, while substantially increasing D2-HG concentration. These alterations are associated with metabolome imbalance, the regulation of the tumour-associated immune system in gliomas, and epigenome modifications such as histone hypermethylation, which leads to aberrant expression of oncogenes and tumour suppressor genes.

It is noteworthy that two other compounds that accumulate from distorted biochemical pathways (i.e. the Krebs' cycle), *succinate* and *fumarate*, also are structural mimetics of α-KG and are pivotal in the initiation and progression of malignant tumours via inducing hypermethylation phenotypes with metabolic reprogramming, and alterations of redox homeostasis [47,48].

In a host of glial tumours, these oncometabolites are closely related to activating oncogenic mechanisms that transpire through the cancer hallmarks. In particular, D-2HG seems to play the first fiddle in glioma genesis. This realisation gained significance in updating the WHO classification in 2016 [19]. Astrocytomas develop under the influence of *IDH* driver mutations, unlike pilocytic tumours and pleomorphic xanthoastrocytoma (PXA) in which *BRAF* alterations are crucial. Similarly, subependymal giant cell astrocytoma (SEGA) arises under the influence of the *TSC1/TSC2* mutations. These observations

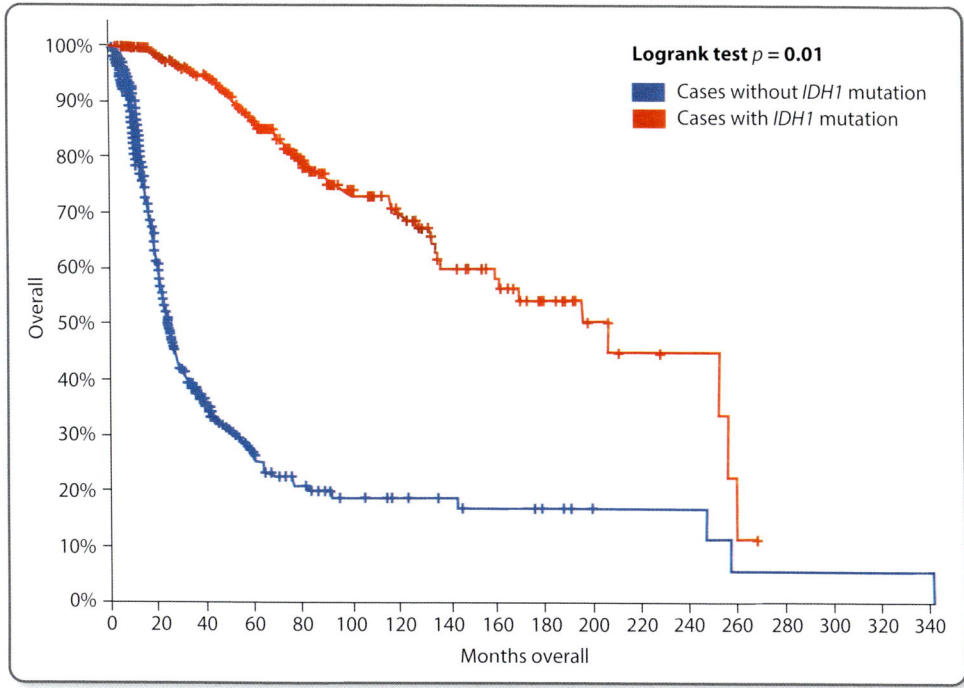

Figure 6.3 Effect of isocitrate dehydrogenase (IDH) mutations on survival. Overall survival curve. The total number of patients included in the overall survival analysis = 921. Number of cases with IDH1 mutation = 312 (number of events = 64; median overall survival (months) = 207). Number of cases without IDH1 mutation = 609 [number of events = 280; median overall survival (months) = 25], $p = 0.01$.

Source: With permission from Murugan AK et al. (2022) [45].

redrew the family tree of astrocytic neoplasms. Patients with a glioma with *IDH* mutations show prolonged survival (**Figure 6.3**), so *IDH* mutation is not only a diagnostic but also a prognostic (and eventually predictive) marker [44].

It seems counterintuitive for an aberrant gene to confer beneficial properties. Detailed analysis of the glioma microenvironment later provided answers to this perplexing observation. Characterisation of immune cells from *IDH*wt and *IDH*mut gliomas showed a marked global depletion of immune (inflammatory) cells in *IDH*mut gliomas, including microglia, macrophages, dendritic cells, B cells, and T cells. Apparently, inhibition of the tumour-associated immune system in gliomas can also result in a survival benefit [34].

Gliomas can be divided into CpG island methylator phenotype (CIMP) and non-CIMP. The mutation of a single gene, *IDH1*, establishes G-CIMP (glioma CIMP) by remodelling the methylome with extensive epigenomic changes and distinct biology [49–51]. On the other hand, canonical mutations, including chromosome gains and losses (ch7+ / ch10–), characterise non-CIMP gliomas [52]. The oncometabolite D-2HG is the driver of the G-CIMP. In *IDH*mut tumours, typically in oligodendrogliomas, a high level of trimethylation of *H3*K9 and *H3*K27 has been observed, which represses gene expression [53]. This established G-CIMP-high and G-CIMP-low glioma types, providing grade and histology-independent glioma stratification [52].

The importance of *H3*K27 methylation status became striking when studies compared cell lineage, stem cell properties, and tumour inductive molecular pathway alterations in paediatric and adult gliomas [54]. Altered methylation of *H3*K27M suppresses expression of *EZH2*. This change leads to abnormal epigenetic repression that interferes with cell differentiation [55]. Diffuse intrinsic pontine gliomas (DIPG), common in children, are rapidly fatal, like GB in adults. However, the pathognomonic histological features of the latter (microvascular proliferation and necrosis) are not characteristic of DIPG [54]. The paediatric high-grade glioma group in the current classification comprises *H3*K27-altered gliomas, *H3* G34-mutant tumours, and *H3/IDH*-wild-type neoplasms. Paediatric diffuse low-grade gliomas are currently subclassified into distinct histomolecular entities including diffuse astrocytoma, MYB- or MYBL1-altered, and diffuse low-grade glioma, MAPK pathway-altered. This illustrates how (oncometabolite induced) methylation contributes to tumour heterogeneity. These examples highlight the importance of various forms of methylation in glioma genesis. The following chart displays examples of oncometabolic interference with methylation.

METHYLOME ANALYSIS COMPLETES GLIOMA CLASSIFICATION

Since the 1970s, DNA methylation is regarded as a "silencing" epigenetic mark. A decisive neuro-oncological example is methylation of the O^6-methylguanine-DNA-methyltransferase (*MGMT*) gene promoter. This suppresses expression of this DNA-repair enzyme, which enhances the efficacy of temozolomide (TMZ) chemotherapy [56]. Methylation changes may involve transcriptional start sites as well as gene bodies. Regulatory elements and repeat sequences may be affected. During the 2010s, a revolution in analytical, statistical, and computational methodology occurred. Genome-wide DNA methylation analysis of gliomas proved to be a promising tool early on [57] and with state-of-the-art bioinformatic approaches a methylome classifier was developed [58]. Currently, DNA methylation status contributes to understanding the 5th Edition of the WHO classification of CNS tumours. Methylome analysis also generates information about copy number variations (CNVs) and helps to pinpoint the cell of origin in various cancers.

A recent study has reported how the methylome classifier (known as the DKFZ/Heidelberg classifier) can be used in clinical practice [59]. **Figure 6.4** illustrates the effects of methylome analysis on glial tumour types, subtypes, and grades. The data show that the methylation pattern helps to confirm or refine histologically ambiguous diagnoses. Methylome characteristics occasionally provided diagnoses substantially different from the original histopathological opinion or single molecular test-based diagnosis. The classifier also suggested previously unrecognised tumour subtypes. Methylation profiling often significantly changed the earlier indicated treatment protocols for several glioma types. Methylation classification does have its limitations. The data might need advanced bioinformatics analysis, and the result might need to be complemented by targeted DNA sequencing, or IHC. methodological issues are DNA purity and the presence of inflammatory cells, which may affect the reliability of the classifier score. A detailed analysis of methylome-based CNS tumour classification has been published [60]. This tool may be beneficial in case of contradictory opinions or when a tumour displays unusual morphological or IHC characteristics. The methylation classifier may change, confirm, or refine the diagnosis with upgrading, downgrading, or grade assignment.

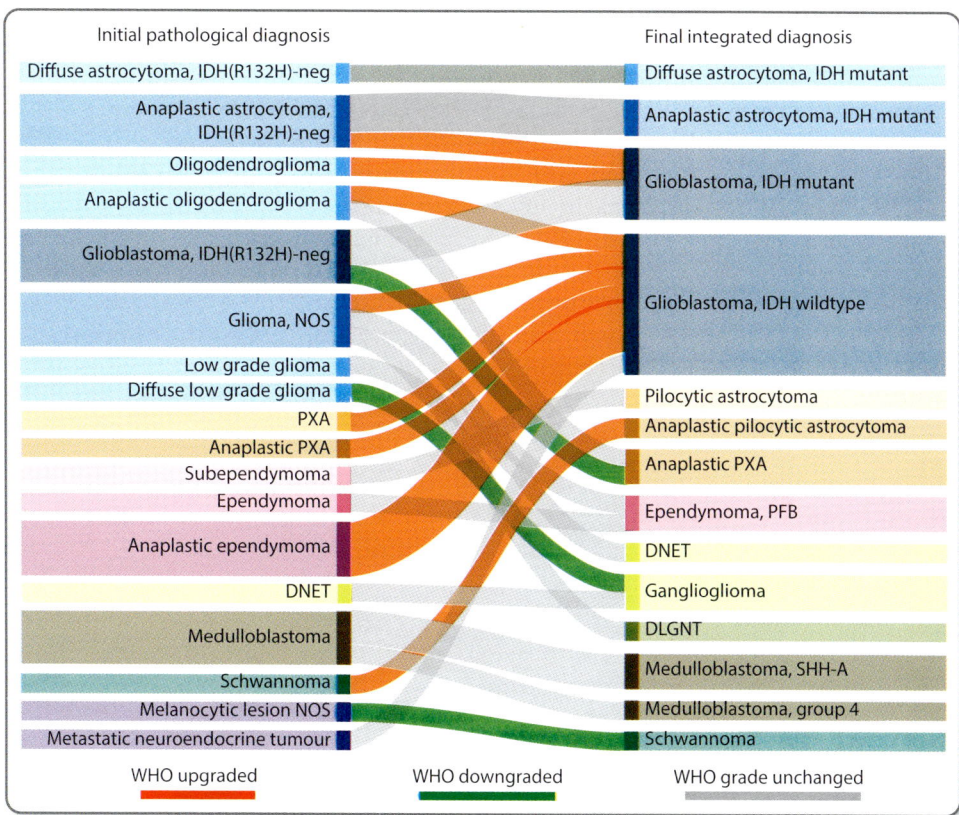

Figure 6.4 Establishing new diagnoses based on methylation profiling of CNS tumours. Methylation profiling led to a change from initial histopathological diagnosis (left) to the final integrated diagnosis (right) or the identification of a new clinically relevant molecular subtype in 29 cases. This subset includes patients with a newly identified diagnosis, a resolved differential diagnosis different from the top initial diagnosis, or a new clinically relevant molecular subtype. WHO grading changes are shown in red (upgrading) and green (downgrading).

DLGNT, diffuse leptomeningeal glioneuronal tumour; DNET, dysembryoplastic neuroepithelial tumour; IDH, isocitrate dehydrogenase; NOS, not otherwise specified; PXA, pleomorphic xanthoastrocytoma

Source: Redrawn with permission Karimi S et al. (2019) [59]

In the context of the 5th Edition of the WHO classification, the perception is that "optimal methodological approaches have yet to be determined" [24]. Like other more advanced and costly methods [DNA and RNA sequencing, DNA FISH, RNA expression profiling, omics analysis, and others], whole genome methylation analysis is not globally available. This will result in frequent use of the NOS designation.

PRESENT STATUS OF GLIOMA CLASSIFICATION

The updated 4th Edition of the WHO classification introduced the NOS designation, and the 5th Edition introduced NEC as a further diagnostic designation. NOS following a pathological diagnosis informs the clinician that the necessary molecular information is not available or that assignment of a specific WHO diagnosis is not possible due to technical reasons. The NEC designation indicates that although all required testing has been completed, the results are incongruent with any specific WHO entity's essential diagnostic criteria. Further studies will contribute to elucidation of NEC designated cases. Global introduction and acceptance of molecular diagnostic methods will support global use of the classification.

The 5th Edition of the WHO classification profoundly rearranged major categories, types, and subtypes of glioneuronal tumours and gliomas, often introducing new names and changing grades as illustrated in **Figure 6.5** [24]. The classification states that the exact cell lineage remains elusive in most CNS tumours. However, significant strides have been made in this respect in glioblastoma research. **Figure 6.6** displays the four molecular glioblastoma types and helps to understand phenotypic plasticity in the most malignant

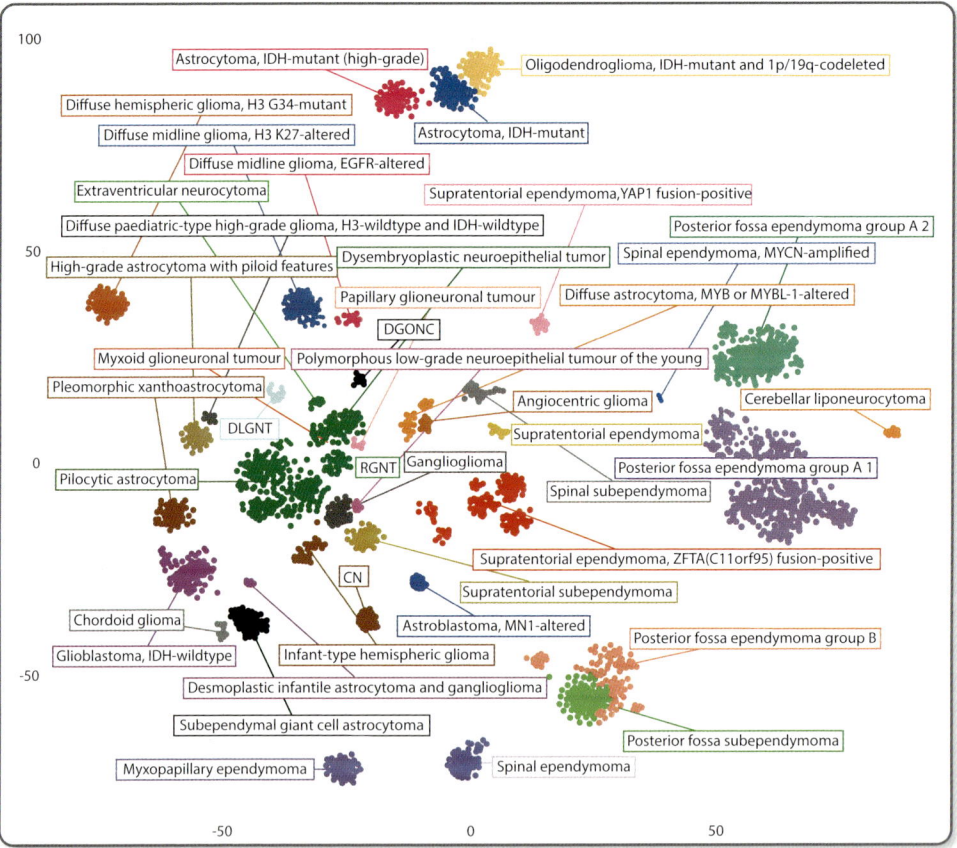

Figure 6.5 Unsupervised, non-linear t-distributed stochastic neighbour embedding (t-SNE) projection of methylation array profiles from 2,632 tumours. Samples were selected from an extensive database of >50,000 brain tumour datasets to serve as reference profiles for training a supervised classification model based on strict criteria: all these samples showed a high calibrated classification score (>0.9) when applying the brain tumour classifier available at https://www.molecularneuropathology.org.

CN, central neurocytoma; DLGNT, diffuse leptomeningeal glioneuronal tumor; DGONC, diffuse glioneuronal tumour with oligodendroglioma-like features and nuclear clusters; RGNT, rosette-forming glioneuronal tumour.

Source: With permission from Martin Sill, Stefan Pfister, Andreas von Deimling. With the kind permission of IARC/WHO.

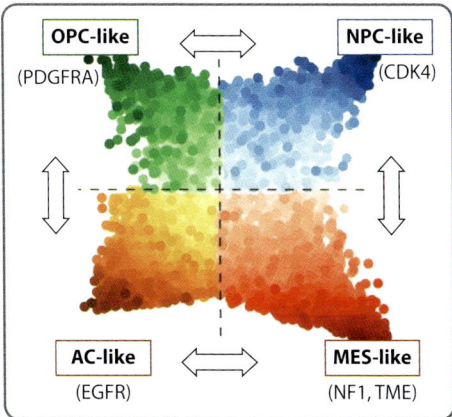

Figure 6.6 There are four subtypes of GB. Combining scRNA-seq and sophisticated computational analysis helped to understand transcriptional and genetic heterogeneity in human and experimental GB. The original work resulted from broad international collaboration and described four dominant glioblastoma cellular states. These states epitomise definitive neural cell types. The evolution of this cellular heterogeneity results from selective copy number amplifications of different genes (*CDK4, EGFR,* and *PDGFRA*) and NF1 mutations. Significant effects of the microenvironment favour defined cellular states. All cell types exhibit marked plasticity. This feature represents a considerable hurdle in identifying the cell of origin in gliomas.

EGFR, epidermal growth factor receptor; GB, glioblastoma; MES, mesenchymal; NF, nuclear factor; NPC, neural precursor; OPC, oligodendrocyte-progenitor; PDGFRA, platelet-derived growth factor receptor alpha; TME, tumour microenvironment.

glioma [24]. As the figure indicates, while there is a clear separation between these GB types, a possible transition between the four groups is also highly likely. It is worth noting that subtype differentiation is impossible with traditional histopathological means, although they may have distinct clinical implications.

Combining scRNA-seq and sophisticated computational analysis helped to understand transcriptional and genetic heterogeneity in human and experimental GB. The original work resulted from broad international collaboration and described four dominant glioblastoma cellular states [61,62], which epitomise definitive neural cell types. The evolution of this cellular heterogeneity results from selective copy number amplifications of different genes (*CDK4, EGFR, PDGFRA*) and *NF1* mutations. Significant effects of the microenvironment favour defined cellular states. All cell types exhibit marked plasticity. This feature represents a considerable hurdle in identifying the cell of origin in gliomas. It is also of note that malignant cells differ between patients to a greater extent than non-malignant cells [61]. These observations directly affect our efforts to develop patient-specific treatments.

CONCLUSION

Hanahan and Weinberg suggested a heuristic approach to unify and simplify the principles responsible for the complexity of cancer phenotypes and genotypes [27–29]. It is possible to address gliomagenesis while adhering to their suggestions. The 5th Edition of the WHO classification details our current concept of glioma classification [24]. It is evident that with the advent of molecular analyses including that of the methylome, the earlier dominance of "lumping" efforts is converting to a novel "splitting" attitude. Newly recognised tumour types abound, and predictably, the tendency will continue to flourish. One recent example is the new paediatric tumour group "*glioneuronal tumour kinase-fused' (GNT-KinF-A)*" that resulted from epigenetic-molecular dissection [63]. Unfortunately, a parallel advancement in treatment regimens startlingly lags, and malignant gliomata remain incurable. A critical balance between splitting and lumping seems highly desirable because only this can elucidate targetable molecular mechanisms. Glioma precision medicine is – and will be – dependent on including artificial intelligence (AI) in ever-broadening "omics" explorations.

Note: The author is unaware of any affiliations, memberships, funding, or financial holdings that might be perceived as affecting the objectivity of this review.

Key points for clinical practice

- Molecular/genetic changes in gliomagenesis occur in a defined order along the progression of low-grade tumours towards high-grade tumours.
- Mutations of the *TP53* gene are an early event preceding loss or modification of PTEN and amplification of EGFR, the latter two events characterising higher-grade tumours.
- Grade 2 oligodendrogliomas are characterised by allelic loss of 1p and 19q.
- Grade 3 oligodendrogliomas contain loss of 9p21 and *PIK3CA* mutation.
- Mutations of the isocitrate dehydrogenase genes (*IDH1* or *IDH2*) are found as an early event in the vast majority of low-grade gliomas and secondary high-grade gliomas.
- In the layered/integrated classification approach the histopathological name comes first, followed by the list of genetic characteristics as adjectives, as, for example, in diffuse midline glioma, *H3* K27M–mutant.
- NOS designation is added to a diagnosis when histological or molecular diagnostic information to assign a more specific WHO diagnosis is not available.
- NEC designation is added to a diagnosis when required diagnostic testing has been successfully performed, but the results do not readily allow for a WHO 2021 diagnosis, due to a mismatch between clinical, histological, immunohistological and/or genetic features or the results supporting an emerging entity not yet included in the WHO classification.

ACKNOWLEDGEMENTS

The author is grateful to IACR Press, Lyon, France, for the permission to use Figures 2.01 and 2.28 from the *WHO Classification of Tumours Editorial Board. Central nervous system tumours. Lyon (France): International Agency for Research on Cancer; 2021. (WHO classification of tumours series, 5th ed.; vol. 6)*. https://publications.iarc.fr/601.

Grateful thanks are due to *Murugan Avaniyapuram Kannan* (Department of Molecular Oncology, King Faisal Specialist Hospital and Research Centre, Riyadh, Saudi Arabia) for the permission to use Figure 1, from his publication entitled "Isocitrate Dehydrogenase IDH1 and IDH2 Mutations in Human Cancer: Prognostic Implications for Gliomas". Br J BioMed Sci 2022; 79:10208. Creative Commons Attribution License (CC BY).

The author is deeply indebted to Kenneth D Aldape and Gelareh Zadeh for their permission to use Figure 1, from their paper entitled "The central nervous system tumour methylation classifier changes neuro-oncology practice for challenging brain tumour diagnoses and directly impacts patient care." Clin Epigenetics 2019; 11:185. doi: 10.1186/s13148-019-0766-2. This article is distributed under the terms of the Creative Commons Attribution 4.0 International License. (http://creativecommons.org/licenses/by/4.0/)

REFERENCES

1. Hajdu IS. A Note From History: Landmarks in History of Cancer, Part 1. Cancer 2011; 117:1097–1102.
2. Virchow R. Die Cellularpathologie in ihrer Begründung auf physiologische und pathologische Gewebelehre. Berlin: Verlag von August Hirschwald, 1859.
3. Bailey H, Cushing H. A Classification of the Tumors of the Glioma Group on a Histogenetic Basis, with a Correlated Study of Prognosis. Philadelphia: J B Lippincott Company, 1926.
4. Coons SW, Johnson PC, Scheithauer BW, et al. Improving diagnostic accuracy and interobserver concordance in the classification and grading of primary gliomas. Cancer 1997; 79:1381–1393.
5. Scheithauer BW. Development of the WHO Classification of Tumors of the Central Nervous System: A Historical Perspective. Brain Pathol 2009; 19:551–564.
6. Dabbs DJ. Diagnostic Immunohistochemistry: Theranostic and Genomic Applications, 5th ed. Philadelphia: Elsevier, 2019.
7. Kleihues P, Burger PC, Scheithauer BW. Histological Typing of Tumours of the Central Nervous System, 2nd ed. Springer-Verlag: Berlin, 1993.
8. Kleihues P, Cavenee WK. World Health Organization Classification of Tumours—Pathology and Genetics. Tumours of the Nervous System. IARC Press: Lyon, 2000.
9. Jaffe ES, Harris NL, Stein H, Vardiman JW (Eds). World Health Organization Classification of Tumours. Pathology and Genetics of Tumours of Haematopoietic and Lymphoid Tissues. IARC Press: Lyon, 2001.
10. Kleihues P, Ohgaki H. Phenotype vs Genotype in the Evolution of Astrocytic Brain Tumors. Toxicologic Pathol 2000; 28:164–170.
11. Louis DN, Ohgaki H, Wiestler OD, Cavenee WK. WHO Classification of Tumours of the Central Nervous System, 4th ed. IARC Press: Lyon, 2007.
12. Dunbar E, Yachnis AT. Glioma diagnosis: immunohistochemistry and beyond. Adv Anat Pathol 2010; 17:187–201.
13. Furnari FB, Fenton T, Bachoo RM, et al. Malignant astrocytic glioma: genetics, biology, and paths to treatment. Genes Dev 2007; 21:2683–2710.
14. Parsons DW, Jones S, Zhang X, et al. An integrated genomic analysis of human glioblastoma multiforme. Science 2008; 321:1807–1812.
15. Ohgaki H, Kleihues P. The Definition of Primary and Secondary Glioblastoma. Clin Cancer Res 2013; 19:764–772.
16. Yan H, Parsons DW, Jin G, et al. IDH1 and IDH2 Mutations in Gliomas. N Engl J Med 2009; 360:765–773.
17. Gravendeel LAM, Kouwenhoven MCM, Gevaert O, et al. Intrinsic Gene Expression Profiles of Gliomas Are a Better Predictor of Survival than Histology. Cancer Res 2009; 69:9065–9072.
18. Masui K, Cloughes TF, Misschel PS. Review: Molecular pathology in adult high-grade gliomas: from molecular diagnostics to target therapies. Neuropathol Appl Neurobiol 2012; 38:271–291.
19. Louis DN, Ohgaki H, Wiestler OD, Cavenee WK. WHO classification of tumours of the central nervous system, Revised 4th edition. IARC Press: Lyon, 2016.
20. Louis DN, Perry A, Burger P, et al. International Society of Neuropathology-Haarlem Consensus Guidelines for Nervous System Tumor Classification and Grading. Brain Pathol 2014; 24:429–435.
21. Louis DN, Perry A, Reifenberger G, et al. The 2016 World Health Organization classification of tumors of the central nervous system: a summary. Acta Neuropathol 2016; 131:803–820.
22. Louis DN, Aldape K, Brat DJ, et al. Announcing cIMPACT-NOW: the Consortium to Inform Molecular and Practical Approaches to CNS Tumor Taxonomy. Acta Neuropath 2017; 133:1–3.
23. Louis DN, Wesseling P, Paulus W, et al. cIMPACT-NOW update 1: Not Otherwise Specified (NOS) and Not Elsewhere Classified (NEC). Acta Neuropathol 2018; 135:481–484.
24. WHO Classification of Tumours Editorial Board. Central Nervous System Tumours. WHO Classification of Tumours, 5th Edition. IARC Press: Lyon, 2021.
25. Iv M, Bisdas S. Neuroimaging in the Era of the Evolving WHO Classification of Brain Tumors. Am J Roentgenol 2021; 217:3–15.
26. Kurokawa R, Kurokawa M, Baba A, et al. Major Changes in 2021 World Health Organization Classification of Central Nervous System Tumors. RadioGraphics 2022; 42:1–20.

27. Hanahan D Weinberg RD. The Hallmarks of Cancer. Cell 2000; 100:57–70.
28. Hanahan D, Weinberg RA. Hallmarks of cancer: the next generation. Cell 2011; 144:646–674.
29. Hanahan D. Hallmarks of cancer: New dimensions. Cancer Discovery 2022; 12:31–46.
30. Petterson SA, Sørensen MD, Burton M, et al. Differential expression of checkpoint markers in the normoxic and hypoxic microenvironment of glioblastomas. Brain Pathol 2023; 33(1):e13111.
31. Mancini A, Xavier-Magalhães A, Woods WS, et al. Disruption of the b1L Isoform of GABP Reverses Glioblastoma Replicative Immortality in a TERT Promoter Mutation-Dependent Manner. Cancer Cell 2018; 34:513–528.
32. Lu Ch, Ward PS, Kapoor GS, et al. IDH mutation impairs histone demethylation and results in a block to cell differentiation. Nature 2012; 483:474–478.
33. Qiu R, Zhong Y, Li Q, et al. Metabolic Remodeling in Glioma Immune Microenvironment: Intercellular Interactions Distinct From Peripheral Tumors. Front Cell Dev Biol 2021; 9:693215.
34. Himes BT, Geiger PhA, Ayasoufi K, et al. Immunosuppression in Glioblastoma: Current Understanding and Therapeutic Implications. Front Oncol 2021; 11:770561.
35. Alghamri MS, McClellan BL, Hartlage CS, et al. Targeting Neuroinflammation in Brain Cancer: Uncovering Mechanisms, Pharmacological Targets, and neuropharmaceutical Developments. Front Pharmacol 2021; 12:680021.
36. Kan LK, Drummond K, Hunn M, et al. Potential biomarkers and challenges in glioma diagnosis, therapy and prognosis. BMJ Neurology Open 2020; 2:e000069.
37. Yanovich-Arad G, Ofek P, Yeini E, et al. Proteogenomics of glioblastoma associates molecular patterns with survival. Cell Rep 2021; 34:108787.
38. Li S, Wang C, Chen J, et al. Signaling pathways in brain tumors and therapeutic interventions. Signal Transduct Targeted Ther 2023; 8:8.
39. Salam R, Saliou A, Bielle F, et al. Cellular senescence in malignant cells promotes tumor progression in mouse and patient Nat Commun 2023; 14:441.
40. Nejman D, Livyatan I, Fuks G, et al. The human tumor microbiome is composed of tumor type specific intracellular bacteria. Science 2020; 368:973–980.
41. Strickland M, Stoll EA. Metabolic Reprogramming in Glioma. Front Cell Dev Biol 2017; 5:43.
42. Shen X, Wu S, Zhang J, et al. Wild-type IDH1 affects cell migration by modulating the PI3K/AKT/mTOR pathway in primary glioblastoma cells. Molecular Med Reports 2020; 22:1949–1957.
43. Han S, Liu Y, Cai SJ, et al. Review article. IDH mutation in glioma: molecular mechanisms and potential therapeutic targets. Br J Cancer 2020; 122:1580–1589.
44. Chou FJ, Liu Y, Lang F, Yang Ch. D-2-Hydroxyglutarate in Glioma Biology. Cells 2021; 10:2345.
45. Murugan AK, Alzahrani AS. Isocitrate dehydrogenase IDH1 and IDH2 Mutations in Human Cancer: Prognostic Implications for Gliomas. Br J Biomed Sci 2022; 79:10208.
46. Liao Ch, Xijuan Liu X, Cheng Zhang Ch, Qing Zhang Q. Tumor hypoxia: From basic knowledge to therapeutic implications. Semin Cancer Biol 2023; 88:172–186.
47. Sulkowski PL, Oeck S, Dow J, et al. Oncometabolites suppress DNA repair by disrupting local chromatin signaling. Nature 2020; 582:586–591.
48. Liu Y, Yang Ch. Oncometabolites in Cancer: Current Understanding and Challenges. Cancer Res 2021; 81:2820–2823.
49. Turacan S, Rohle D, Goenka A, et al. IDH1 mutation is sufficient to establish the glioma hypermethylator phenotype. Nature 2012; 483:479–483.
50. Ammendola S, Caldonazzi N, Simbolo M, et al. H3K27me3 immunostaining is diagnostic and prognostic in diffuse gliomas with oligodendroglial or mixed oligoastrocytic morphology. Virchows Archiv 2021; 479:987–996.
51. Noushmehr H, Weisenberger DJ, Diefes K, et al. Identification of a CpG island methylator phenotype that defines a distinct subgroup of glioma. Cancer Cell 2010; 17:510–522.
52. Malta T, de Souza CF, Sabedot TS, et al. Glioma CpG island methylator phenotype (G-CIMP): biological and clinical implications. Neuro-Oncol 2018; 20:608–620.
53. Sturm D, Bender S, Jones DTW, et al. Paediatric and adult glioblastoma: multiform (epi)genomic culprits emerge. Nature Rev Cancer 2014; 14:92–107.
54. Buczkowicz P, Bartels U, Bouffet E, et al. Histopathological spectrum of paediatric diffuse intrinsic pontine glioma: diagnostic and therapeutic implications. Acta Neuropathologica 2014; 128:573–581.

55. Venneti S, Garimella MT, Sullivan LM, et al. Evaluation of histone 3 lysine 27 trimethylation (H3K27me3) and enhancer of Zest 2 (EZH2) in pediatric glial and glioneuronal tumors shows decreased H3K27me3 in H3F3A K27M mutant glioblastomas. Brain Pathol 2013; 23:558–564.
56. Hegi ME, Diserens AC, Gorlia Th, et al. MGMT Gene Silencing and Benefit from Temozolomide in Glioblastoma. N Engl J Med 2005; 352:997–1003.
57. Wiestler b, Capper D, Still M, et al. Integrated DNA methylation and copy-number profiling identify three clinically and biologically relevant groups of anaplastic gliomata. Acta Neuropathologica 2014; 128:561–571.
58. Capper D, Jones DTW, Sill M, et al. DNA methylation-based classification of central nervous system tumours. Nature 2018; 555:469–474.
59. Karimi S, Zuccato JA, Mamatjan Y, et al. The central nervous system tumor methylation classifier changes neuro-oncology practice for challenging brain tumor diagnoses and directly impacts patient care. Clin Epigenetics 2019; 11:185.
60. Wu Z, Abdullaev Z, Pratt D, et al. Impact of the methylation classifier and ancillary methods on CNS tumor diagnostics. Neuro-Oncol 2022; 24:571–581.
61. Verhaak RGW, Hoadley KA, Purdom E, et al. An integrated genomic analysis identifies clinically relevant subtypes of glioblastoma characterized by abnormalities in PDGFRA, IDH1, EGFR and NF1. Cancer Cell 2010; 17:98–110.
62. Puram SV, Tirosh I, Parikh AS, et al. Single-Cell Transcriptomic Analysis of Primary and Metastatic Tumor Ecosystems in Head and Neck Cancer. Cell 2017; 171:1611–1624.
63. He X, Liu X, Zuo F, et al. Artificial intelligence-based multi-omics analysis fuels cancer precision medicine. Semin Cancer Biol 2023; 88:187–200.

Chapter 7

Chromatin regulatory complexes-associated cancers: The emerging landscapes of switch/sucrose non-fermenting (complex)-deficient and NUTM1-rearranged malignancies

Abbas Agaimy

INTRODUCTION

Traditionally, neoplasms have been classified by their presumable line of differentiation. This can be achieved either morphologically (presence of cytological, architectural, or stromal characteristics or variable combinations thereof) or utilising available diagnostic immunohistochemistry (IHC) using antibodies recognising subtle differentiation features not readily identifiable by microscopy. These include intermediate filament proteins (to identify epithelial cells, smooth muscle cells, etc.) cell surface receptors (haematolymphoid malignancies), transcription factors (e.g. primitive rhabdomyoblastic differentiation) and others. Albeit technically complex and not widely available, electron microscopy represented another powerful historical tool used to identify morphological features of differentiation at the ultrastructural level (e.g. neuroendocrine granules, intermediate filaments, premelanosomes, and other tissue-specific organelles).

It is noteworthy that historical lumping of unclassified neoplasms in vaguely defined (e.g. fibroblastic, mesenchymal, epithelial etc.) categories gave the false impression that the fraction of histogenetically unclassified tumours is rather small. However, with the increasing use of more reliable next generation antibodies for IHC, and the gradually increasing use of new sequencing technologies, it became evident that the fraction of neoplasms not fitting in the traditional histogenetic categories is ever increasing, at the expense of phenotypically classifiable entities. These "histogenetically indeterminate" neoplasms encompass two major categories: (1) tumours with distinct phenotypes sharing same (convergent) genetic abnormality/driver genotype and (2) neoplasms with

Abbas Agaimy MD, Institute of Pathology, Friedrich-Alexander-University Erlangen-Nürnberg, University Hospital, Erlangen, Germany.
Email: abbas.agaimy@uk-erlangen.de (for correspondence)

overlapping immuno-phenotypes having divergent genetic landscape. This emerging notion as well as the increasingly recognised distinct biological behaviour of tumours sharing the same phenotype or genotype, including discrepant responsiveness to different therapeutic approaches, all underpin the need for an aetiology- and/or genome-based approach to classify such neoplasms of indeterminate histogenesis. For example, in the upper aerodigestive tract, the mere combination of basaloid morphology with epithelial immunophenotype and variable squamous cell marker expression is no longer considered sufficient evidence for a diagnosis of squamous cell carcinoma. This review highlights how emerging new knowledge stimulates the emergence of new approaches in the diagnosis and classification of neoplasms, using SWI/SNF-deficient and *NUTM1*-rearranged carcinomas as an example.

THE SWITCH/SUCROSE NON-FERMENTING COMPLEX

The switch/sucrose non-fermenting (SWI/SNF) complex is a subfamily of adenosine triphosphate (ATP)-dependent chromatin remodelling complexes, conserved from yeast to man. It represents a highly co-ordinated system composed of >20 biochemically distinct subunits, including among others the SMARC family (*SMARCA2, SMARCA4, SMARCB1, SMARCC1, SMARCC2, SMARCE1, SMARCD1, SMARCD2,* and *SMARCD3*), the ARID family (*ARID1A* and *ARID1B*) and *PBRM1*. The encoding genes are localised to different chromosomes but the contributing peptides function in a co-ordinated manner as a single complex. The various combinatorial assemblies are thought to support context-dependent activities of the complex [1–3]. The complex functions in an ATP-ase-dependent manner to regulate vital cellular processes via chromatin remodelling and hence closely influences the regulation of transcription [1–3]. The highly complex function of the SWI/SNF complex is facilitated via enrichment of its components at the sites of promoters and enhancers of active genes [1–3]. The ultimate consequences of this are regulatory effects on cell differentiation and cell proliferation.

The switch/sucrose non-fermentable complex and cancer

In early studies, SWI/SNF subunits were frequently found to be absent in cancer cell lines. Subsequent studies showed that genes encoding subunits of the complex, including *ARID1A, ARID2, SMARCB1, SMARCA4* and *PBRM1* are frequently mutated in human malignancies. Based on its fundamental role in regulating cell differentiation and hence tightly controlling cell renewal, loss or collapse of the SWI/SNF complex essentially results in lack of cell differentiation and enhanced self-renewal capabilities. This characteristic represents an almost universal feature of SWI/SNF deficiency and is reflected in the fact that the vast majority of SWI/SNF-deficient malignancies tend to display a non-descript undifferentiated looking cell phenotype with poor cell cohesion [4,5]. This common feature is responsible for significant diagnostic difficulties and under-recognition of several types of SWI/SNF-deficient malignancies across different organs. However, as is the rule with most gene abnormalities, exceptions do exist and a small subset of SWI/SNF-deficient neoplasms display a well-differentiated organotypical morphology [4,5] (**Table 7.1**).

Although the exact function of most individual SWI/SNF complex subunits is still largely obscure, it has been widely accepted that the complex functions collectively as a

Table 7.1 Comparison of the major clinicopathological features of de novo (primary) and secondary (dedifferentiated) switch/sucrose non-fermenting (SWI/SNF)-deficiency-associated neoplasms		
Features	**de novo SWI/SNF-deficient neoplasms**	**Secondary SWI/SNF-deficient neoplasms**
Age	Any but children>>>adults>>elderly	Adults and elderly
Sites of involvement	Any, mainly CNS, kidney, soft tissue, sinonasal	Any, mainly uterus, kidney, bladder, GI tract, lung
Differentiated component	Absent	Mostly present, may be absent*
Cell morphology	Monotonous	Frequently bizarre, sarcomatoid and heterogeneous populations
Bizarre smudge nuclei	Usually absent	Usually present
Rhabdoid cell component	Varies from 0% to 100%	Varies from 0% to 100%
Basaloid/small cell morphology	May be present (ovary, soft tissue, sinonasal)	Uncommon
Organotypical differentiation	Rare (subsets of NSCLC and GI carcinomas)	Common in the differentiated primary component
Teratoid morphology	Common in sinonasal tract (TCS, rare in other sites)	Rare to absent
Yolk sac-like morphology	Common in the kidney (RMC), uncommon in sinonasal tract**, much rare in other sites***	Rare
MMR deficiency	Rare	Frequent in uterine and GI carcinomas
Vimentin	Uniformly positive	Uniformly positive in the dedifferentiated component
Pankeratins	Mostly positive but variable	In dedifferentiated clone mostly positive but variable to complete loss may be seen
Neuroendocrine markers	Frequently variably positive (mostly synaptophysin)	Frequently variably positive (mostly synaptophysin)
Aggressiveness/biology	Variable, highly aggressive (CNS, kidney, ovary), benign or low-grade in some soft-tissue entities	Uniformly aggressive
Most frequently involved genes	SMRACB1 (CNS, kidney, soft tissue) SMARCA4 (thorax, ovary)	ARID1A>>SMARCA2>SMARCA4>SMARCB1
Heredity	0% up to ~40% (organ-dependent)	0%

*lack of differentiated component is largely dependent on the extent of sampling so that dedifferentiated and undifferentiated neoplasms are on the spectrum of same process and are defined by sampling and time point when the secondary genetic hit has occurred.
**Mostly in SMARCB1-deficient adenocarcinomas.
***Only rare reports have described yolk sac-like features in CNS and soft tissue/vulvar rhabdoid tumours.
CNS, central nervous system; GI, gastrointestinal; NSCLC, non-small cell lung cancer; RMC, renal medullary carcinoma; TCS, teratocarcinosarcoma.

tumour suppressor pathway [1–3]. This is reflected by the fact that biallelic inactivation of any of its subunits (either as a somatic event or a germline disease) results in development of diverse neoplastic entities in different organs [3]. Almost all the known SWI/SNF subunits have been implicated in the pathogenesis of neoplasms in different organs, either as primary drivers or as secondary events leading to dedifferentiation (**Table 7.1**). The overall frequency of SWI/SNF subunit alterations across all cancers is remarkably high (in the range of ~20%), comparable to that of *TP53* mutations [1–3]. The presence or absence of coexistent driver mutations in other genes is largely dependent on the nature of the SWI/SNF mutation (primary driver event versus secondary alteration superimposed on a primary driver). This aspect also has impact on the morphological pattern of the neoplasm (monomorphic as in most of primarily SWI/SNF-driven entities, versus biphasic or composite in those with secondary SWI/SNF loss) [4,5].

Mutation variability in different SWI/SNF component across organs

In decreasing order of frequency, the SWI/SNF subunits *SMARCB1, SMARCA4, SMARCA2, ARID1A, SMARCA2* and *PBRM1* have received much attention and have been well studied. Notably, a remarkable variation in the frequency of mutated SWI/SNF subunits is observed across organs (**Table 7.2**).

Table 7.2 Site-associated neoplastic entities and their related SWI/SNF genes			
Organ	**Entity**	**Lost SWI/SNF protein/%***	**Heredity**
CNS	ATRT	*SMARCB1* (98%)	>~30%
	ATRT	*SMARCA4* (2%)	~20%
	CRINET	*SMARCB1* (100%)	No sufficient
	Desmoplastic myxoid pineal tumour	*SMARCB1* (100%)	data
Soft tissue	Epithelioid sarcoma	*SMARCB1* (100%)	No
	Malignant rhabdoid tumour	*SMARCB1* (98%)	~30%
	Epithelioid schwannoma	*SMARCB1* (75%)	No
	Epithelioid MPNST	*SMARCB1* (50%)	Rare case reports
Sinonasal	*SMARCB1*-deficient carcinoma NST	*SMARCB1* (100%)	No
	SMARCB1-deficient adenocarcinoma	*SMARCB1* (100%)	No
	SMARCA4-deficient undifferentiated carcinoma	*SMARCA4* (100%)	No
	Sinonasal teratocarcinosarcoma	*SMARCA4* (82%)	No
Lung/thorax	*SMARCA4*-deficient adenocarcinoma	*SMARCA4* (5.5%)	No
	SMARCA4-deficient SCC	*SMARCA4* (5.2%)	
	SMARCA2-deficient adenocarcinoma	*SMARCA2* (6.4)	
	SMARCA2-deficient SCC	*SMARCA2* (1.7%)	
	SMARCA2-deficient undifferentiated carcinoma	*SMARCA2* (33%)	
	SMARCA4-deficient undifferentiated thoracic tumour*	*SMARCA4* (100%)	
GI tract	Adenocarcinoma/undifferentiated carcinoma	ARID1A	No
Kidney	Malignant rhabdoid tumour	*SMARCB1* (98%)	>30
	RMC (100%)	*SMARCB1* (100%)	Not
	ccRCC	*PBRM1* (40–60%)	hereditary
	Dedifferentiated/undifferentiated RCC	Diverse SWI/SNF subunits lost in 65%	Rare families No

Continues opposite

Organ	Entity	Lost SWI/SNF protein/%**	Heredity
Urinary bladder	Dedifferentiated/undifferentiated urothelial carcinoma	Diverse SWI/SNF subunits lost in 71% (*SMARCA2, ARID1A, INI1, SMARCA4*)	No
Uterus	Undifferentiated *SMARCA4*-deficient neoplasms (sarcomas!)	*SMARCA4* (100%)	No sufficient data
	Dedifferentiated/undifferentiated carcinoma endometrioid adenocarcinoma	Diverse SWI/SNF subunits lost in 66% (*ARID1A, SMARCA4, SMARCB1*)	No
Ovary	Small cell carcinoma of ovary, hypercalcemic type	*SMARCA4* (100%)	~40%

*Cases declared as with 100% are by definition deficient for the respective gene.
ATRT, atypical teratoid and rhabdoid tumour; ccRCC, clear cell renal cell carcinoma; CRINET, cribriform neuroepithelial tumour; NST, no special type; SCC, squamous cell carcinoma; SWI/SNF, switch/sucrose non-fermenting

SMARCB1-DEFICIENT NEOPLASMS

SMARCB1 (SWI/SNF Related, Matrix Associated, Actin Dependent Regulator of Chromatin, Subfamily B, Member 1, also known as integrase interactor-1/*INI1; BAF47, hSNF5*, etc.) is one of the main core subunits of the complex, mapping to chromosome 22q11.2 [6]. Like other subunits of the SWI/SNF complex, *SMARCB1* is evolutionarily highly conserved and hence is expressed in all normal cell types of human tissues. Biallelic inactivation of *SMARCB1* results in complete protein loss by IHC, irrespective of the exact underlying genetic or epigenetic mechanism [6–8].

Loss of *SMARCB1* has emerged as a defining diagnostic feature for several neoplastic entities (**Table 7.2**). These include [6–8]:
- True epithelial malignancies
  - *SMARCB1*-deficient sinonasal carcinoma
  - Renal medullary carcinoma
- Primitive paediatric malignancies
  - Intracranial and extracranial malignant rhabdoid tumours
  - So-called atypical teratoid/rhabdoid tumours (AT/RT)
- Soft-tissue neoplasms
  - Classical and proximal-type epithelioid sarcoma.

In addition to these, a heterogeneous group of other entities may display secondary *SMARCB1* loss in the context of dedifferentiation [9,10].

SMARCB1 deficiency in a subset of poorly or undifferentiated sinonasal carcinomas was first recognised in 2014 [11,12]. These tumours may display either a nondescript or undifferentiated morphology of no special type (NST, mostly showing basaloid and less frequently eosinophilic cell features) or may feature variable glandular differentiation, hence qualifying as adenocarcinomas [13,14]. The distinction between the two categories (NST versus adenocarcinoma) is rather morphological as their immunophenotypes largely overlap [13,14] (**Figure 7.1**). However, expression of yolk sac associated markers [alpha-fetoprotein (AFP)] and the presence of prominent yolk-sac-like morphological

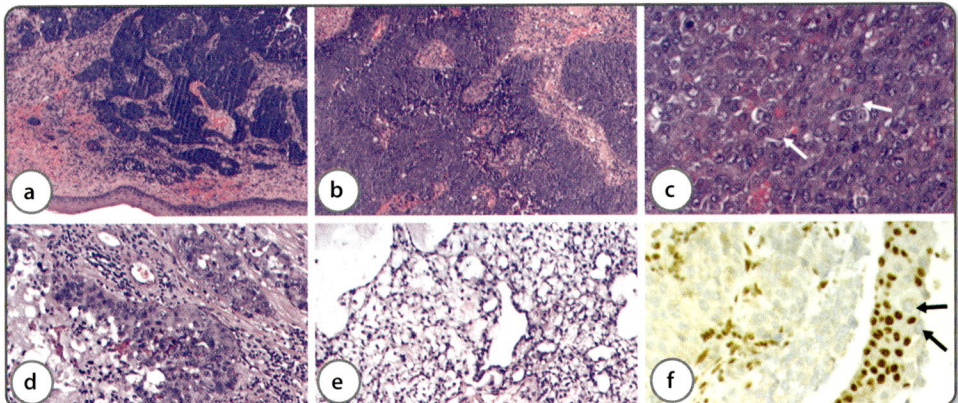

Figure 7.1 Examples of the morphology of *SMRACB1* (INI1)-deficient sinonasal carcinomas. (a and b) Most cases display non-descript basaloid monomorphic morphology indistinguishable from basaloid non-keratinising squamous cell carcinoma. (c) Anaplastic large cell morphology with scattered rhabdoid cells (white arrows). *SMARCB1*-deficient adenocarcinoma displays high-grade glandular elements (d) or reticular microcystic (e) or other yolk sac-like patterns. (f) Loss of *SMARCB1* is definitional, note pagetoid intraepithelial neoplastic cells highlighted by *SMARCAB1* loss (black arrows).

patterns are characteristic of the adenocarcinoma category (**Table 7.1**). A prerequisite for diagnosing these uncommon neoplasms is the exclusion of other molecularly defined specific types (NUT carcinoma and others) in the spectrum of poorly differentiated/undifferentiated sinonasal carcinomas and of other high-grade intestinal or non-intestinal adenocarcinomas [15].

Renal medullary carcinoma is a rare type of renal-cell carcinoma defined by characteristic clinical (almost all cases are associated with sickle-cell trait or sickle-cell disease), morphological (infiltrating cords, nests, microcysts, sheets and tubules with a myxoid desmoplastic reaction containing a mononuclear cell infiltrate) and immunophenotypic (invariably *SMARCB1* loss) features [16] (**Figure 7.2**). The diagnosis can only be made when other RCC subtypes with secondary *SMARCB1* deficiency (such as clear cell RCC with sarcomatoid differentiation, collecting duct carcinoma with secondary *SMARCB1* loss or fumarate hydratase-deficient RCC with secondary *SMARCB1* loss) have been excluded.

Epithelioid sarcoma of soft tissue represents the prototype of *SMARCB1*-deficient neoplasms in adults. The disease predominantly affects young adults and two distinct subtypes have been identified with defining clinicopathological and anatomic characteristics. The classical type occurs at distal extremity sites, usually as multinodular/multilobulated granuloma-like epithelioid malignancy expressing epithelial markers and displaying loss of *SMARCB1* [17]. The proximal type, which also displays loss of *SMARCB1*, shows a highly anaplastic large cell or rhabdoid morphology and occurs predominantly at proximal extremity locations and in the pelviperineal region [17,18]. This lesion can easily be confused with primary or metastatic undifferentiated carcinoma (**Figure 7.3**).

At molecular level, these primarily *SMARCB1*-driven malignancies have surprisingly stable genomes as next generation sequencing (NGS) frequently fails to identify any additional mutations, and thus often lack other concurrent driver events. Moreover, it is

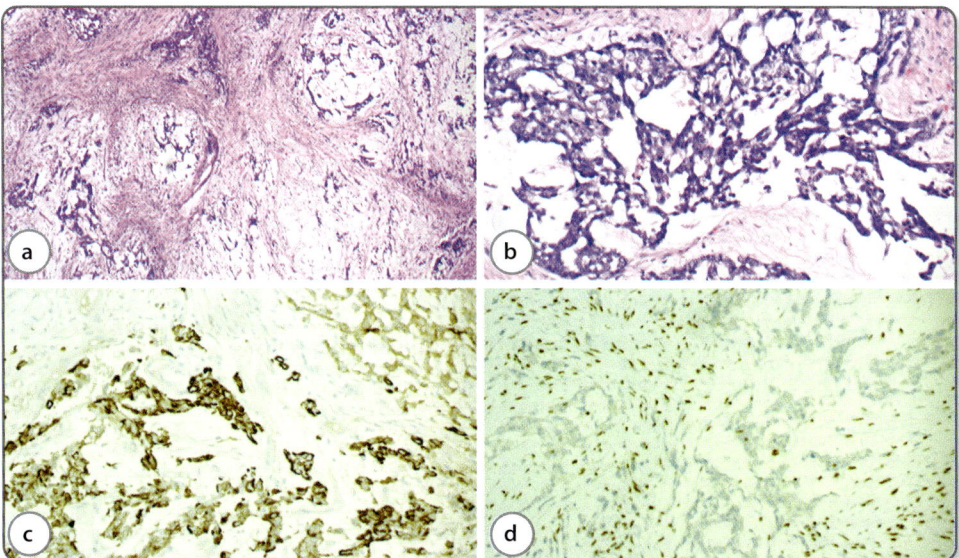

Figure 7.2 Renal medullary carcinoma more frequently displays reticular yolk-sac-like morphology (a and b), expresses uniformly pankeratin (c) and shows complete *SMARCB1* loss (d).

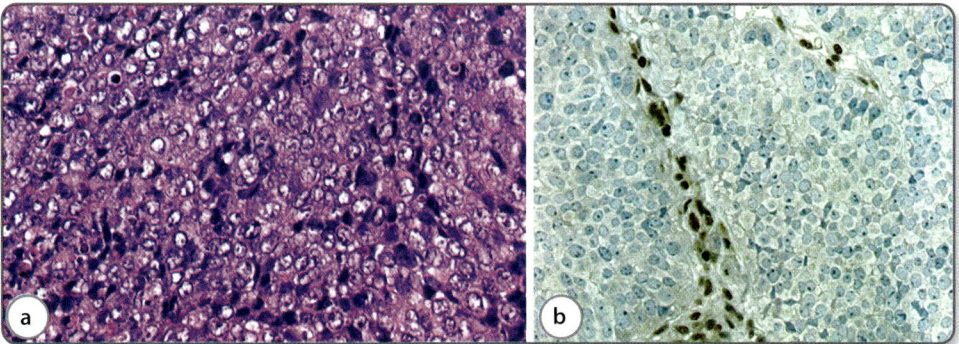

Figure 7.3 Proximal-type epithelioid sarcoma shows a non-descript large cell epithelioid/rhabdoid morphology indistinguishable from anaplastic carcinoma by histology alone (a) and is defined by *SMARCB1* loss (b).

cautious to avoid molecular profiling as single diagnostic tool, as cases may show false negative results based on the type of mutation and the platform used. *SMARCB1* loss proved to be the most reliable (highly sensitive and highly specific) tool to identify them in the appropriate clinicopathological and morphological context.

TREATMENT AND PROGNOSIS

Currently, there is no universal treatment strategy for these heterogeneous entities based on genotype only. Site of origin, histopathological diagnosis (carcinoma versus sarcoma) and disease stage guide local-surgical and oncological therapy strategies. However, anecdotal cases point to a potentially enhanced response to platinum-based chemotherapy of *SMARCB1*-deficient sinonasal carcinoma compared to other poorly differential carcinomas at this site without *SMARCB1* loss [19]. The prognosis of these neoplasms varies greatly, based on site and stage. Renal medullary carcinoma has the most aggressive course while sinonasal carcinomas and epithelioid sarcomas display an aggressive but heterogeneous course with occasional long-term survival after multimodal therapy of non-metastatic, albeit locally advanced, disease [17–19].

DIFFERENTIAL DIAGNOSIS AND TERMINOLOGIES

The terminology used for these entities is admittedly biased by tumour site and other clinicopathological features. Therefore, they cannot always be distinguished based on pure morphological and/or immunophenotypic characteristics only. Notably, they all share yolk-sac-like morphology with variable reticular-microcystic features, albeit with highly variable frequency (**Table 7.1**). Accordingly, in some cases, it may be impossible to distinguish primary from metastatic disease. Consequently, for some sites, it may be difficult to distinguish carcinoma versus sarcoma without incorporating clinical history, anatomic site, and other relevant criteria. However, detailed differential diagnostic considerations as defined by tumour site and morphology in a given case are beyond the objectives of this review, and the readers are referred to detailed papers devoted to this aspect published elsewhere.

SMARCA4-DEFICIENT NEOPLASMS

SMARCA4 (*BRG1*, mapped to 19p13.2) encodes a major catalytic subunit of the SWI/SNF complex that functions in a mutually exclusive manner with *SMARCA2*, another catalytic subunit of the complex [1–3]. This gene has been the topic of extensive research in the last decade, which resulted in better understanding of its biological properties and its involvement in oncogenesis. *SMARCA4* deficiency is the primary driver in a variety of highly aggressive malignancies of different histogenetic origin in different organs and affecting different age groups. While *SMARCB1*-deficient neoplasms show site-dependent morphotypic variations, most *SMARCA4*-deficient malignancies share a highly anaplastic morphotype composed of either monotonous small cells, large epithelioid/rhabdoid cells or a mixture of both. These neoplasms segregate into two major subgroups:

1. Primarily undifferentiated malignancies originating in different organs [ovary, mediastinum, lung, sinonasal tract (20–22)].
2. Composite dedifferentiated malignancies featuring a defined differentiated component with secondary morphological shift to an anaplastic phenotype [digestive tract lung, uterus, genitourinary, kidney, others (9,10)].

A minority (1–2%) of paediatric atypical teratoid/rhabdoid tumours (AT/RTs) with an intact *SMARCB1* gene locus are driven alternatively by *SMARCA4* loss [23]. Except for this rare subset of paediatric rhabdoid tumours, *SMARCA4*-deficient malignancies are diseases of adults; the age range, however, varies greatly depending on the site of origin (younger in the ovary, sinonasal tract and the thorax; middle age to elderly in the digestive, genitourinary, and gynaecological tract).

Histologically, *SMARCA4*-deficient malignancies display large undifferentiated, epithelioid or rhabdoid cells arranged into irregularly communicating nests, lobules or trabeculae set within a sparse to prominent reactive myxoid/oedematous or desmoplastic stroma. In contrast to their *SMARCB1*-deficient counterparts, *SMARCA4*-related malignancies only rarely show a basaloid (blue cell) pattern, which is almost restricted to a subset of small cell carcinoma of the ovary, hypercalcaemic type (SCCOHT) [4]. The nuclei mostly show vesicular chromatin with prominent macronuclei, brisk mitotic activity, and extensive geographic coagulative necrosis (**Figure 7.4**). IHC shows variable reactivity for low-molecular weight keratins, EMA, CD34 and SALL4, but all lineage-specific markers are negative, indicating a primitive cell phenotype. Most ovarian and variable subsets of *SMARCA4*-deficient tumours in other organs show concomitant loss of *SMARCA2* [21,22]. Variable, usually patchy to moderate reactivity with synaptophysin, CD56 and rarely chromogranin represents another frequent feature of these malignancies, and this should not be misinterpreted as evidence of genuine neuroendocrine differentiation [24].

SMARCA4-deficient primitive "teratoid" malignancies

Although the term "atypical teratoid tumours" has been historically introduced to *SMRACB1*-deficient central nervous system tumours of childhood [23], this terminology is rather a misnomer, as these tumours only rarely display genuine morphological teratoid features. Recent studies point to the existence of rare subsets of neoplasms driven by *SMARCA4*-deficiency and displaying a primitive polyphenotypic/multilineage differentiation.

Sinonasal teratocarcinosarcoma is a highly aggressive rare teratoid somatic malignancy featuring triphasic morphology with variable admixtures of embryonal-type epithelium (squamous, glandular, and respiratory), mesenchymal/stromal elements and neuro-epithelial structures [25]. Recently, the majority of sinonasal teratocarcinosarcomas (82%) was found to harbour biallelic *SMARCA4* inactivation, associated with *SMARCA4* loss as the sole molecular driver with total loss detected in 68% and variable partial loss being observed in 14% of cases [26] (**Figure 7.4**).

Finally, rare somatic teratoid tumours harbouring *SMARCA4* loss have been reported in non-sinonasal sites [27].

Prognosis and treatment

SMARCA4-deficient malignancies are highly aggressive diseases that result in extensive dissemination or recurrences soon after initial diagnosis or treatment. For these malignancies, specific therapeutic regimens have not been established. Treatment is usually a combination of radical surgery and aggressive multimodal adjuvant therapy. Most patients succumb to disease within 1 year.

Differential diagnosis and terminologies

How to classify *SMARCA4*-deficient undifferentiated malignancies is still a topic of controversy. In the ovary, however, the SCCOHT terminology has been widely accepted. Admittedly, a large proportion of ovarian *SMARCA4*-deficient undifferentiated malignancies does not show the prototypical small cells, but an epithelioid/rhabdoid large cell pattern instead. However, such "variant" patterns are well recognised in almost all neoplasms across all organs and sites and therefore this is not a valid argument against the original diagnostic terminology SCCOHT for ovarian cases. The same reasoning applies to the lack of paraneoplastic hypercalcaemia in a subset of ovarian cases [28].

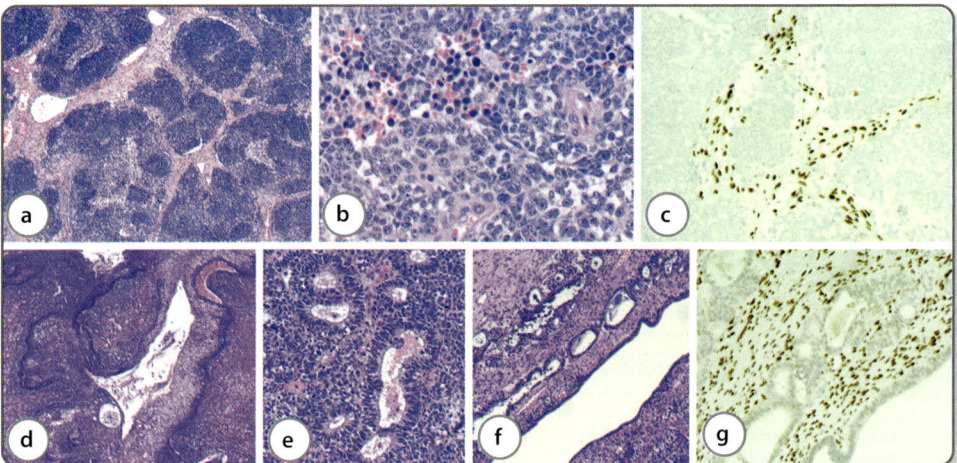

Figure 7.4 *SMRACA4*-deficient sinonasal carcinoma showing prominent microlobular growth (a) of large undifferentiated cells (b). (c) Loss of *SMARCA4* is diagnostic. Sinonasal teratocarcinosarcoma as a frequently *SMARCA4*-deficent malignancy displays variable combination of embryonal-looking clear-cell squamous epithelium (d), primitive neuroepithelial tubules merging with undifferentiated neuroectodermal cells (e) and more mature looking cystic respiratory epithelial glands (f). *SMRACA4* loss is observed in majority of cases, note loss in the bland-looking cystic respiratory glands as well with retained nuclear expression in the reactive stromal cells (g).

In the sinonasal tract, by consensus *SMARCA4*-deficient neoplasms are divided into two major groups:

1. *SMARCA4*-deficient undifferentiated carcinomas
2. *SMARCA4*-deficient but morphologically readily defined teratocarcinosarcoma [14]. Although to differentiate between these two in limited biopsy material might be impossible in some cases, in resection specimens or larger biopsies real morphological overlap between the two categories is not seen. This argues against the notion that the two might represent two morphotypes within the same disease spectrum, and instead is in line with two distinctive morphologically separable entities sharing the same genetic defect. Large cell neuroendocrine carcinoma is another consideration in sinonasal sites, given that variable neuroendocrine markers may be expressed in *SMARCA4*-deficient sinonasal carcinomas. However, these tumours usually lack cytological characteristics of neuroendocrine cells so that their separation from large cell neuroendocrine carcinomas is mostly morphology-based [24].

A major controversy regarding *SMARCA4*-deficient malignancies has arisen for intrathoracic and gynaecological cases. In the thorax and the mediastinum, these tumours were initially proposed as sarcomas related to BAF-deficient neoplasms [22]. However, several later studies confirmed clinicopathological, aetiological (heavy smoking), morphological (occasional biphasic features or presence of differentiated carcinoma component), and molecular (smoking mutational signature) features, closely related to non-small cell lung cancer [29,30]. These observations justified modification of the original sarcoma terminology to the descriptive term "*SMARCA4*-deficient undifferentiated thoracic tumour" in the most recent WHO classification of thorax tumours.

A similar controversy arose for gynaecological tumours which are morphologically not distinguishable from undifferentiated endometrial carcinoma variants, as the features are ill-defined and do not allow reproducible classification [31]. At this point, it is noteworthy that the mere lack of keratin expression does not exclude an epithelial origin; the reverse is also true: Strong keratin expression is not invariably indicative of an epithelial origin. Similar arguments apply to other adjunct markers of epithelial tissue such as claudin-4 [32]. In ambiguous cases, molecular profiling to identify the underlying mutational signature may prove helpful in the classification of these challenging tumours [29–31].

Therapeutic implications of SWI/SNF deficiency

To date, no entity-specific therapy has been established for these rare, but frequently highly aggressive malignancies. In addition to the above-mentioned higher responsiveness of some *SMARCB1*- or *SMARCA4*-deficient neoplasms to platinum-based chemotherapy regimens, accumulating observations suggest promising results of immune therapy. New therapeutic opportunities utilising enhancer of zeste homolog-2 (*EZH2), CDK4/6* and other SWI/SNF complex-associated vulnerabilities are still emerging in clinical trials [19,33–36]. All these issues can only be better resolved, and the related questions be well answered if these neoplasms are properly recognised and separated from their many mimics in daily surgical pathology practice.

NUTM1-REARRANGED NEOPLASMS

NUT Midline Carcinoma Family Member-1 (*NUTM1*, also known as *NUT*) has been implicated in the molecular pathogenesis of a paediatric midline (thymic/mediastinal) carcinoma with a t(15;19) translocation, a rare highly aggressive malignancy first described in 1991 [37]. This was followed by the discovery of the *BRD4-NUT* fusion in 2003 [38]. A valuable morphological clue to the diagnosis is the characteristic abrupt squamous differentiation/abrupt keratinisation, which however is observed in no >43% of cases [40]. A highly specific and sensitive anti-NUT monoclonal antibody was developed [39], applicable in IHC tests, and since then NUT carcinoma was increasingly diagnosed in daily and consultation practice, also in cases lacking the characteristic morphology (**Figure 7.5**).

The increasing use of NUT-IHC to further characterise unclassified poorly differentiated malignancies, and the increasing application of next generation sequencing tools using RNA-seq platforms, have led to the following major developments in the rapidly emerging field of *NUTM1*-rearranged neoplasia:

- Increased recognition of non-midline anatomic locations in several lateralised organs including lungs, salivary glands, kidneys as well as other non-midline sites such as pancreas and soft tissue (justifying removal of the modifier "midline" from current WHO classifications).
- Increased recognition of a wider age range, ranging from paediatric cases to the elderly
- Expansion of the immunoprofile of NUT carcinoma, with recognition of keratin-poor/keratin-negative and p63-negative tumours that would otherwise not have been correctly diagnosed.
- Increased identification of a plethora of novel fusion gene partners that have enabled deeper insight into their emerging pathobiology landscapes
- The emerging notion that some *NUTM1*-rearranged neoplasms might be of mesenchymal origin (in the sense of NUT sarcomas)
- Recognition of the unexpected occurrence of *NUTM1* rearrangements in fully benign skin adnexal neoplasms (e.g. poroma), challenging the historical dogma of *NUTM1* rearrangements as a hallmark of lethal disease and aggressiveness.

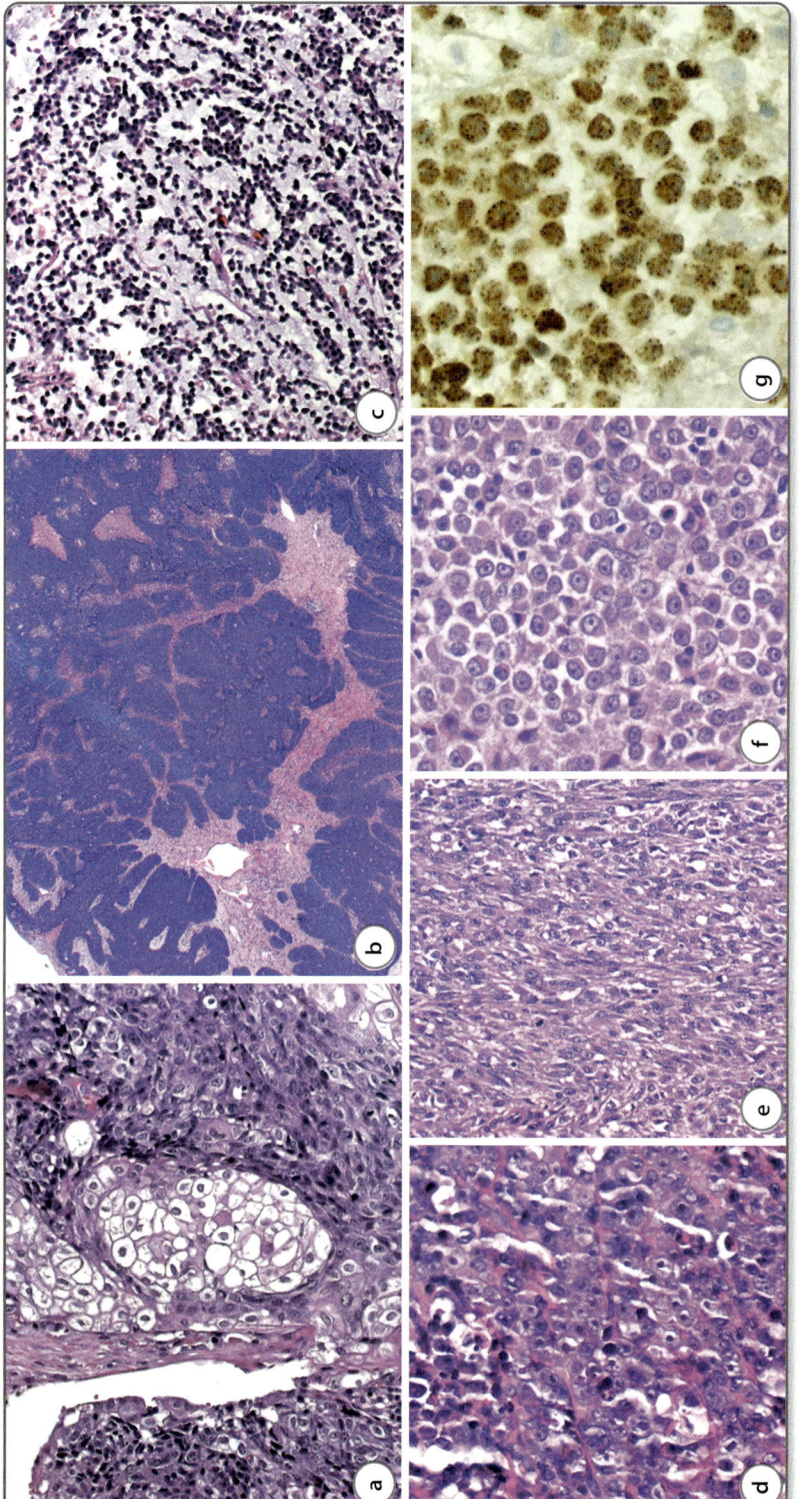

Figure 7.5 Morphological diversity of *NUTM1*-rerranged malignancies. (a) The characteristic basaloid morphology with abrupt squamous foci/abrupt keratinisation is seen in no >43% of all cases (this tumour had an *NSD3::NUTM1* fusion). (b) Pure basaloid morphology may be mistaken for basaloid squamous cell carcinoma (case with *BRD3::NUTM1* fusion). (c) Small cell (lymphoid-looking) cell morphology (case with *BRD4::NUTM1* fusion). (d) Large epithelioid cell morphology (case with *BRD4::NUTM1* fusion). (e and f) Mixed spindled and epithelioid/round cell morphology in colorectal NUT sarcoma with *MXD4::NUTM1 fusion*. (g) Punctate nuclear NUT immunoreactivity highlighting the megadomains.

This final part of this review will highlight and discuss in brief the emerging clinicopathological, immunophenotypic, histogenetic and molecular landscapes of *NUTM1*-rearranged neoplasia that emerged through the widespread use of NUT-IHC and NGS technologies during the last two decades (**Table 7.3**). Details of the individual entities are beyond the scope of this review, and the readers are referred to more detailed original studies and review articles on the topic elsewhere.

NUTM1-rearranged malignancies: Carcinomas versus sarcomas

With the expanding family of NUT malignancies and their rapidly evolving morphological and genotypic landscapes, a key question is whether to classify these neoplasms uniformly, or differentially as carcinomas, sarcomas or malignancies of unknown histogenesis. The issue is further complicated by the finding of *NUTM1* rearrangements also in rare haematological malignancies [41]. Such observations open up the question whether phenotypic and genotypic features exist that might be helpful to define histogenetic categories for these rare aggressive diseases [42,43].

Table 7.3 Major genetic subgroups of *NUTM1*-rearranged neoplasms				
Fusion partner	**Entity**	**Biology**	**Proposed histogenetic origin**	**Comments**
BRD4	NUT carcinoma	Aggressive	Epithelial	Most frequent genotype in NUT carcinoma
BRD3	NUT carcinoma	Aggressive	Epithelial	Second frequent genotype in NUT carcinoma[1]
NSD3	NUT carcinoma	Aggressive	Epithelial	Second frequent genotype in NUT carcinoma[1,2]
ZNF532, ZNF592	NUT carcinoma	Aggressive	Epithelial[3]	Rare genotype in NUT carcinoma
YAP1	Poroma Porocarcinoma	Ranges from fully benign to aggressive	Skin adnexa	Frequent in both benign poroma and porocarcinoma
WWTR1	Poroma	Benign	Skin adnexa	Rare genotype
MGA, CIC, MXD4	NUT sarcoma[4]	Aggressive	Likely mesenchymal	MXD4 mostly colorectal or visceral
BCORL1, MXD1, AXTN1	Undifferentiated soft tissue and visceral malignancies	Aggressive	Uncertain	Heterogenous category
BRD9, IKZF1, CUX1, AFF1, ZNF618, SLC12A6, ACIN1	Paediatric B-cell acute lymphoblastic leukaemia	More favourable prognosis	Immature B-cell precursors	

[1]The frequency of the BRD-3 and NSD-3 fusions is comparable in unselected cases.
[2]NSD-3 fused tumours tend to be overrepresented in non-midline pulmonary, non-sinonasal head, and neck cases.
[3]Some cases have been reported from non-epithelialised bone sites so their histogenesis is not clear yet.
[4]CIC-rearranged cases have been included in the CIC sarcoma category.

Genetic landscape of NUT malignancies

Irrespective of their anatomic site, morphology, phenotype or exact genotype, NUT malignancies are defined by rearrangements involving the *NUTM1* gene (mapped to 15q14). The bromodomain containing 4 (*BRD4*) gene (mapped to 19p13.12) is the most frequent fusion partner (characterises two-thirds of cases). In the remaining one-third of cases variant fusions with *BRD3* (mapped to 9q34.2) and the nuclear receptor binding SET domain protein 3 (*NSD3* mapped to 8p11.23) are encountered as alternate fusion partners with almost similar frequency [40,42,43]. However, recently, two members of the "Z4" transcriptional coregulator zinc finger (ZNF) protein complex (ZNF532 and ZNF592) have been recognised as a fourth fusion partner category in NUT carcinomas [44–49]. These novel fusion proteins co-localise and closely interact with the BRD4-NUT oncogenic complex [44].

Chromatin regulatory complexes are formed by *BRD4* via interaction with *BRD3, NSD3, ZNF532,* and *ZNF592*. NUT chimeric proteins induce an abnormal association between NUT and the BRDs/ZNFs chromatin regulatory complexes, which ultimately leads to formation of large histone hyperacetylation domains via interaction between NUT and the histone acetyltransferase p300 [44–46]. It has been shown experimentally that not only *BRD4,* but other fusion partner variants (*BRD3, NSD3, ZNF532* and *ZNF592*) bind to *BRD4* and lead to similarly abnormal associations between NUT and the BRDs/ZNFs chromatin regulatory complexes [44–46]. In terms of function, these aberrant NUT, p300 and *BRD4* regulatory complexes drive mistargeting of active chromatin. The bromodomains of the BRDs drive the oncogenic potential of these fusion proteins. Experimental studies have illustrated that the five major fusion variants (*BRD4-NUTM1, BRD3-NUTM1, NSD3-NUTM1, ZNF53- NUTM-* and *ZNF592-NUTM1*), resulting in variant *NUTM1* chimeric fusion proteins, share biological and pharmacological properties. This led to the current notion that neoplasms carrying any of these fusion variants probably represent a spectrum in a single entity, namely NUT carcinoma [44–46]. Although this concept is supported by the fact that most of these tumours do indeed originate within epithelial organs (lung, thymus, and mucosal head and neck sites), it remains obscure which cell of origin gives rise to the ZNF rearranged variants which have been reported to originate within bones [44–49]. On the other hand, *NUTM1-ZNF532* knockdown was shown to be associated with cell differentiation and induced expression of the terminal squamous cell differentiation marker involucrin [44–46]. This argues for the carcinoma concept of the ZNF-fused variant, similar to the canonical *BRD4-NUTM1* cases. Current data are in line with the variant fusions being homologous to the canonical *BRD4* variant, and suggest that all these disease subgroups might be treatable by bromodomain or p300 inhibitors, irrespective of the exact fusion partner among the five fusions [46]. Bromodomain (BET) inhibitors bind to the bromodomains of *BRD2, BRD3* and *BRD4* proteins, which block their capacity to interact with chromatin and thus abolish their oncogenic function. BET inhibitors hold great promise as targeted treatment for NUT malignancies.

Several other fusion gene partners have been identified recently, including *MGA, CIC, MXD4, MXD1, BCORL1,* and *AXTN1* [42,50–54]. These fusion partners characterise malignancies of probable mesenchymal or unknown histogenetic origin [51–53]. *CIC* and *BCORL1* as *NUTM1* fusion partners likely de-repress transcriptional targets similar to *CIC-DUX4* and *CREBBP-BCORL1,* through NUT possibly converting these transcriptional repressors into transcriptional activators via recruitment of p300 [54]. In addition, fusions between *NUTM1* and *MYC* dominant-negative factors (*MGA, MYXD1,* and *MXD4)*, likely act to de-repress MYC targets via the recruitment of p300 through NUT [46,51–55]. As the latter transcriptional repressors are associated with sarcomas and not involved in the BRD-NUT assembly, response of these neoplasms (tentatively called here "NUT sarcomas") to BET inhibitors is uncertain and remains to be verified in future experimental studies.

Recently described *NUTM1*-rearranged benign and malignant epithelial neoplasms

NUTM1 rearrangements have been recently recognised in a high proportion of skin adnexal neoplasms, specifically in benign poromas and porocarcinomas [56,57]. These tumours differentiate similar to poroid neoplasms in general and the underlying *NUTM1* fusion cannot be suspected on morphological grounds, in contrast to the classical NUT carcinomas. Finally, 38% of thyroid NUT carcinomas displayed a thyroid follicular carcinoma-like morphology and expressed a follicular-like immunophenotype (PAX8+, TTF1+) [58]. Moreover, these organotypical tumours had a more protracted clinical course compared to classical NUT carcinoma in the thyroid. The thyroid-typical morphology in a subset of NUT carcinomas of the thyroid and the well-known well-differentiated morphology in a subset of *SMARCA4*-deficient lung adenocarcinoma are two striking examples highlighting the occasional capacity of these two genotypes to permit cell differentiation under not yet understood molecular conditions of the cell [58,59].

Key points for clinical practice

- Distinct biological behaviour of tumours sharing the same phenotype or genotype, including discrepant responsiveness to different therapeutic approaches, requires aetiology- and/or genome-based classification.
- Heretofore, difficult-to-classify and undifferentiated malignancies appear to be driven by SWI/SNF deficiency and *NUTM1* rearrangements, which alter chromatin regulatory complexes.
- SWI/SNF-deficient malignancies tend to display a non-descript undifferentiated looking cell phenotype with poor cell cohesion.
- Loss of *SMARCB1*, a core subunit of the SWI/SNF complex, defines the following neoplastic entities:
  - True epithelial malignancies
    - SMARCB1-deficient sinonasal carcinoma
    - Renal medullary carcinoma
  - Primitive paediatric malignancies
    - Intracranial and extracranial malignant rhabdoid tumours
    - So-called atypical teratoid/rhabdoid tumours
  - Soft-tissue neoplasms
    - Classical and proximal-type epithelioid sarcoma.
- Loss of *SMARCA4*, a major catalytic subunit of the SWI/SNF complex, is the primary driver in a variety of highly aggressive malignancies of different histogenetic origin in different organs and affecting different age groups.

- *NUT* gene fusions characterise a category of until recently unclassified poorly differentiated malignancies.
- About 50% of NUT carcinomas is characterised histologically by abrupt squamous differentiation/abrupt keratinisation.
- Specific NUT antibodies facilitate the recognition of NUT carcinomas.
- Non-midline anatomic locations of NUT carcinomas include lungs, salivary glands, kidneys and pancreas.
- The genetic landscape of *NUTM1*-rearranged neoplasms points to a heterogeneous category of neoplasms of true epithelial origin (benign or malignant), probable mesenchymal origin (NUT sarcomas), haematolymphoid origin (leukaemias) and neoplasms of yet uncertain histogenesis.

REFERENCES

1. Wang X, Haswell JR, Roberts CW. Molecular pathways: SWI/SNF (BAF) complexes are frequently mutated in cancer--mechanisms and potential therapeutic insights. Clin Cancer Res 2014; 20:21–27.
2. Kadoch C, Crabtree GR. Mammalian SWI/SNF chromatin remodeling complexes and cancer: Mechanistic insights gained from human genomics. Sci Adv 2015; 1:e1500447.
3. Wang L, Tang J. SWI/SNF complexes and cancers. Gene 2023; 870:147420.
4. Agaimy A. SWI/SNF Complex-Deficient Soft Tissue Neoplasms: A Pattern-Based Approach to Diagnosis and Differential Diagnosis. Surg Pathol Clin 2019; 12:149–163.
5. Agaimy A, Bishop JA. SWI/SNF-deficient head and neck neoplasms: An overview. Semin Diagn Pathol 2021; 38:175–182.
6. Judkins AR. Immunohistochemistry of INI1 expression: a new tool for old challenges in CNS and soft tissue pathology. Adv Anat Pathol 2007; 14:335–339.
7. Hollmann TJ, Hornick JL. INI1-deficient tumors: diagnostic features and molecular genetics. Am J Surg Pathol 2011; 35:e47–e63.
8. Agaimy A. The expanding family of SMARCB1(INI1)-deficient neoplasia: implications of phenotypic, biological, and molecular heterogeneity. Adv Anat Pathol 2014; 21:394–410.
9. Agaimy A, Daum O, Märkl B, et al. SWI/SNF Complex-deficient Undifferentiated/Rhabdoid Carcinomas of the Gastrointestinal Tract: A Series of 13 Cases Highlighting Mutually Exclusive Loss of SMARCA4 and SMARCA2 and Frequent Co-inactivation of SMARCB1 and SMARCA2. Am J Surg Pathol 2016; 40:544–553.
10. Agaimy A, Cheng L, Egevad L, et al. Rhabdoid and Undifferentiated Phenotype in Renal Cell Carcinoma: Analysis of 32 Cases Indicating a Distinctive Common Pathway of Dedifferentiation Frequently Associated With SWI/SNF Complex Deficiency. Am J Surg Pathol 2017; 41:253–262.
11. Agaimy A, Koch M, Lell M, et al. SMARCB1(INI1)-deficient sinonasal basaloid carcinoma: a novel member of the expanding family of SMARCB1-deficient neoplasms. Am J Surg Pathol 2014; 38:1274–1281.
12. Bishop JA, Antonescu CR, Westra WH. SMARCB1 (INI-1)-deficient carcinomas of the sinonasal tract. Am J Surg Pathol 2014; 38:1282–1289.
13. Shah AA, Jain D, Ababneh E, et al. SMARCB1 (INI-1)-Deficient Adenocarcinoma of the Sinonasal Tract: A Potentially Under-Recognized form of Sinonasal Adenocarcinoma with Occasional Yolk Sac Tumor-Like Features. Head Neck Pathol 2020; 14:465–472.
14. Agaimy A. Proceedings of the North American Society of Head and Neck Pathology, Los Angeles, CA, March 20, 2022: SWI/SNF-deficient Sinonasal Neoplasms: An Overview. Head Neck Pathol 2022; 16:168–178.
15. Agaimy A, Franchi A, Lund VJ, et al. Sinonasal Undifferentiated Carcinoma (SNUC): From an Entity to Morphologic Pattern and Back Again-A Historical Perspective. Adv Anat Pathol 2020; 27:51–60.

16.   Ohe C, Smith SC, Sirohi D, et al. Reappraisal of Morphologic Differences Between Renal Medullary Carcinoma, Collecting Duct Carcinoma, and Fumarate Hydratase-deficient Renal Cell Carcinoma. Am J Surg Pathol 2018; 42:279–292.

17:   Chbani L, Guillou L, Terrier P, et al. Epithelioid sarcoma: a clinicopathologic and immunohistochemical analysis of 106 cases from the French sarcoma group. Am J Clin Pathol 2009; 131:222–227.

18.   Hornick JL, Dal Cin P, Fletcher CD. Loss of INI1 expression is characteristic of both conventional and proximal-type epithelioid sarcoma. Am J Surg Pathol 2009; 33:542–550.

19.   Agaimy A, Hartmann A, Antonescu CR, et al. SMARCB1 (INI-1)-deficient Sinonasal Carcinoma: A Series of 39 Cases Expanding the Morphologic and Clinicopathologic Spectrum of a Recently Described Entity. Am J Surg Pathol 2017; 41:458–471.

20.   Witkowski L, Carrot-Zhang J, Albrecht S, et al. Germline and somatic SMARCA4 mutations characterize small cell carcinoma of the ovary, hypercalcemic type. Nat Genet 2014; 46:438–443.

21.   Conlon N, Silva A, Guerra E, et al. Loss of SMARCA4 Expression Is Both Sensitive and Specific for the Diagnosis of Small Cell Carcinoma of Ovary, Hypercalcemic Type. Am J Surg Pathol 2016; 40:395–403.

22.   Le Loarer F, Watson S, Pierron G, et al. SMARCA4 inactivation defines a group of undifferentiated thoracic malignancies transcriptionally related to BAF-deficient sarcomas. Nat Genet 2015; 47:1200–1205.

23.   Cai C. SWI/SNF deficient central nervous system neoplasms. Semin Diagn Pathol 2021; 38:167–174.

24.   Kasajima A, Konukiewitz B, Schlitter AM, et al. Mesenchymal/non-epithelial mimickers of neuroendocrine neoplasms with a focus on fusion gene-associated and SWI/SNF-deficient tumors. Virchows Arch 2021; 479:1209–1219.

25.   Heffner DK, Hyams VJ. Teratocarcinosarcoma (malignant teratoma?) of the nasal cavity and paranasal sinuses A clinicopathologic study of 20 cases. Cancer 1984; 53:2140–2154.

26.   Rooper LM, Uddin N, Gagan J, et al. Recurrent Loss of SMARCA4 in Sinonasal Teratocarcinosarcoma. Am J Surg Pathol 2020; 44:1331–1339.

27.   de Kock L, Fahiminiya S, Fiset PO, et al. Infantile Pulmonary Teratoid Tumor. N Engl J Med 2018; 378:2238–2240.

28.   Young RH, Oliva E, Scully RE. Small cell carcinoma of the ovary, hypercalcemic type. A clinicopathological analysis of 150 cases. Am J Surg Pathol 1994; 18:1102–1116.

29.   Agaimy A, Fuchs F, Moskalev EA, et al. SMARCA4-deficient pulmonary adenocarcinoma: clinicopathological, immunohistochemical, and molecular characteristics of a novel aggressive neoplasm with a consistent TTF1neg/CK7pos/HepPar-1pos immunophenotype. Virchows Arch 2017; 471:599–609.

30.   Rekhtman N, Montecalvo J, Chang JC, et al. SMARCA4-Deficient Thoracic Sarcomatoid Tumors Represent Primarily Smoking-Related Undifferentiated Carcinomas Rather Than Primary Thoracic Sarcomas. J Thorac Oncol 2020; 15:231–247.

31.   Tessier-Cloutier B, Coatham M, Carey M, et al. SWI/SNF-deficiency defines highly aggressive undifferentiated endometrial carcinoma. J Pathol Clin Res 2021; 7:144–153.

32.   Schaefer IM, Agaimy A, Fletcher CD, Hornick JL. Claudin-4 expression distinguishes SWI/SNF complex-deficient undifferentiated carcinomas from sarcomas. Mod Pathol 2017; 30:539–548.

33.   Bell EH, Chakraborty AR, Mo X, et al. SMARCA4/BRG1 Is a Novel Prognostic Biomarker Predictive of Cisplatin-Based Chemotherapy Outcomes in Resected Non-Small Cell Lung Cancer. Clin Cancer Res 2016; 22:2396–2404.

34.   Wang Y, Chen SY, Karnezis AN, et al. The histone methyltransferase EZH2 is a therapeutic target in small cell carcinoma of the ovary, hypercalcaemic type. J Pathol 2017; 242:371–383.

35.   Xue Y, Meehan B, Fu Z, et al. SMARCA4 loss is synthetic lethal with CDK4/6 inhibition in non-small cell lung cancer. Nat Commun 2019; 10:557.

36.   Abou Alaiwi S, Nassar AH, Xie W, et al. Mammalian SWI/SNF Complex Genomic Alterations and Immune Checkpoint Blockade in Solid Tumors. Cancer Immunol Res 2020; 8:1075–1084.

37.   Kubonishi I, Takehara N, Iwata J, et al. Novel t(15;19)(q15;p13) chromosome abnormality in a thymic carcinoma. Cancer Res 1991; 51:3327–3328.

38.   French CA, Kutok JL, Faquin WC, et al. Midline carcinoma of children and young adults with NUT rearrangement. J Clin Oncol 2004; 22:4135–4139.

39. Haack H, Johnson LA, Fry CJ, et al. Diagnosis of NUT midline carcinoma using a NUT-specific monoclonal antibody. Am J Surg Pathol 2009; 33:984–991.

40. Chau NG, Ma C, Danga K, et al. An Anatomical Site and Genetic-Based Prognostic Model for Patients With Nuclear Protein in Testis (NUT) Midline Carcinoma: Analysis of 124 Patients. JNCI Cancer Spectr 2019; 4:pkz094.

41. Cheng Z, Luo Y, Zhang Y, et al. A novel NAP1L4/NUTM1 fusion arising from translocation t(11;15) (p15;q12) in a myeloid neoplasm with eosinophilia and rearrangement of PDGFRA highlights an unusual clinical feature and therapeutic reaction. Ann Hematol 2020; 99:1561–1564.

42. Luo W, Stevens TM, Stafford P, et al. NUTM1-Rearranged Neoplasms-A Heterogeneous Group of Primitive Tumors with Expanding Spectrum of Histology and Molecular Alterations-An Updated Review. Curr Oncol 2021; 28:4485–4503.

43. McEvoy CR, Fox SB, Prall OWJ. Emerging entities in NUTM1-rearranged neoplasms. Genes Chromosomes Cancer 2020; 59:375–385.

44. Shiota H, Elya JE, Alekseyenko AA, et al. "Z4" Complex Member Fusions in NUT Carcinoma: Implications for a Novel Oncogenic Mechanism. Mol Cancer Res 2018; 16:1826–1833.

45. Chien YW, Hsieh TH, Chu PY, et al. Primary malignant epithelioid and rhabdoid tumor of bone harboring ZNF532-NUTM1 fusion: the expanding NUT cancer family. Genes Chromosomes Cancer 2019; 58:809–814.

46. Alekseyenko AA, Walsh EM, Zee BM, et al. Ectopic protein interactions within BRD4-chromatin complexes drive oncogenic megadomain formation in NUT midline carcinoma. Proc Natl Acad Sci U S A 2017; 114:E4184–E4192.

47. Agaimy A, Haller F, Renner A, et al. Misleading Germ Cell Phenotype in Pulmonary NUT Carcinoma Harboring the ZNF532-NUTM1 Fusion. Am J Surg Pathol 2022; 46:281–288.

48. Chen M, Zhao S, Liang Z, et al. NUT carcinoma of the parotid gland: report of two cases, one with a rare ZNF532-NUTM1 fusion. Virchows Arch 2022; 480:887–897.

49. Abreu RF, Oliveira TB, Hertzler H, et al. NUT carcinoma, an under-recognized malignancy: a clinicopathologic and molecular series of 6 cases showing a subset of patients with better prognosis and a rare ZNF532:NUTM1 fusion. Hum Pathol 2022; 126:87–99.

50. Stevens TM, Morlote D, Xiu J, et al. NUTM1-rearranged neoplasia: a multi-institution experience yields novel fusion partners and expands the histologic spectrum. Mod Pathol 2019; 32:764–773.

51. Tamura R, Nakaoka H, Yoshihara K, et al. Novel MXD4-NUTM1 fusion transcript identified in primary ovarian undifferentiated small round cell sarcoma. Genes Chromosomes Cancer 2018; 57:557–563.

52. Le Loarer F, Pissaloux D, Watson S, et al. Clinicopathologic Features of CIC-NUTM1 Sarcomas, a New Molecular Variant of the Family of CIC-Fused Sarcomas. Am J Surg Pathol 2019; 43:268–276.

53. Van Treeck BJ, Thangaiah JJ, Torres-Mora J, et al. NUTM1-rearranged colorectal sarcoma: a clinicopathologically and genetically distinctive malignant neoplasm with a poor prognosis. Mod Pathol 2021; 34:1547–1557.

54. Eagen KP, French CA. Supercharging BRD4 with NUT in carcinoma. Oncogene 2021; 40:1396–1408.

55. Grayson AR, Walsh EM, Cameron MJ, et al. MYC, a downstream target of BRD-NUT, is necessary and sufficient for the blockade of differentiation in NUT midline carcinoma. Oncogene 2014; 33:1736–1742.

56. Sekine S, Kiyono T, Ryo E, et al. Recurrent YAP1-MAML2 and YAP1-NUTM1 fusions in poroma and porocarcinoma. J Clin Invest 2019; 129:3827–3832.

57. Agaimy A, Tögel L, Haller F, et al. YAP1-NUTM1 Gene Fusion in Porocarcinoma of the External Auditory Canal. Head Neck Pathol 2020; 14:982–990.

58. Barletta JA, Gilday SD, Afkhami M, et al. NUTM1-rearranged Carcinoma of the Thyroid: A Distinct Subset of NUT Carcinoma Characterized by Frequent NSD3-NUTM1 Fusions. Am J Surg Pathol 2022; 46:1706–1715.

59. Herpel E, Rieker RJ, Dienemann H, et al. SMARCA4 and SMARCA2 deficiency in non-small cell lung cancer: immunohistochemical survey of 316 consecutive specimens. Ann Diagn Pathol 2017; 26:47–51.

Chapter 8

Papillary renal cell carcinoma: A review of the past, present and future

Oluwayomi Oyedeji, Sean R Williamson, Khaleel I Al-Obaidy

INTRODUCTION

Papillary renal cell carcinomas (PRCC) account for up to 15% of all renal cell carcinomas (RCC). Over the last 30 some years, PRCC has been recognized as the second most common type of renal malignancy and as a tumor that has unique clinicopathologic features. However, increased interest in this issue provided also novel data indicating that this neoplastic entity includes several subtypes. Advances in molecular biology provided additional data about these tumors indicating that not all controversies have been resolved. Discussions are still going on about the pathogenesis of these tumors, the validity and criteria for their classification and clinical implication of all these morphologic and subcellular findings. In this review article, we will highlight some of these contentious issues and touch upon the discussions about these interesting tumors using questions and answers format.

PRCC account for up to 15% of all RCC. This diagnosis became accepted in the late 1990s. What is the history of renal cell carcinoma classification and how the PRCC was accepted as a distinct entity?

Papillary architecture is a morphology seen in both malignant and benign lesions in many organs, and many are named in reference to this architecture. The term "papillary carcinoma" as a subtype of RCC dates back to late 1960s when reports of renal papillary-tubular adenocarcinomas emerged as tumours with distinctive radiologic and histologic

Oluwayomi Oyedeji MD, Department of Pathology and Laboratory Medicine, Henry Ford Hospital, Detroit, MI, USA
Email: Oyedejioluwayomi@gmail.com

Sean R Williamson MD, Pathology and Laboratory Medicine Institute, Cleveland Clinic Foundation, Cleveland, OH, USA
Email: williamson.sean@outlook.com

Khaleel I Al-Obaidy MD, Department of Pathology and Laboratory Medicine, Henry Ford Health, Detroit, MI, USA
Email: dr.khaleel.alobaidy@gmail.com (for correspondence)

appearances [1]. However, the 1986 study by Thoenes et al was a major landmark for the foundation and identification of the now-established classifications of renal tumours. This renal tumour classification was based on the architectural and cytomorphological features, and the putative part of the nephron from which these tumours were thought to be derived [2]. The discoveries of Thoenes et al set the template for the 1996 Heidelberg and 1997 Rochester consensus classifications of the current renal epithelial tumours that led to the recognition of different renal tumours including PRCC [3–7].

Epidemiologic data may contribute to our understanding of the pathogenesis PRCC, but are the sex, race, and familial predisposition data important for diagnosis of PRCC in daily clinical practice?

Kidney and renal pelvic tumours are the 6th and 9th leading site of new cancer diagnosis for men and women, respectively, according to the American Cancer Society statistics [8,9]. PRCC shows a slight male predominance with a male-to-female ratio ranging from 2:1 to 3.5:1. A recently published multi-centred collaborative research study on renal tumours showed an overall 0.6-times lower prevalence of PRCC in women [8,10]. Additionally, in a pan-cancer analysis study of the cancer statistics in the United States, there was a general male predominance and worse prognosis of malignancies involving the kidney [9]. Several studies have shown a racial predisposition to PRCC, where African–Americans have a higher predisposition to developing PRCC [11,12]. The study from the Surveillance, Epidemiology, and End Results Program of the National Cancer Institute (SEER) data showed a higher incidence of PRCC in patients of African ancestry as well as higher mortality than in Caucasians [9].

Are PRCC more often multifocal or bilateral or linked to certain hereditary conditions than other renal cancers?

The majority of PRCC are sporadic; however, clusters of familial and hereditary forms of PRCC exist in which tumours are likely to show multifocality and/or bilaterality as well as higher tendencies for earlier age presentation than sporadic PRCC. The most common example of these is the hereditary papillary renal carcinoma syndrome (HPRC) which results from a germline mutation in the *c-MET* proto-oncogene at chromosome 7q31, leading to predisposition to the development of numerous and often bilateral PRCC [13,14]. In this syndrome, there is approximately 90% likelihood of developing PRCC by the age of 80 years [15]. Therefore, the presence of bilateral and multifocal tumours may prompt a consideration of hereditary germline mutations in the appropriate clinical settings [16,17]. However, multiple PRCC is also relatively common in the setting of end-stage renal disease/chronic renal disease, which is likely much more common than HPRC.

PRCC were for some time subdivided into two groups and reported as type 1 or 2 PRCC. Are there important differences between type 1 and 2 PRCC? Why was that classification abandoned?

In 1997, Dr Delahunt and Dr Eble studied 105 PRCC and divided them into two groups, types 1 and type 2, based on their morphologic characteristics (**Figure 8.1**). Type 1 tumours

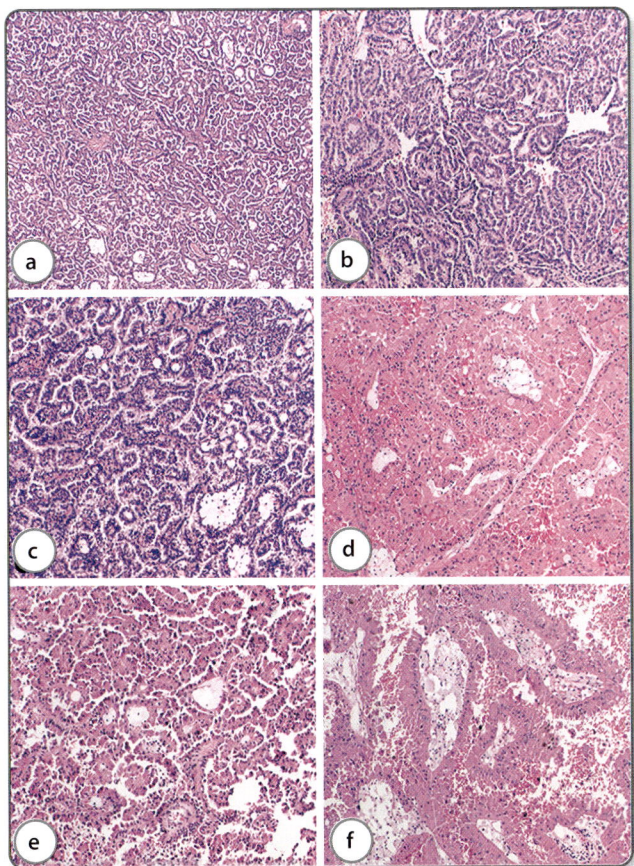

Figure 8.1 Classic papillary renal cell carcinoma. (a to c) Representative images showing the classic papillary renal cell carcinoma "type 1" morphology where there are multiple papillae that are covered by a single layer of basophilic appearing neoplastic cells with scant amount of pale cytoplasm and small nuclei. Few of the fibrovascular core contains tight aggregates of foamy macrophages. (d to f) Representative images showing the classic papillary renal cell carcinoma "type 2" with numerous papillary and compact tubular architectures that are formed of larger neoplastic cells with abundant eosinophilic cytoplasm and enlarged hyperchromatic nuclei. Foamy histiocytes are present within the fibrovascular cores as well.

were noted to have papillary architecture, lined by a single layer of cells with scanty basophilic cytoplasm containing a low nuclear grade. Type 2 tumours were noted to have complex papillary architecture, lined by pseudostratified layers of cells with abundant eosinophilic cytoplasm, typically with higher nuclear grade [18]. PRCCs show frequent copy number alterations including gain of chromosome 7 and 17 and/or, loss of Y chromosome as well as c-*MET* mutations [19]. It is worth knowing that distinction between type 1 and 2 may be difficult to make because of the occurrence of mixture of type 1 and 2 architectural and cytological patterns in some tumours [20].

In the recent years, there was a continuous debate regarding the true prognostic significance of subtyping PRCC into type 1 and 2. Many studies including the original study by Drs Delahunt and Eble support the notion that PRCC type 2 has more aggressive clinical course when compared to PRCC type 1 [20–22]. However, recent studies have shown that subtyping of the PRCC into type 1 and 2 is not an independent risk factor for overall survival, whereas the nuclear grade and pathological stage of the tumour are more important prognosticators than the morphologic subtype [20,23,24]. Additionally, advancement in the approach of diagnosing renal tumours has been developed in recent years and it is now known that RCCs with papillary architecture show significant tumour heterogeneity in both architectural patterns and cytologic features. A number of tumours that were once considered PRCC type 2 are now considered independent types of RCCs, including the prime example of fumarate hydratase deficient RCC and MITF family translocation renal cell carcinomas (*TFE3*-rearranged or *TFEB*-rearranged/amplified) family translocation carcinomas [25,26]. Therefore, it is no longer recommended to subdivide PRCC into types 1 and 2 [26–28].

These changes have been recognised in current 2022 WHO classification of renal tumours, however, many tumours have been regarded as part of the morphological spectrum of PRCCs, including: Papillary renal neoplasm with reverse polarity (PRNRP) **(Figure 8.2)** (with characteristic recurrent *KRAS* mutations), biphasic hyalinising psammomatous RCC **(Figure 8.3)** (with characteristic recurrent *NF2* mutations), Warthin-like PRCC **(Figure 8.4)**, and biphasic PRCC (also known as alveolar/squamoid PRCC, **Figure 8.5**) [29–35]. It is also worth noting that some of these will likely become distinct entities given their unique molecular alterations in future classification schemes. Ultimately, not all kidney masses with papillary or tubular-papillary growth patterns are PRCCs, and alternative diagnostic consideration of other types of RCC should always be entertained in the context of overall clinical, morphological, immunophenotypic, and molecular profiles.

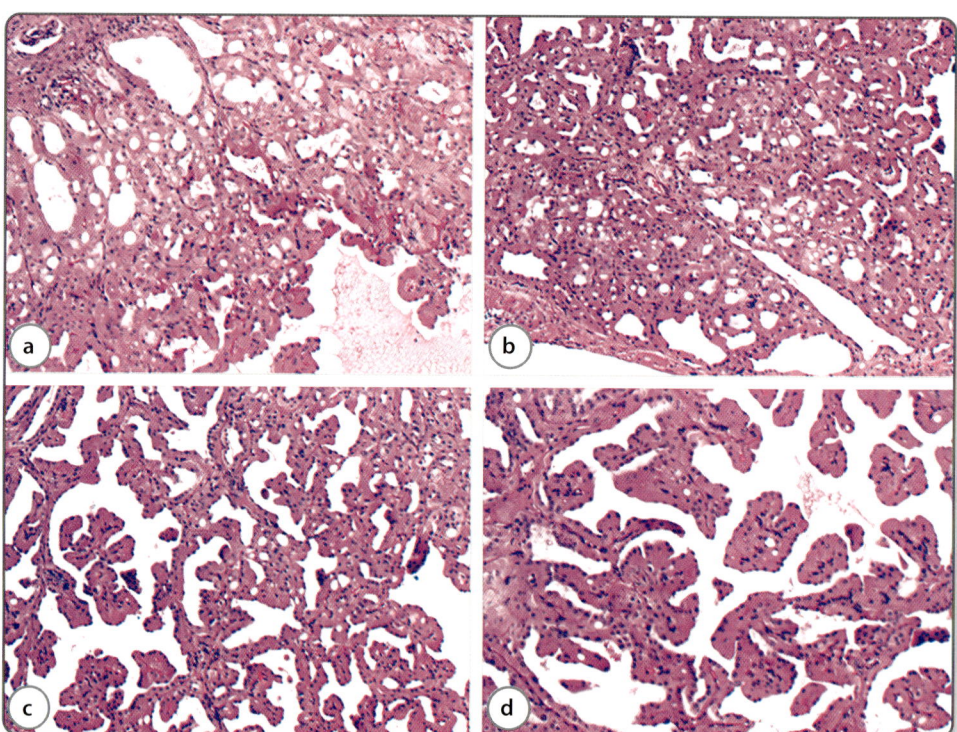

Figure 8.2 Papillary renal neoplasm with reverse polarity. (a to d) Representative images showing a low-grade tumour, formed of thin papillary and tubular structures composed of cuboidal cells with eosinophilic finely granular cytoplasm and the nuclei that are characteristically well spaced and located at the apical surface opposite to the basement membrane.

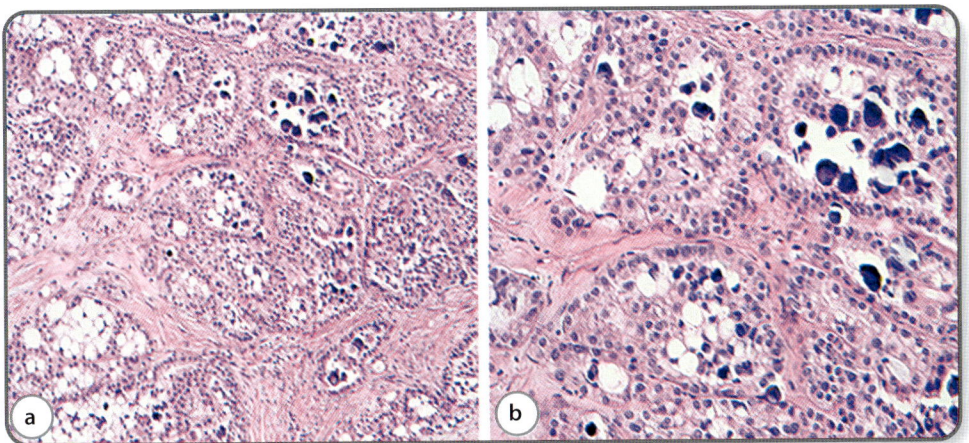

Figure 8.3 Biphasic hyalinising psammomatous renal cell carcinoma. (a and b) Representative images showing the tumour demonstrating tubular and small papillary structures, separated by hyalinised stroma. A biphasic appearance formed of larger epithelial cells with vesicular chromatin and well-developed pale cytoplasm and smaller cells with darker condensed chromatin and minimal cytoplasm. Psammomatous calcifications are readily seen.

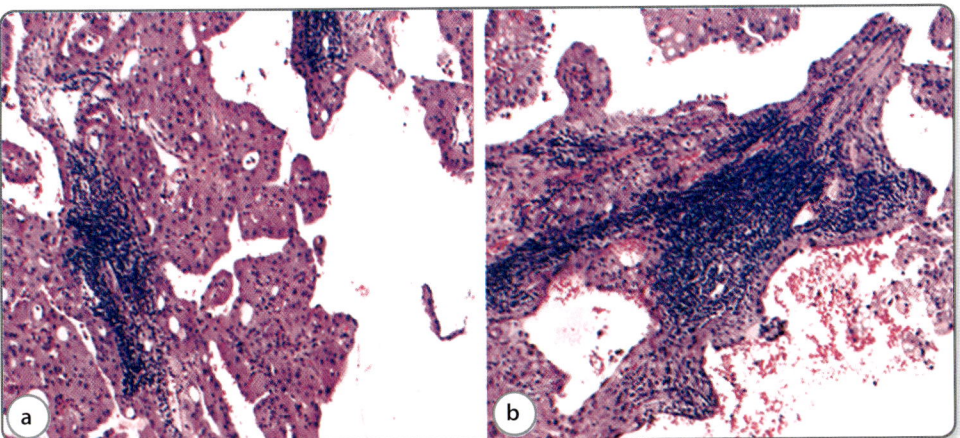

Figure 8.4 Warthin-like papillary renal cell carcinoma. (a and b) Representative images showing a tumour with papillary architecture that has dense lymphoid infiltrate within the fibrovascular cores. The cells covering the papillae are large, oncocytic and polygonal reminiscent to that seen in salivary gland Warthin tumour.

What is the diagnostic importance of other microscopic findings such as psammoma bodies, foamy macrophages, and similar secondary changes?

Closely and densely packed papillae/tubules can be interpreted as a solid pattern of PRCC, which may mimic metanephric adenoma. However, the presence of uniformly low-grade small nuclei and positive reactions for WT1 and CD57 help to confirm the diagnosis of the

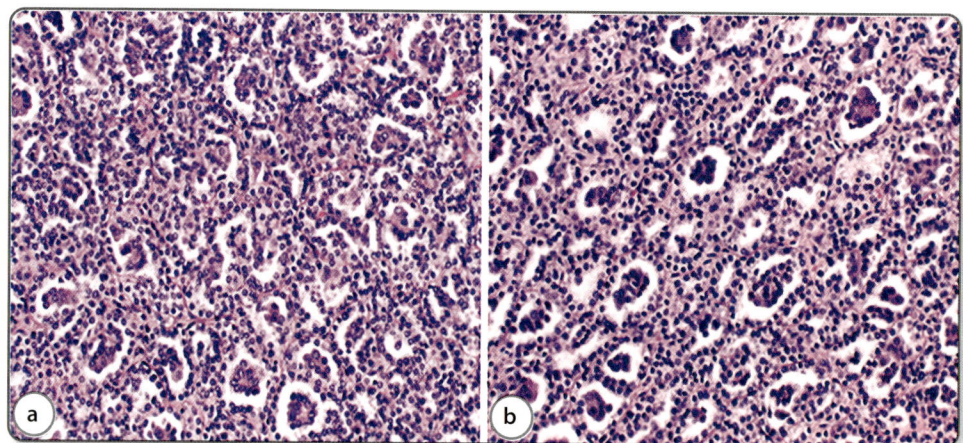

Figure 8.5 Biphasic squamoid alveolar renal cell carcinoma. (a and b) Representative images showing distinctly biphasic cell populations formed of compact papillary architecture displaying dual squamoid nests surrounded by smaller cells with uniform nuclei, in what appears to be an alveolar or glomeruloid structures. *Note:* True squamous cell differentiation is not present.

latter. Similarly, psammomatous calcifications, foamy macrophages, hemosiderin-laden macrophages, hemosiderin deposition in tumour cells can occur in other renal tumours, therefore, although these might be helpful for the diagnosis of PRCC, they are not entirely specific and their presence is not required for PRCC diagnosis [20]. Additionally, a recent study also suggested that the presence microcystic architecture (characterised by multiple epithelial-lined cystic spaces containing papillary tumour) in the classic type 1 PRCC may potentially correspond to an aggressive histologic morphology in PRCC [28].

Are papillary renal cell carcinomas routinely graded, using WHO/ISUP (International Society of Urological Pathology)?

The old-grading system (Fuhrman grading), which evaluates nuclear size, nuclear shape and nucleolar features, has been in use for many years. However, Fuhrman grading suffered drawbacks by having a low-to-moderate intra- and inter-observer reproducibility and a questionable clinical utility in prognosticating tumour outcomes [5,36–38]. The new WHO/ISUP grading system, introduced at the conclusion of the ISUP consensus meeting in Vancouver in 2012 and adopted by the WHO, hence the name WHO/ISUP, is recommended for grading of clear cell and papillary RCC [39]. This grading system correlates well with prognosis for clear cell and papillary PRCC. It is a four-tier grading system (Grade 1 to 4), which includes degree of nucleolar prominence at different power field and the presence of extreme pleomorphism, sarcomatous or rhabdoid morphology that defines grade 4 [39]. The WHO/ISUP grading has an edge over the Fuhrman grading due to its better reproducibility among pathologists and its better clinical relevance [25]. The prognostic utility of WHO/ISUP grading in the emerging and new tumour entities with papillary lesions are still being studied due to the impurity of cases that have been once included under the umbrella of PRCC, resulting in conflicting outcomes and therefore more studies are needed to assess the grading system utility.

Minor papillary components can be found in other RCC. Which RCC most often have a papillary component? Is that important in practice? Are there actually hybrid tumours composed of PRCC and other types of renal carcinomas?

Papillary architectural pattern is neither sensitive nor specific to PRCC and can be seen in many renal tumours when generously sampled [17,20,40]. Some of these tumours were acknowledged by the 2022 WHO classification of renal tumours as distinct entities, whereas others were included as subtypes of PRCC. These include most of the molecularly defined renal carcinomas such as *TFE3*-rearranged RCC, *TFEB*-rearranged/amplified RCC, *ALK*-rearranged RCCs, *ELOC* (*TCEB1*)-mutated RCC, FH-deficient RCC or *SMARCB1*-deficient renal medullary carcinoma. Other renal tumours with papillary architecture but showing features of other recognised subtypes of RCC, such as clear cell papillary renal cell tumour, acquired cystic disease-associated RCC, tubulocystic RCC, collecting duct carcinoma and PRNRP, do commonly have papillary morphology [20]. All these tumours could cause diagnostic challenges/pitfalls as they possess different biologic behaviours that span the indolent/low-grade to low malignant potential to highly aggressive clinical behaviour [17].

What are the common immunohistochemical features of PRCCs? How common are PRCC that do not show such predominant or expected immunohistochemical features?

Immunohistochemistry is an important supplementary study that could help in differentiating the subtypes of PRCC including the emerging variants. PRCC tumours are frequently immunoreactive for low molecular weight keratin and CD10 in >90% of tumours. Keratin-7 is positive in >80% of what has traditionally been classified as the classical PRCC type 1, but only around 20% of the historic PRCC type 2, given the variable morphologic features of the latter and tendency of eosinophilic tumours to show minimal or negative keratin-7 [28].

Alpha-methylacyl-CoA racemase (AMACR) and vimentin immunoreactivity are also identified in the majority of PRCC [33,41]. Other pertinent negative markers include carbonic anhydrase-9, GATA3, and fumarate hydratase (normal/retained staining), as well as other molecular specific markers, such as TFE3 immunohistochemistry, are important to rule out other diagnoses.

Are the cytogenetic data such as gain and loss of some chromosomes important for the diagnosis in dubious cases?

No cytogenetic alterations are entirely sensitive or specific to all types of PRCC. However, PRCCs often show frequent chromosomal alterations that could assist in differentiating PRCC from other tumours with papillary morphology, in tandem with appropriate morphological evaluation. Historically, gain of chromosome-17 was reported in approximately 70% of sporadic historic PRCC type 1, whereas aberrations in chromosome 1p, 3p, 5q, monosomy 2, and loss of 9p were more often seen in historic PRCC type 2 [42–45]. Therefore, cytogenetic analysis can be helpful in cases that have ambiguous papillary morphology. Additionally, some examples of clear cell RCC with high-grade morphology may show papillary like structures. In such cases, finding these chromosomal alterations will support the diagnosis of PRCC, whereas finding a deletion or loss of heterozygosity (LOH) of chromosome 3p will support the diagnosis of clear cell renal cell carcinoma (ccRCC) [42,46].

Are the molecular pathology findings of importance for distinguishing PRCCs from other RCC, or for that matter subclassifying PRCC?

Historic PRCC type 1 shows frequent alteration of the *c-MET* pathway, whereas PRCC type 2 has more complex molecular profiles, without specific molecular alterations [47]. However, *MET* alterations are more common in the HPRC setting and less frequent in the sporadic setting. Molecular alterations seen in PRCC type 2 include *CDKN2A, SETD2, BAP1, PBRM1* mutations as well as CpG Island methylator phenotype. Based on these molecular data, it was suggested that type 2 consists of at least three subtypes [19,47]. Additionally, in a study by Saleeb et al where integrated morphology, immunophenotypes and molecular approach was utilised, PRCCs were divided into four subtypes. PRCC type 1 was enriched in *WNT,* Hedgehog, and Notch signalling pathway alteration and PRCC type 2 showed alterations in *MTOR, VEGF* and *HIF* signalling pathways, PRCC NOS showed alteration in the *ABCC2* pathway and finally PRCC-oncocytic low-grade subtype [48]. The latter was then found to have distinctive morphologic, immunohistochemical and molecular profile than classic PRCC as described by Al-Obaidy et al, and was relabelled "papillary renal neoplasm with reverse polarity (PRNRP)" and included as provisional entity (**Figure 8.2**) [31–33]. This diversity in molecular alterations has led to the recommendation against the historic subtyping of PRCC into types 1 and 2 by the current 2022 WHO classification system. However, finding a recurrent genetic alteration is a helpful diagnostic tool in supporting the diagnosis of some of the tumour entities included in the spectrum of PRCC in the current 2022 WHO classification system, such as recurrent *KRAS* mutations in PRNRP and recurrent *NF2* mutations in the biphasic hyalinising psammomatous RCC.

Overall, do PRCCs have a better prognosis than classical clear cell RCCs? Is that true for the variants as well?

According to the most recent 2022 WHO classifications of renal tumours, PRCC is known to have a favourable biological behaviour and prognosis when compared to other histological subtypes of RCC such as clear cell RCC; however, the heterogeneous nature of PRCC with its different subtypes, variable clinicopathologic features, and genetic changes makes it difficult to prognosticate. When PRCC was first subdivided into types 1 and 2, it was observed that type 1 has a better prognosis than type 2, and many studies have shown that clinically localised type 2 has unfavourable prognosis and higher metastatic potential when compared to type 1 PRCC [18,23,49,50]. These findings are now being debated, and recent studies have shown that what has been historically categorised as type 2, had overall higher WHO/ISUP nucleolar grade which may explain the worse prognosis, and therefore, subtyping PRCC into types 1 and 2 has no influence on patients' outcome when adjusting for disease stage and other classical prognostic features [24]. This discrepancy may, in part, reflect that a fraction of the historical type 2 PRCC represents FH-deficient RCC, which is highly aggressive and associated with the inherited hereditary leiomyomatosis and RCC syndrome.

CONCLUSION

The evolving classification of renal neoplasia has touched many tumor entities, including the papillary renal cell carcinoma, which has been subclassified into types 1 and 2 based on the histomorphologic features. This sub-classification was no longer recommended by the current 2022 WHO classification of renal tumors as many tumors were no longer considered part of the PRCC classification. However, four morphological patterns were recognized, including two provisional entities, papillary renal neoplasm with reverse polarity and biphasic hyalinization and psammomatous renal cell carcinoma, which both have distinct morphologic and molecular (*KRAS* and *NF2*, respectively) characteristics.

Key points for clinical practice

- Current renal tumour classification is based on architectural and cytomorphological features, relative to the putative part of the nephron from which these tumours were thought to be derived. This has now been extended and completed using molecular (genetic) criteria.
- Most PRCC are sporadic; however, clusters of familial and hereditary forms of PRCC exist.
- The diversity in molecular alterations in PRCC has led to the 2022 WHO recommendation against previously used subtyping of PRCC.
- The subdivision of PRCC into types 1 and 2 has been abandoned in WHO 2022; newly identified variants are PRNRP, biphasic hyalinising psammomatous RCC, Warthin-like PRCC, and biphasic PRCC.
- Papillary architectural pattern is neither sensitive nor specific to PRCC and can be seen in many renal tumours (including molecularly defined renal carcinomas such as *TFE3*-rearranged RCC, *TFEB*-rearranged/amplified RCC, *ALK*-rearranged RCCs, *ELOC* (*TCEB1*)-mutated RCC, FH-deficient RCC or SMARCB1-deficient renal medullary carcinoma, and tuberous sclerosis-associated RCC).
- The WHO/ISUP grading system is recommended for grading of clear cell and papillary RCC.
- PRCC has a more favourable biological behaviour and prognosis than other histological subtypes of RCC; however, variable clinicopathologic features and genetic changes of various subtypes of PRCC have not allowed clear indications as to prognosis.

REFERENCES

1. Weiss RM, Becker JA, Davidson AJ, et al. Angiographic appearance of renal papillary-tubular adenocarcinomas. J Urol 1969; 102:661–664.
2. Thoenes W, Storkel S, Rumpelt HJ, et al. Cytomorphological typing of renal cell carcinoma--a new approach. Eur Urol 1990; 18:6–9.
3. Kovacs G, Akhtar M, Beckwith BJ, et al. The Heidelberg classification of renal cell tumours. J Pathol 1997; 183:131–133.
4. Storkel S, Eble JN, Adlakha K, et al. Classification of renal cell carcinoma: Workgroup No. 1. Union Internationale Contre le Cancer (UICC) and the American Joint Committee on Cancer (AJCC). Cancer 1997; 80:987–989.
5. Delahunt B. Histopathologic prognostic indicators for renal cell carcinoma. Semin Diagn Pathol 1998; 15:68–76.

6.   Delahunt B, Velickovic M, Grebe SK. Evolving classification of renal cell neoplasia. Expert Rev Anticancer Ther 2001; 1:576–584.
7.   Delahunt B, Eble JN, Board of Education of the Royal College of Pathologists of A. Renal cell neoplasia. Pathology 2002; 34:13–20.
8.   Siegel RL, Miller KD, Fuchs HE, et al. Cancer Statistics, 2021. CA Cancer J Clin 2021; 71:7–33.
9.   Dong M, Cioffi G, Wang J, et al. Sex Differences in Cancer Incidence and Survival: A Pan-Cancer Analysis. Cancer Epidemiol Biomarkers Prev 2020; 29:1389–1397.
10.   May M, Aziz A, Zigeuner R, et al. Gender differences in clinicopathological features and survival in surgically treated patients with renal cell carcinoma: an analysis of the multicenter CORONA database. World J Urol 2013; 31:1073–1080.
11.   Schmidt LS, Nickerson ML, Angeloni D, et al. Early onset hereditary papillary renal carcinoma: germline missense mutations in the tyrosine kinase domain of the met proto-oncogene. J Urol 2004; 172:1256–1261.
12.   Olshan AF, Kuo TM, Meyer AM, et al. Racial difference in histologic subtype of renal cell carcinoma. Cancer Med 2013; 2:744–749.
13.   Lubensky IA, Schmidt L, Zhuang Z et al. Hereditary and sporadic papillary renal carcinomas with c-met mutations share a distinct morphological phenotype. Am. J. Pathol. 1999; 155; 517–526.
14.   Comperat E, Cheng L. Urologic Surgical Pathology, 4th edition. Amsterdam, Netherlands, Elsevier; 2020.
15.   Al-Obaidy KI, Alruwaii ZI, Williamson SR, et al. The pathological and molecular genetic landscape of the hereditary renal cancer predisposition syndromes. Histopathology 2022; 81:15–31.
16.   Tickoo SK, Reuter VE. Differential diagnosis of renal tumors with papillary architecture. Adv Anat Pathol 2011; 18:120–132.
17.   Athanazio DA, Amorim LS, da Cunha IW, et al. Classification of renal cell tumors – current concepts and use of ancillary tests: recommendations of the Brazilian Society of Pathology. Surg Exper Pathol 2021; 4:4.
18.   Delahunt B, Eble JN. Papillary renal cell carcinoma: a clinicopathologic and immunohistochemical study of 105 tumors. Mod Pathol 1997; 10:537–544.
19.   Cancer Genome Atlas Research Network, Linehan WM, Spellman PT, et al. Comprehensive Molecular Characterization of Papillary Renal-Cell Carcinoma. N Engl J Med 2016; 374:135–145.
20.   Lobo J, Ohashi R, Helmchen BM, et al. The Morphological Spectrum of Papillary Renal Cell Carcinoma and Prevalence of Provisional/Emerging Renal Tumor Entities with Papillary Growth. Biomedicines 2021; 9:1418.
21.   Allory Y, Ouazana D, Boucher E, et al. Papillary renal cell carcinoma. Prognostic value of morphological subtypes in a clinicopathologic study of 43 cases. Virchows Arch 2003; 442:336–342.
22.   Fernandes DS, Lopes JM. Pathology, therapy and prognosis of papillary renal carcinoma. Future Oncol 2015; 11:121–132.
23.   Wong ECL, Di Lena R, Breau RH, et al. Morphologic subtyping as a prognostic predictor for survival in papillary renal cell carcinoma: Type 1 vs. type 2. Urol Oncol 2019; 37:721–726.
24.   Murugan P, Jia L, Dinatale RG, et al. Papillary renal cell carcinoma: a single institutional study of 199 cases addressing classification, clinicopathologic and molecular features, and treatment outcome. Mod Pathol 2022; 35:825–835.
25.   Warren AY, Harrison D. WHO/ISUP classification, grading and pathological staging of renal cell carcinoma: standards and controversies. World J Urol 2018; 36:1913–1926.
26.   Moch H, Amin MB, Berney DM, et al. The 2022 World Health Organization Classification of Tumours of the Urinary System and Male Genital Organs-Part A: Renal, Penile, and Testicular Tumours. Eur Urol 2022; 82:458–468.
27.   Alaggio R, Amador C, Anagnostopoulos I, et al. The 5th edition of the World Health Organization Classification of Haematolymphoid Tumours: Lymphoid Neoplasms. Leukemia 2022; 36:1720–1748.
28.   Chan E, Stohr BA, Butler RS, et al. Papillary Renal Cell Carcinoma With Microcystic Architecture Is Strongly Associated With Extrarenal Invasion and Metastatic Disease. Am J Surg Pathol 2022; 46:392–403.

29. Argani P, Reuter VE, Eble JN, et al. Biphasic Hyalinizing Psammomatous Renal Cell Carcinoma (BHP RCC): A Distinctive Neoplasm Associated With Somatic NF2 Mutations. Am J Surg Pathol 2020; 44:901–916.

30. Skenderi F, Ulamec M, Vanecek T, et al. Warthin-like papillary renal cell carcinoma: Clinicopathologic, morphologic, immunohistochemical and molecular genetic analysis of 11 cases. Ann Diagn Pathol 2017; 27:48–56.

31. Al-Obaidy KI, Saleeb RM, Trpkov K, et al. Recurrent KRAS mutations are early events in the development of papillary renal neoplasm with reverse polarity. Mod Pathol 2022; 35:1279–1286

32. Al-Obaidy KI, Eble JN, Nassiri M, et al. Recurrent KRAS mutations in papillary renal neoplasm with reverse polarity. Mod Pathol 2020; 33:1157–1164.

33. Al-Obaidy KI, Eble JN, Cheng L, et al. Papillary Renal Neoplasm With Reverse Polarity: A Morphologic, Immunohistochemical, and Molecular Study. Am J Surg Pathol 2019; 43:1099–1111.

34. Petersson F, Bulimbasic S, Hes O, et al. Biphasic alveolosquamoid renal carcinoma: a histomorphological, immunohistochemical, molecular genetic, and ultrastructural study of a distinctive morphologic variant of renal cell carcinoma. Ann Diagn Pathol 2012; 16:459–469.

35. Denize T, Just PA, Sibony M, et al. MET alterations in biphasic squamoid alveolar papillary renal cell carcinomas and clinicopathological features. Mod Pathol 2021; 34:647–659.

36. Fuhrman SA, Lasky LC, Limas C. Prognostic significance of morphologic parameters in renal cell carcinoma. Am J Surg Pathol 1982; 6:655–663.

37. Medeiros LJ, Jones EC, Aizawa S, et al. Grading of renal cell carcinoma: Workgroup No. 2. Union Internationale Contre le Cancer and the American Joint Committee on Cancer (AJCC). Cancer 1997; 80:990–991.

38. Al-Aynati M, Chen V, Salama S, et al. Interobserver and intraobserver variability using the Fuhrman grading system for renal cell carcinoma. Arch Pathol Lab Med 2003; 127:593–596.

39. Srigley JR, Delahunt B, Eble JN, et al. The International Society of Urological Pathology (ISUP) Vancouver Classification of Renal Neoplasia. Am J Surg Pathol 2013; 37:1469–1489.

40. Saleeb RM, Brimo F, Farag M, et al. Toward Biological Subtyping of Papillary Renal Cell Carcinoma With Clinical Implications Through Histologic, Immunohistochemical, and Molecular Analysis. Am J Surg Pathol 2017; 41:1618–1629.

41. Tretiakova MS, Sahoo S, Takahashi M, et al. Expression of alpha-methylacyl-CoA racemase in papillary renal cell carcinoma. Am J Surg Pathol 2004; 28:69–76.

42. Quddus MB, Pratt N, Nabi G. Chromosomal aberrations in renal cell carcinoma: An overview with implications for clinical practice. Urol Ann 2019; 11:6–14.

43. Corless CL, Aburatani H, Fletcher JA, et al. Papillary renal cell carcinoma: quantitation of chromosomes 7 and 17 by FISH, analysis of chromosome 3p for LOH, and DNA ploidy. Diagn Mol Pathol 1996; 5:53–64.

44. Jiang F, Richter J, Schraml P, et al. Chromosomal imbalances in papillary renal cell carcinoma: genetic differences between histological subtypes. Am J Pathol 1998; 153:1467–1473.

45. Kovacs G, Fuzesi L, Emanual A, et al. Cytogenetics of papillary renal cell tumors. Genes Chromosomes Cancer 1991; 3:249–255.

46. Togo Y, Yoshikawa Y, Suzuki T, et al. Genomic profiling of the genes on chromosome 3p in sporadic clear cell renal cell carcinoma. Int J Oncol 2016; 48:1571–1580.

47. Alaghehbandan R, Perez Montiel D, Luis AS, et al. Molecular Genetics of Renal Cell Tumors: A Practical Diagnostic Approach. Cancers 2019; 12:85.

48. Saleeb RM, Plant P, Tawedrous E, et al. Integrated Phenotypic/Genotypic Analysis of Papillary Renal Cell Carcinoma Subtypes: Identification of Prognostic Markers, Cancer-related Pathways, and Implications for Therapy. Eur Urol Focus 2018; 4:740–748.

49. Simone G, Tuderti G, Ferriero M, et al. Papillary type 2 versus clear cell renal cell carcinoma: Survival outcomes. Eur J Surg Oncol 2016; 42:1744–1750.

50. Kim KH, You D, Jeong IG, et al. Type II papillary histology predicts poor outcome in patients with renal cell carcinoma and vena cava thrombus. BJU Int 2012; 110:E673–E678.

Chapter 9

Breast implant related lymphomas

Mario L Marques-Piubelli, Sofia A Garces, Roberto N Miranda

INTRODUCTION

How common are lymphomas of the breast?

Lymphomas of the breast are rare. In perspective, out of 1.5 million of malignancies excluding cutaneous carcinomas, that are diagnosed each year in the United States, approximately 5%, or 80,000 patients are affected with lymphoma, which is the seventh most common malignancy [1] and some 2,000 patients are affected by breast lymphoma. In comparison, almost 300,000 women are diagnosed with breast cancer in the USA each year. The breast can be the site of primary lymphoma but it can also be involved and secondary or disseminated lymphomas and leukaemias. When we say "the breast" we usually are referring to the breast parenchyma, that is breast ducts and lobules. During the last two decades a new subset of lymphomas has taken the limelight: Breast implant associated (BIA) lymphomas, which develop around the breast implants and are usually contained by a fibrous capsule [2–4].

What are the most common histopathologic forms of lymphoma involving the breast?

The vast majority (~90%) of lymphomas affecting primarily the breast are lymphomas derived from B lymphocytes, while lymphomas derived from T lymphocytes account for <10% of cases [5]. The most frequent lymphomas are diffuse large B-cell lymphoma and extranodal marginal zone lymphoma [5]. Secondary involvement by systemic lymphomas includes a wide array of histologic subtypes including precursor B-cell and T-lymphoblastic

Mario L Marques-Piubelli MD, Department of Translational Molecular Pathology, The University of Texas MD Anderson Cancer Center, Houston, TX, USA
Email: MLPiubelli@mdanderson.org

Sofia A Garces MD, Department of Hematopathology, The University of Texas MD Anderson Cancer Center, Houston, TX,USA
Email: SGarces@mdanderson.org

Roberto N Miranda MD, Department of Hematopathology, The University of Texas MD Anderson Cancer Center, Houston, TX, USA
Email: Roberto.miranda@mdanderson.org (for correspondence

leukaemia/lymphomas, as well as mature B- and T-cell lymphomas such as follicular lymphoma, Burkitt lymphoma and marginal zone lymphoma.

SILICONE BREAST IMPLANT RELATED LYMPHOMAS

Silicone implant related lymphomas are a relatively new iatrogenic clinicopathologic entity. How common are these lymphomas?

The initial estimate of incidence of this lymphoma in 2008 was 1 in 300,000 persons [6]. However, this figure was reassessed in 2018, and the current estimates of its incidence are 1 in 10,000 to 1 in 30,000 [7]. Thus, this lymphoma that was considered as extremely rare a decade ago, has been recognised more frequently, and currently, its descriptive frequency is considered as "uncommon". Estimates vary in different parts of the world because of the variability of factors involved in assessing risk and diagnosis. It has been estimated that approximately 35 million women have breast implants world-wide and 1,200 of these will be diagnosed with breast implant associated anaplastic large cell lymphoma (BIA-ALCL). Using simple mathematics, one may calculate that 1:30,000 persons with implants may get BIA-ALCL. Essentially, all of these neoplasms were found in association with textured but not smooth shell implants, more accurate estimates should consider the surface of implants. In this context, the incidence of BIA-ALCL has been as high as 1:350 among women who received textured implants, usually for reconstructive surgery, who in addition were also followed closely [8]. There are no bona fide cases of BIA-ALCL arising around smooth breast implants.

A few historical facts: How were breast silicone implant related lymphomas initially discovered? When were they defined as a specific clinicopathologic entity?

BIA-ALCL was first reported in 1997 [9,10] although we believe the first case was inadvertently published in 1996 as a primary effusion lymphoma, an human herpesvirus-8 (HHV-8) associated lymphoma [11]. Keech and Creech [9] reported a 41-year-old woman who received saline-filled textured implants 5 years prior, with unilateral periprosthetic mass and axillary lymphadenopathy, classified as ALCL and treated with chemotherapy (CHOP). A short follow-up showed complete remission. The authors wondered whether ALCL was caused by the implant. Less than 10 cases were published in the next 10 years. Roden et al. [12] published the first series of cases. It included four patients who presented with periprosthetic effusion but no mass. All had capsulectomy, one received chemotherapy, one radiation therapy, and one did not receive adjuvant therapy. After a follow-up period of 13 months for three patients, all achieved complete remission, and Roden et al [12] suggested that the disease is indolent and only reminiscent of a lymphoproliferative disorder. The first estimate on the incidence of this lymphoma was published in 2008 by De Jong et al [6]. The United States Food and Drug Administration (US-FDA) in 2011 published an excerpt alerting of the possible association between breast implants and ALCL [13]. The World Health Organization included BIA-ALCL as a provisional entity in 2017 [14], and as a definitive entity in 2019 [2], which was then confirmed in 2022 [15].

Do these lymphomas develop more often following cosmetic implant surgery or post cancer treatment reconstructive implant placement?

There is no consensus because of the lack of firm epidemiologic data. However, it is suspected that the lymphoma occurs equally in patients who received the implant for cosmetic reasons or in patients with reconstructive surgery after breast cancer.

What are the identifiable risk factors in women with breast implants? Does the risk of lymphoma depend on the type of breast implant?

There are no known risk factors for developing this form of lymphoma. Germ-line *BRCA* and *TP53* mutations have been detected in a small subset of patients, but an inherently higher risk for developing BIA-ALCL in these patients has not been established. On the other hand, cancer susceptibility is an undefined term for BIA-ALCL at this time, for which we lack criteria to assign risk to defined populations.

Texturing of the surface of the implant has been established as a determining risk factor for developing BIA-ALCL [16]. Some researchers claim the roughest the implant surface, the most likely patients may develop BIA-ALCL [17]. By contrast, no bona fide cases of BIA-ALCL have been reported in patients who had only smooth implants.

How much time after implantation do such lymphomas develop?

The range is between 2 years and >30 years, and the median time is 8–10 years [3]. Approximately 95% of tumours are unilateral, and it is extremely rare that both breasts are clinically affected. However, when the contralateral implant and capsule are removed, up to 5% of patients may have BIA-ALCL on that side as well. Therefore, cases reported as bilateral result from unilateral clinically manifest disease and the contralateral disease is mostly an incidental finding.

How do BIA-ALCL present clinically?

The most common presentation is a periprosthetic effusion, wrongly called "seroma", which occurs in approximately 70% of cases. About 20% present with a tumour mass, many of which also have regional lymphadenopathy, and approximately 5% of cases are discovered incidentally while patients are evaluated for other reasons [3,18]. It is also possible that some cases present with effusion and tumour, but many patients presenting with tumour only, have a history of effusion.

How should effusions around the implants be treated and surveyed to detect lymphoma in early stages?

Since most patients present with effusion, the most effective imaging is ultrasound. Fine-needle aspiration (FNA) of the fluid is the most effective way to diagnose the disease (**Figure 9.1**). The aspirated fluid is subjected to cytologic examination and if an immediate assessment yields suspicious cells, flow cytometry immunophenotype is recommended [19]. We recommend that the cytologic handling should include direct smear of the fluid, and if only few cells are found, we proceed with a concentration

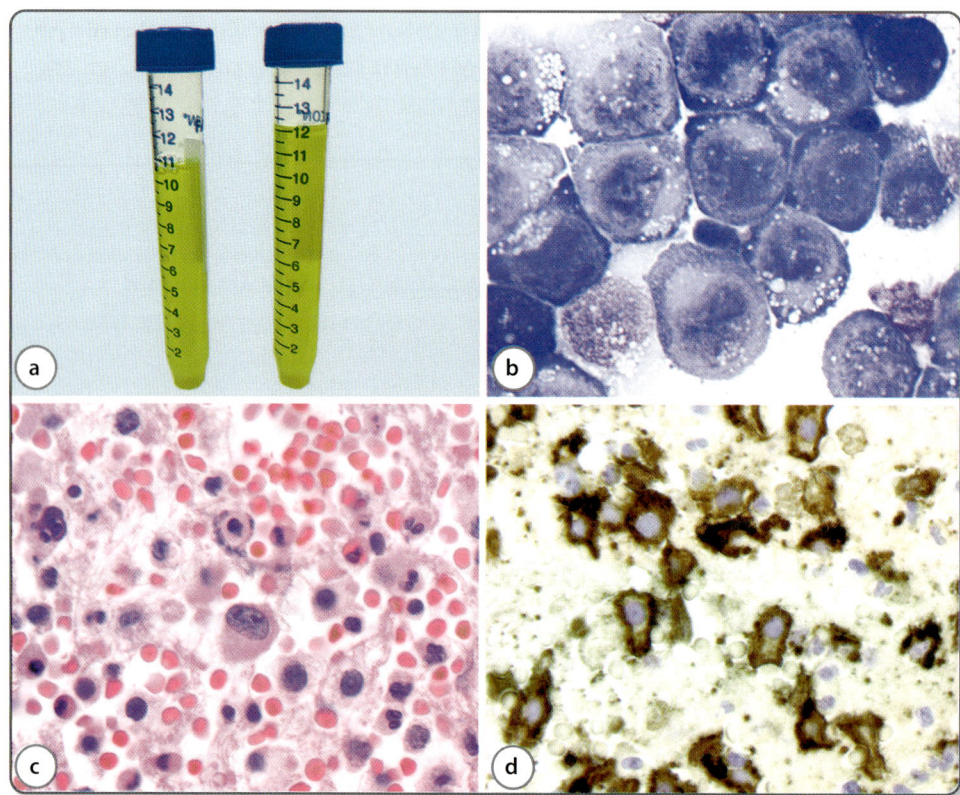

Figure 9.1 Cytologic handling and processing of periprosthetic fluids, and cytologic features of breast implant-associated anaplastic large cell lymphoma (BIA-ALCL). The periprosthetic fluid is aspirated with fine needle under ultrasound guidance. (a) Falcon tube is filled with yellowish fluid. Ideally 15 mL are sent for cytologic examination, 15 mL for flow cytometry and 15 mL for molecular testing. (b) Cytologic smear stained with Wright Giemsa shows large pleomorphic cells with abundant cytoplasm, central large, oval to lobated nuclei with prominent nucleoli. It is common the presence of small vacuoles in the cytoplasm. Wright Giemsa, 1000×. (c) Cell block section shows red cells and scattered mononuclear cells with karyorrhexis and a large cell with moderately abundant cytoplasm and oval nucleus. Haematoxylin and eosin, 400×. (d) Immunohistochemistry for CD30 in a cell block highlights numerous cells positive for CD30, consistent with ALCL. The reason many more lymphoma cells are highlighted with CD30 when compared with haematoxylin and eosin stain (c) is because dying lymphoma cells shrink and morphologically can be difficult to recognise with routine stains. Immunohistochemistry for CD30 with haematoxylin counterstain, 400×.

method. Cytologic smears are best stained with Wright Giemsa, searching for large, atypical cells (**Figure 9.1**). Cell block is recommended as a way to look for atypical cells (**Figure 9.1**). Immunohistochemical stains with the antibody to CD30 may be used to highlight any large cell (**Figure 9.1**). Flow cytometry immunophenotype is tailored to evaluate for abnormal phenotypes of T cells and their expression with CD30. The evaluation of tumour masses can also be subjected to FNA or needle core biopsy. The purpose of the initial work up is getting the diagnosis, that is followed by staging of the disease and planning for therapy [20,21].

On gross examination it is customary to classify silicone implant related lymphomas as in situ lesions and invasive lymphoma. Are these two forms of disease interrelated? Does the in-situ form progress to the invasive tumour?

It is not entirely clear whether the in-situ disease progresses to infiltrative disease or whether these are two distinct entities that carry separate risks of dissemination. However, we think that the disease has different pathologic stages of progression. We believe the disease begins around the textured breast implant while the capsule is firmly attached to the implant. When a critical number of tumour cells is reached, the capsule is detached from the implant leading to the formation of effusion [4]. This is the earliest manifestation of disease and it consists of lymphoma cells floating in the effusion in the middle of abundant necrosis that grossly appears as a fibrinoid fluid **(Figure 9.1)**. Sometimes these cells get trapped on the luminal surface of the capsule and we consider this a pathologic stage T1, or a non-invasive stage, since the lymphoma cells are clearly demarcated by stroma **(Figure 9.2)**. Some investigators call this in situ lymphoma. It is very difficult to state that the disease will remain as such or will progress if we leave the effusion untouched, or if we observe the fate of an effusion. We do not know yet if some lymphomas have an entirely benign course and will remain as effusion if we leave them untouched, or some lymphomas are deemed to become invasive or progressive. Evans et al [22] reported 10 patients who had a missed diagnosed of BIA-ALCL when they presented with effusion and had fluid examination or capsule biopsies. Upon follow up of 0.5–4 years, three patients remained with the same pathologic stage, while at least five showed progression to invasive disease. As noted above, we currently cannot determine which patients diagnosed at a non-invasive stage will develop an aggressive form of lymphoma.

Should resection of silicone implant and the breast lymphoma be accompanied by lymph node resection? How frequent is invasive BIA-ALCL accompanied by lymph node involvement?

The optimal therapy of BIA-ALCL is complete resection of the capsule and implants [20]. If the tumour is complete resected, the patient can be considered cured, even in invasive cases, as long as margins of resection are negative after complete capsulectomy. Patients with invasive disease who do not have a complete excision of disease, may need adjuvant chemotherapy. Suspicious lymph nodes should be removed and thoroughly examined searching for lymphoma. If lymph nodes are not enlarged or are not suspicious of involvement by imaging studies, there is no need to remove them, and there is no need for axillary dissection [20]. The chance that lymph nodes are involved increases with disease invasive through the capsule. Lymph nodes are rarely involved while the capsule shows non-invasive disease. In such cases, we recommend thorough gross examination of the capsule, cutting it serially while looking for and sampling areas of nodularity [23]. Invasion confined to capsule is associated with 12% chance of lymph node involvement, while invasion beyond capsule (pathologic stage T4) is associated with 38% chance of lymph node involvement [18].

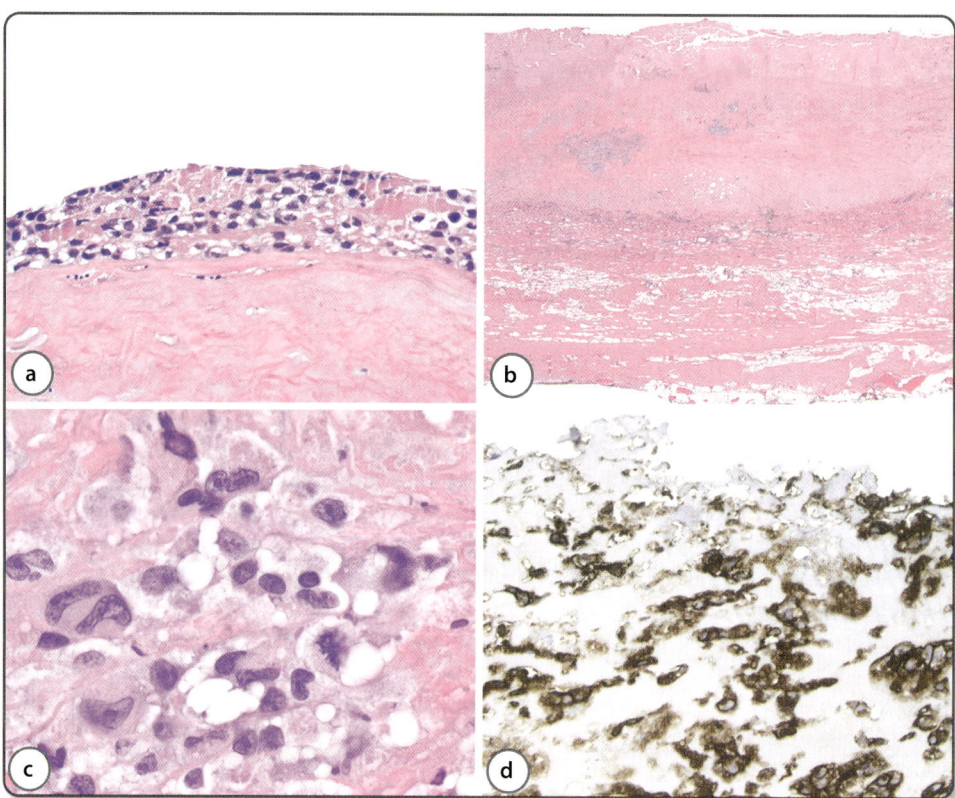

Figure 9.2 Histopathologic features of BIA-ALCL. (a) Pathologic stage I: 'On edge' section of capsule shows the luminal surface of non-invasive BIA-ALCL where a layer of lymphoma cells is distinctly separated from underlying stroma. Haematoxylin and eosin, 200×. (b) Pathologic stage III: "On edge" section of capsule shows the luminal side with extensive necrosis and scattered clusters of lymphoma cells invading into the thickness of periprosthetic capsule. The bottom of the figure shows underlying skeletal muscle and adipose tissue, which are not involved by lymphoma; inked resection at the bottom is away from lymphoma cells. (c) High magnification of ALCL cells shows that the cells are pleomorphic and surrounded by necrotic debris. Haematoxylin and eosin, 1000×. (d) Immunohistochemistry for CD30 highlights numerous lymphoma cells, strongly reactive with CD30, surrounded by acellular necrosis. Immunohistochemistry for CD30 with haematoxylin counterstain.

HISTOPATHOLOGY, IMMUNOHISTOCHEMISTRY, AND MOLECULAR BIOLOGY OF BIA-ALCL

What are the typical histopathologic features of silicone implant related breast lymphomas?

The most common histologic type of lymphomas associated with breast implants is the anaplastic large cell lymphoma (ALCL), which comprises >90% of lymphomas associated with implants [24]. Other less common histologic types include diffuse large B-cell lymphoma, marginal zone lymphoma [25], Epstein–Barr virus associated large B-cell lymphoma [26], and extranodal T/NK cell lymphoma [27]. BIA-ALCL can be identified cytologically or in tissue biopsies or capsule resections. Cytologically, the cells are large, pleomorphic, with abundant cytoplasm and central lobated, vesicular nuclei with frequent prominent nucleoli (**Figure 9.1**). The background shows necrotic debris and karyorrhexis. Histologically, the neoplastic cells appear in small clusters surrounded by necrotic debris when non-invasive. In general, <10% of cells on the luminal surface are viable, and the majority appear as ghost cells. In some cases, all the lymphoma cells are necrotic and the disease is only identified in the cytologic specimen. We denominate pathologic stage T1 to the non-invasive stage (**Figure 9.2**). The tumour cells are seen progressively into the thickness of the capsule, commonly surrounded by small lymphocytes and histiocytes in pathologic stages T2 and T3 (**Figure 9.2**). The cells are large, with moderately abundant cytoplasm, central, lobated nuclei with frequent distinct nucleoli, mitosis and karyorrhexis. Abundant ghost cells are noted (**Figure 9.2**). The most advanced pathologic stage is T4 characterised by large nodules or masses with central necrosis and viable cells at the advancing edge. In the invasive stages, there is more sclerosis and necrosis as well as more inflammatory cells including abundant eosinophils [4,20,24].

What are the typical immunohistochemical features of BIA-ALCL? Are there any outliers and how often does one encounter lymphomas that do not have the expected typical immunoprofile?

CD30 is the best marker to detect BIA-ALCL (**Figure 9.2**) and it complements a good histologic evaluation for large, atypical cells. Optimal conditions for performing this marker are recommended to avoid overdiagnosis and underdiagnosis. Scattered small CD30 positive cells are not unusual in inflammatory capsules. There is a need to complement CD30 with T-cell lineage markers such as CD3, CD4 or CD43, as well as CD45 [3,4,24]. It is interesting that >70% of cases lack the T-cell marker CD3, and almost 80% lack expression of the T-cell receptors alpha-beta (βF1 antibody) or delta. If all the T-cell markers are negative, B cell markers CD20, CD79 or PAX5, or NK cell markers CD56, CD2 or CD7 are recommended. Polymerase chain reaction (PCR) searching for monoclonal rearrangements of the T-cell receptors gamma or beta may be the ultimate means of demonstrating T-cell lineage. ALK is not necessary for cases of BIA-ALCL, since there are no bona fide cases of ALK (+) ALCL reported in the literature.

What are the typical molecular biologic features of BIA-ALCL? Any novel data?

Approximately 90% of cases demonstrate monoclonal rearrangements of the T-cell receptor genes, encoding either the gamma or beta chain. When the tumour is definitive by histologic or immunophenotypic features, it may not be necessary to perform PCR for T-cell receptors. However, PCR is necessary when the evidence is incomplete or doubtful [24].

Molecular studies such as next generation sequencing have revealed mutations of *STAT3* and *JAK1* in approximately 20–30% of cases [28]. RNA sequencing studies have demonstrated the overexpression of hypoxia associated genes including carbonic anhydrase, that can be demonstrated by CA9 immunohistochemistry [29].

Do the molecular biology data and immunologic studies of various T cell types (TH1, TH2, and TH17) provide any clues about the histogenesis of BIA-ALCL?

Although there are no uniform data, immunologic studies have demonstrated overexpression of cytokines related with TH1, TH2 and TH17 response, that can be associated with allergy or with a yet unknown pro-inflammatory antigen [30]. These cytokines also suggest activation of the innate immune response [30]. The nature of the inciting substance in the implants has not been yet identified but postulated derived from the microbiome colonising breast implants [31]. This theory is controversial and has not been confirmed.

Does the BIA-ALCL differ from other ALCL that may involve breasts?

Currently, there are four groups of disorders that histologically are classified as ALCL, and then subclassified as systemic or localised: (1) ALK+ ALCL and (2) ALK-ALCL which are systemic lymphomas; and (3) BIA-ALCL and (4) Primary cutaneous ALCL which are localised lymphomas. The systemic ALCLs require chemotherapy to control the disease, while local management is required for the latter two [32]. All the four groups of ALCL can be indistinguishable histologically, in that are composed of large pleomorphic cells, including a subset of large cells with folded, kidney-shaped nuclei deemed as "hallmark cells", and all are strongly positive for CD30 in a membrane and Golgi pattern. ALK+ ALCL is characterised by the expression of ALK or by translocations involving ALK of which *ALK-NPM1* is the most common [32]. Systemic ALK-ALCL is an aggressive lymphoma, which lacks ALK, but may have translocations of *DUSP22* and *TP53*, similar to primary cutaneous ALCL, which is characterised by single or multiple masses confined to the skin [33,34].

DIFFERENTIAL DIAGNOSIS OF BIA-ALCL

Which other lymphomas and lymphoproliferative disorders must be considered in the differential diagnosis of BIA-ALCL?

The differential diagnosis is wide and includes reactive periprosthetic effusions [35] as well as neoplasms involving the periprosthetic capsule **(Table 9.1)** [35]. Systemic lymphomas such as follicular lymphoma or small lymphocytic lymphoma may affect the breast in patients with breast implants, but the tumours may be away from the capsule [36]. Patients with reconstructive surgery including implants can have recurrence of breast carcinoma located to the implant, including periprosthetic effusion [37]. Other tumours associated with breast implants include squamous cell carcinoma [38], a highly aggressive malignancy once is invasive. Fibromatosis can also be a cause of mass in breast capsules; it can be recurrent if removed incompletely [39].

    The differential diagnosis of lymphomas that involve the capsule include those of B-cell lineage such as diffuse large B-cell lymphoma [40], marginal zone lymphoma and EBV(+) large B-cell lymphoma associated with breast implants [26]. These lymphomas may be clinically similar to BIA-ALCL; however, the histologic features may be different, in that EBV+ large B cell lymphoma has more calcification and necrosis, and the neoplastic cells are of B-cell lineage and are positive for EBV [26]. Other T-cell lymphomas involving the capsules are much rarer and include extranodal T/NK cell lymphoma [27] a case

Table 9.1 Differential diagnosis of breast implant-associated anaplastic large cell lymphoma

	BIA-ALCL	PC-ALCL	sALCL-ALK (−)	sALCL-ALK (+)	Implant EBV (+) LBCL	Implant DLBCL, NOS
Association with breast implants	Yes	No	No	No	Yes	Yes
Clinical features						
Sites affected	Breast	Skin of head and neck or extremities	Nodal and extranodal sites	Nodal and extranodal sites	Breast	Breast
Clinical presentation	Effusion, mass or LAD	Skin mass with ulceration	LAD, extranodal mass	LAD, extranodal mass	Implant induration	Effusion or mass
Pathologic features						
Gross	Periprosthetic fluid or mass	Mass	LAD, extranodal mass	LAD, extranodal mass	Periprosthetic necrosis	Periprosthetic fluid or mass
Histology	Large pleomorphic cells	Large pleomorphic cells	Large pleomorphic cells	Large pleomorphic cells	Large pleomorphic cells	Large pleomorphic cells
Cell predominant	Oval or multilobated	Oval or multilobated	Oval or multilobated	Oval or multilobated	Oval or multilobated	Large centroblastic
Hallmark cells	Detected	Detected	Detected	Detected	No	No
Necrosis	Massive	Variable	Variable	Variable	Massive	Variable
Immunophenotype						
Positive markers	CD30, bright, CD4, CD43	CD30, bright, CD4, CD43	CD30, bright, CD4, CD43	CD30, bright, CD4, CD43, ALK	CD30 var, EBER, CD20, CD79	CD20, CD79
Negative markers	EBER	EBER	EBER, ALK	CD20, CD79	CD3, CD4, CD5	CD3, CD4, CD5, EBER
Genetic features						
Cytogenetics	Del20q	DUSP22-R, P63-R	DUSP22-R, P63-R	ALK-R	NA	NA
Clinical stage	Mostly stage IE	Mostly stage IE	Stage III and IV	Stage III and IV	Mostly stage IE	Mostly stage IE
Therapy						
Mainstay therapy	Surgery	Surgery	Chemotherapy	Chemotherapy	Surgery	Surgery
Vedotin brentuximab indication	Non-resectable disease	Recurrent disease	Yes	Yes	No	No
Prognosis						
5-year OS	89%	90%	60%	85%	NA	NA

ALCL, anaplastic large cell lymphoma; ALK, anaplastic lymphoma kinase, BIA-ALCL, breast implant-associated ALCL; DLBCL, diffuse large B-cell lymphoma; EBV, Epstein–Barr virus; LAD, lymphadenopathy; LBCL, Large B-cell lymphoma; NA, not available; NOS, not otherwise specified; OS, overall survival; PC-ALCL, primary cutaneous ALCL; R, rearranged gene; sALCL, systemic ALCL.

that presented as an invasive mass, and also was subjected to complete excision and chemotherapy to achieve complete remission. Primary cutaneous ALCL may arise in the skin of a patient with implants or as a secondary extension from other skin sites. It is important to carefully assess the underlying implant to exclude that the cutaneous lesion is not an extension of an underlying BIA-ALCL.

We are not aware of classic Hodgkin lymphoma arising in a breast implant; however, we observed that nodal involvement of BIA-ALCL may mimic nodular sclerosis Hodgkin lymphoma (NSHL) [18]. Thus, it is important to inquiry about the presence of breast implants in a woman presenting with axillary NSHL for the possibility that LN involvement as the first manifestation of BIA-ALCL [18].

TREATMENT AND PROGNOSIS

What is the clinical role of various X-ray diagnostic modalities?

The most sensitive imaging technique to detect periprosthetic effusions is the ultrasound [41,42]. For optimal preoperative staging, PET-CT is the most appropriate, since it lights up any area of invasion, where the surgeon will try to go around and removed entirely. Mammography that is a widely used technique used for screening for breast carcinoma, is suboptimal to assess BIA-ALCL in patients with implants [41], since the implants tend to interfere with landmarks, and in addition carry the risk of causing implant rupture. For postoperative follow-up, PET-CT is advised as a highly sensitive technique [21] although there is controversy if this has to be done in asymptomatic patients as well [43].

What is the role of fine-needle aspiration biopsy?

Since most patients present with effusion, the fluid can be tapped by FNA, which is the most effective way to diagnose BIA-ALCL. The ideal volume is 50 mL or more if suitable. Tumour masses are also susceptible of FNA to sample tumour cells. It is a common practice to perform needle core biopsies in tumour masses for the possibility to perform flow cytometry immunophenotype or immunohistochemistry for CD30.

How to handle the periprosthetic effusion fluid?

The aspirated fluid is subjected to cytologic examination as soon as possible and if an immediate assessment yields suspicious cells, flow cytometry immunophenotyping is recommended [19,44].

We recommend direct examination of the cytologic specimen, and if only few cells are found, we recommend concentration of cells such as Ficoll concentration, and then use that pellet to prepare a smear and cell block if possible. Cytologic smears can be stained with Wright Giemsa or with Papanicolaou, searching for large, atypical cells with moderately abundant cytoplasm and lobated vesicular nuclei. Cell block is recommended to evaluate for large, atypical cells and stain with CD30 to highlight any large cell for further evaluation [22,24]. Flow cytometry immunophenotyping is recommended in all specimens with suspicious cells or with uncertain preliminary cytologic evaluation, looking for abnormal phenotypes of T cells and their expression with CD30 [19].

How to handle the contralateral breast?

Estimates are that only 5% of BIA-ALCL are bilateral. The recommendation of the National Comprehensive Cancer Network [21] is to consider removal of the contralateral capsule and implant in a patient with diagnosis of BIA-ALCL. Approximately 5% of patients will harbour an asymptomatic ALCL. However, informed consent of the patient is recommended before proceeding with capsulectomy and implant removal.

How to handle capsulectomies in the dissection room?

We recommend that handling of capsulectomies should follow strategic planning by review of preoperative evaluation to determine the location of any suspicious lesions and communicate to the surgeon to indicate the suspicious areas in the operative specimen. An "en bloc" resection indicates an intact capsulectomy containing the implant, with or without fluid (**Figure 9.3**). This is particularly useful for cases where a grossly identifiable lesion is not detected. Lyapichev et al [23] detail on how to designate the landmarks for proper orientation of the surgical specimen. They also describe how to open the capsule looking for any periprosthetic fluid to be aspirated and handled for cytopathology and flow cytometry evaluation. Once the capsule is opened and the implant removed (**Figure 9.3**) and examined, additional incisions are made through the capsule, in a way to display it flat, proceed to careful examination and pin flat on a wax block for overnight fixation in formalin. The next day, the specimen is rinsed and inked on the outer surface according to orientation, like the specimen is a cube and six aspects are inked each with a different colour (**Figure 9.3**). Random sections are taken of each part of the aspect of the capsule, at least 2-cm in length sections for each aspect and submitted to processing and cutting sections "on edge" (**Figure 9.3**) so that all tissue sections show the luminal surface on one side and the inked margin on the other side. If the capsule is pliable, long sections can be taken and rolled into a cassette, to be cut "on edge" (**Figure 9.3**). This procedure allows us for a comprehensive examination of the capsule and the likelihood of finding most possible lesions in the capsule [23].

How to handle transgender women with breast implants?

There are reports of transgender women with breast implants who developed BIA-ALCL. The diagnostic evaluation, therapy and handling of pathologic specimen is identical to female patients [45].

What is the prognosis after surgical treatment and chemotherapy? And what is the overall mortality?

The prognosis of a completely removed BIA-ALCL, that is complete capsulectomy with implant removal is excellent, or in other words, the patient can be considered cured if the procedure is performed by an experienced surgeon or by a surgical oncologist [20,21]. However, several conditions lead to additional morbidity or mortality. If the diagnosis is not suspected, and patient has removal of the implant with partial capsulectomy, and the diagnosis is postoperative, the patient optimally may need removal of the entire remaining capsule to avoid recurrence of disease [22]. If complete resection is not possible, adjuvant

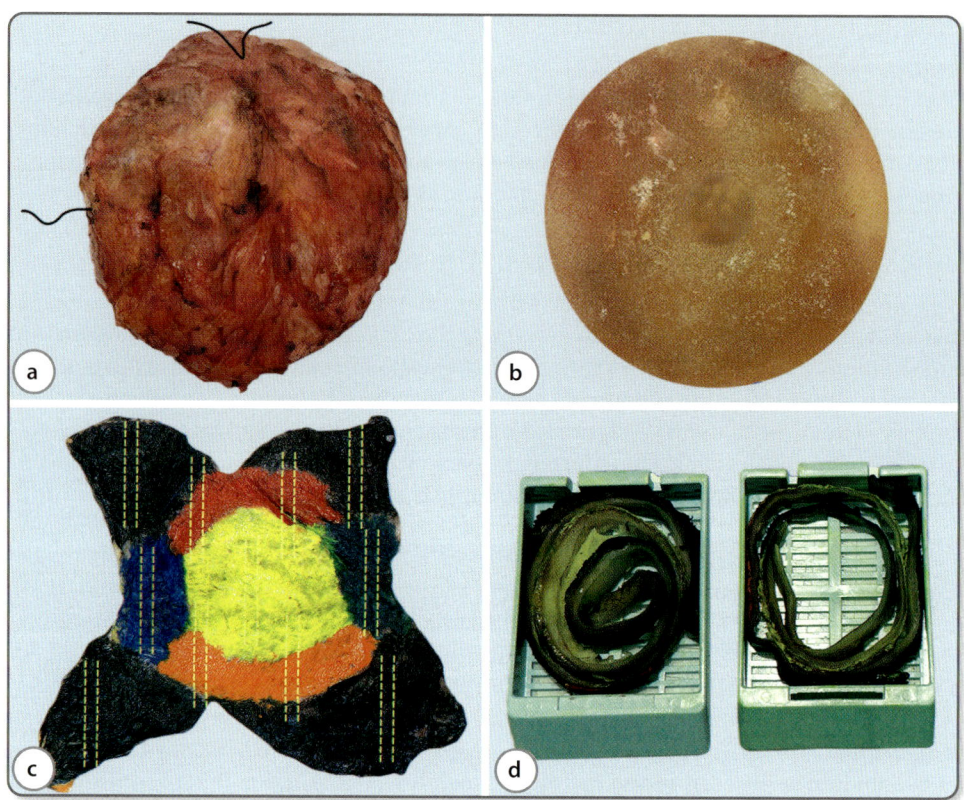

Figure 9.3 Fixation and processing of "en bloc" specimen with a preoperative diagnosis of BIA-ALCL. (a) "En bloc" specimen shows intact capsule containing implant with stitches denoting the orientation: long stitch is lateral margin and short stiches denote superior margin. (b) Upon opening of the capsule, the implant is removed. In this case a textured implant is shown. The striae were areas of calcification. (c) Post-fixation capsulectomy. After overnight fixation in formalin on a wax block, the capsule is flat and inked according to six aspects of an imaginary cube. The specimen is now optimal for sampling, either in 2-cm sections per each of the aspects, or in long strips if the capsule is pliable. (d) Cassettes with long strips of capsule suspicious of BIA-ALCL. The sections are "on edge" to allow the perfect visualisation of the luminal side for lesions, and the inked resection margins to assess for the proximity or involvement of surgical margins.

therapy is recommended [20]. CHOP chemotherapy in light of incomplete surgery may lead to up to 60% recurrence after 1-year follow-up [20]. Vedotin brentuximab (anti-CD30 monoclonal antibody) has led to complete remission in some patients, however, more experience is needed to determine the spectrum of benefit. The role of radiation therapy has not been defined.

Survival is almost 100% for patients with non-invasive disease, and the overall survival (OS) for the entire cohort is 89% at 5 years [20]. Survival progressively decreases to 75% for patients with non-resectable disease, or with lymphadenopathy despite the use of chemo- or immunotherapy. In 2020, it was estimated that 36 patients died because of BIA-ALCL.

CONCLUSION

BIA-ALCL is a recently recognized lymphoma, that arises around textured breast implants. This lymphoma is considered as uncommon, and affects patients with textured breast implants. The most common presentation is an effusion, that if diagnosed early can be cured with complete capsulectomy and removal of implant, while 20% present with regional lymphadenopathy and may be nonresectable, and require adjuvant therapy. The 5-year overall survival is approximately 90%.

> **Key points for clinical practice**
>
> - Breast implant-associated anaplastic large cell lymphoma (BIA-ALCL) is a newly recognised form of localised lymphoma with an estimated incidence of 1: 30,000 women with breast implants.
> - Essentially all BIA-ALCL were diagnosed in breasts containing textured rather than smooth-shelled implants.
> - More than 90% of all reported cases were pathologically classified as diffuse large B-cell lymphomas.
> - BIA-ALCL are typically accompanied with pericapsular fluid effusion which can readily be sampled by fine-needle aspiration biopsy.
> - The diagnostic approach to BI-ALCL includes ultrasound and PET-CT examination, sampling of the fluid for cytopathology, and removal of the implants, and axillar lymph nodes if indicated.
> - Only 5% all BIA-ALCL are bilateral.
> - Proper treatment that includes capsulectomy is accompanied by excellent results.
> - Survival is almost 100% for patients with non-invasive disease, and the overall survival (OS) for the entire cohort is 89% at 5 years.

REFERENCES

1. Siegel RL, Miller KD, Fuchs HE, Jemal A. Cancer statistics, 2022. CA Cancer J Clin 2022; 72:7–33.
2. Miranda RN, Feldman AL, Soares FA. Breast implant-associated anaplastic large cell lymphoma. In: Allison KH, Edi B, Ellis IO, et al., (eds). World Health Organization Breast Tumours, 5th. edition. Lyon: IARC; 2019:245–248.
3. Miranda RN, Aladily TN, Prince HM, et al. Breast implant-associated anaplastic large-cell lymphoma: long-term follow-up of 60 patients. J Clin Oncol 2014; 32:114–120.
4. Aladily TN, Medeiros LJ, Amin MB, et al. Anaplastic large cell lymphoma associated with breast implants: a report of 13 cases. Am J Surg Pathol 2012; 36:1000–1008.
5. Talwalkar SS, Miranda RN, Valbuena JR, et al. Lymphomas involving the breast: a study of 106 cases comparing localized and disseminated neoplasms. Am J Surg Pathol 2008; 32:1299–1309.
6. de Jong D, Vasmel WL, de Boer JP, et al. Anaplastic large-cell lymphoma in women with breast implants. JAMA 2008; 300:2030–2035.
7. de Boer M, van Leeuwen FE, Hauptmann M, et al. Breast Implants and the Risk of Anaplastic Large-Cell Lymphoma in the Breast. JAMA Oncol 2018.
8. Cordeiro PG, Ghione P, Ni A, et al. Risk of breast implant associated anaplastic large cell lymphoma (BIA-ALCL) in a cohort of 3546 women prospectively followed long term after reconstruction with textured breast implants. J Plast Reconstr Aesthet Surg 2020; 73:841–846.

9.   Keech JA, Jr, Creech BJ. Anaplastic T-cell lymphoma in proximity to a saline-filled breast implant. Plast Reconstr Surg 1997; 100:554–555.

10.   Miranda RN, Medeiros LJ, Ferrufino-Schmidt MC, et al. Pioneers of Breast Implant-Associated Anaplastic Large Cell Lymphoma: History from Case Report to Global Recognition. Plast Reconstr Surg 2019; 143:7s–14s.

11.   Lyapichev KA, Medeiros L, Clemens M, et al. Reconsideration of the first recognition of breast implant-associated anaplastic large cell lymphoma: A critical review of the literature. Ann Diag Pathol 2020; 45:151474.

12.   Roden AC, Macon WR, Keeney GL, et al. Seroma-associated primary anaplastic large-cell lymphoma adjacent to breast implants: an indolent T-cell lymphoproliferative disorder. Mod Pathol 2008; 21:455–463.

13.   Center for Devices and Radiological Health U.S. Food and Drug Administration. (2011). Anaplastic Large Cell Lymphoma (ALCL) in Women with Breast Implants: Preliminary FDA Findings and Analyses. [online] Available from https://www.nvpc.nl/uploads/stand/NVPC110126DOC-FN-ASPS_Final_ALCL_White_Paper_Clean_Version_1-18-1177.pdf [Lastaccessed August, 2023],

14.   Feldman AL, Harris NL, Stein H, et al. Breast implant-associated anaplastic large cell lymphoma. In: Swerdlow SH, Campo E, Harris NL, et al., (eds). WHO Classification of Tumours of Haematopoietic and Lymphoid Tissues, Revised 4th edn. Lyon: International Agency for Research on Cancer, 2017:421–422.

15.   Alaggio R, Amador C, Anagnostopoulos I, et al. The 5th edition of the World Health Organization Classification of Haematolymphoid Tumours: Lymphoid Neoplasms. Leukemia 2022; 36:1720–1748.

16.   Doren EL, Miranda RN, Selber JC, et al. U.S. Epidemiology of Breast Implant-Associated Anaplastic Large Cell Lymphoma. Plast Reconstr Surg 2017; 139:1042–1050.

17.   Jones P, Mempin M, Hu H, et al. The Functional Influence of Breast Implant Outer Shell Morphology on Bacterial Attachment and Growth. Plast Reconstr Surg 2018; 142:837–849.

18.   Ferrufino-Schmidt MC, Medeiros LJ, Liu H, et al. Clinicopathologic Features and Prognostic Impact of Lymph Node Involvement in Patients With Breast Implant-associated Anaplastic Large Cell Lymphoma. Am J Surg Pathol 2018; 42:293–305.

19.   Jaffe ES, Ashar BS, Clemens MW, et al. Best Practices Guideline for the Pathologic Diagnosis of Breast Implant-Associated Anaplastic Large-Cell Lymphoma. J Clin Oncol 2020; 38:1102–1111.

20.   Clemens MW, Medeiros LJ, Butler CE, et al. Complete Surgical Excision Is Essential for the Management of Patients With Breast Implant-Associated Anaplastic Large-Cell Lymphoma. J Clin Oncol 2016; 34:160–168.

21.   Clemens MW, Jacobsen ED, Horwitz SM. 2019 NCCN Consensus Guidelines on the Diagnosis and Treatment of Breast Implant-Associated Anaplastic Large Cell Lymphoma (BIA-ALCL). Aesthet Surg J 2019; 39:S3–S13.

22.   Evans MG, Medeiros LJ, Marques-Piubelli ML, et al. Breast implant-associated anaplastic large cell lymphoma: clinical follow-up and analysis of sequential pathologic specimens of untreated patients shows persistent or progressive disease. Mod Pathol 2021; 34:2148–2153.

23.   Lyapichev KA, Pina-Oviedo S, Medeiros LJ, et al. A proposal for pathologic processing of breast implant capsules in patients with suspected breast implant anaplastic large cell lymphoma. Mod Pathol 2020; 33:367–379.

24.   Quesada AE, Medeiros LJ, Clemens MW, et al. Breast implant-associated anaplastic large cell lymphoma: a review. Mod Pathol 2019; 32:166–188.

25.   Evans MG, Miranda RN, Young PA, et al. B-cell lymphomas associated with breast implants: Report of three cases and review of the literature. Ann diagn pathol 2020; 46:151512.

26.   Medeiros LJ, Marques-Piubelli ML, Sangiorgio VFI, et al. Epstein-Barr-virus-positive large B-cell lymphoma associated with breast implants: an analysis of eight patients suggesting a possible pathogenetic relationship. Mod Pathol 2021; 34:2154–2167.

27.   Aladily TN, Nathwani BN, Miranda RN, et al. Extranodal NK/T-cell lymphoma, nasal type, arising in association with saline breast implant: expanding the spectrum of breast implant-associated lymphomas. Am J Surg Pathol 2012; 36:1729–1734.

28. Oishi N, Brody GS, Ketterling RP, et al. Genetic subtyping of breast implant–associated anaplastic large cell lymphoma. Blood 2018; 132:544–547.

29. Oishi N, Hundal T, Phillips JL, et al. Molecular profiling reveals a hypoxia signature in breast implant-associated anaplastic large cell lymphoma. Haematologica 2021; 106:1714–1724.

30. Kadin ME. What Cytokines Can Tell Us About the Pathogenesis of Breast Implant-Associated Anaplastic Large Cell Lymphoma (BIA-ALCL). Aesthetic Surg J 2019; 39:S28–S35.

31. Hu H, Johani K, Almatroudi A, et al. Bacterial Biofilm Infection Detected in Breast Implant-Associated Anaplastic Large-Cell Lymphoma. Plast Reconstr Surg 2016; 137:1659–1669.

32. Medeiros LJ, Elenitoba-Johnson KS. Anaplastic Large Cell Lymphoma. Am J Clin Pathol 2007; 127:707–722.

33. Feldman AL, Dogan A, Smith DI, et al. Discovery of recurrent t(6;7)(p25.3;q32.3) translocations in ALK-negative anaplastic large cell lymphomas by massively parallel genomic sequencing. Blood 2011; 117:915–919.

34. Parrilla Castellar ER, Jaffe ES, Said JW, et al. ALK-negative anaplastic large cell lymphoma is a genetically heterogeneous disease with widely disparate clinical outcomes. Blood 2014; 124:1473–1480.

35. Di Napoli A, Pepe G, Giarnieri E, et al. Cytological diagnostic features of late breast implant seromas: From reactive to anaplastic large cell lymphoma. PLoS One 2017; 12:e0181097.

36. Cook PD, Osborne BM, Connor RL, Strauss JF. Follicular lymphoma adjacent to foreign body granulomatous inflammation and fibrosis surrounding silicone breast prosthesis. Am J Surg Pathol 1995; 19:712–717.

37. Roubaud MJ, Kulber DA. A malignant late seroma 20 years after breast cancer and saline implants. Plast Reconstr Surg 2013; 131:655e–657e.

38. Olsen DL, Keeney GL, Chen B, Visscher DW, Carter JM. Breast implant capsule-associated squamous cell carcinoma: a report of 2 cases. Hum Pathol 2017; 67:94–100.

39. Balzer BL, Weiss SW. Do biomaterials cause implant-associated mesenchymal tumors of the breast? Analysis of 8 new cases and review of the literature. Hum Pathol 2009; 40:1564–1570.

40. Smith BK, Gray SS. Large B-cell lymphoma occurring in a breast implant capsule. Plast Reconstr Surg 2014; 134:670e–671e.

41. Adrada BE, Miranda RN, Rauch GM, et al. Breast implant-associated anaplastic large cell lymphoma: sensitivity, specificity, and findings of imaging studies in 44 patients. Breast Cancer Res Treat 2014; 147:1-14.

42. Noreña-Rengifo BD, Sanín-Ramírez MP, Adrada BE, et al. MRI for Evaluation of Complications of Breast Augmentation. Radiographics 2022; 42:929–946.

43. O'Connell RL, Sharma B, Van Kerckhoven L, et al. Cost and clinical benefit of imaging surveillance after treatment for breast implant-associated anaplastic large cell lymphoma (BIA-ALCL). Eur J Surg Oncol 2022; 48:748–751.

44. Santanelli di Pompeo F, Clemens MW, Atlan M, et al. 2022 Practice Recommendation Updates from the World Consensus Conference on BIA-ALCL. Aesth surg j/Am Soc Aesth Plast surg 2022.

45. Zaveri S, Yao A, Schmidt H. Breast Implant-Associated Anaplastic Large Cell Lymphoma Following Gender Reassignment Surgery: A Review of Presentation, Management, and Outcomes in the Transgender Patient Population. Eur J Breast Health 2020; 16:162–166.

Chapter 10

T- and NK-cell lymphomas of gastrointestinal tract: A practical approach

Anamarija M Perry

INTRODUCTION

Gastrointestinal tract (GI) is a frequent site of lymphoma involvement, accounting for 30–40% of all extranodal lymphoma cases [1]. Overwhelming majority of lymphomas involving the GI tract are of B-cell lineage (the most common being diffuse large B-cell lymphoma and extranodal marginal zone lymphoma of mucosa-associated lymphoid tissue), while T- and NK-cell lymphomas are infrequent and comprise approximately 15% of all GI lymphomas [2]. T- and NK-cell lymphomas most commonly involve small and large intestine, however, virtually any site from oral cavity to anus can be involved. This review will focus on T- and NK-lymphomas that primarily involve the GI tract. These entities include enteropathy-associated T-cell lymphoma (EATL), monomorphic epitheliotropic intestinal T-cell lymphoma (MEITL), intestinal T-cell lymphoma, not otherwise specified (NOS), indolent clonal T-cell lymphoproliferative disorder (LPD) of the gastrointestinal tract, and indolent NK-cell LPD of the gastrointestinal tract. However, some typically nodal and other systemic lymphomas (e.g. extranodal NK-/T-cell lymphoma, nasal type, adult T-cell leukaemia/lymphoma, and anaplastic large cell lymphoma) can involve GI tract either primarily or secondarily in advanced stages [3].

Clinical course, response to therapy and prognosis of T- and NK-cell lymphomas involving the GI tract vary from extremely aggressive to indolent with protracted clinical course. As in the lymph node, these lymphomas are frequently challenging to diagnose and/or subclassify, especially on a small biopsy. This paper will cover diagnostic approach and ancillary studies useful in diagnosis of these entities.

ENTEROPATHY-ASSOCIATED T-CELL LYMPHOMA AND REFRACTORY COELIAC DISEASE

Enteropathy associated T-cell lymphoma

It is a primary intestinal lymphoma derived from intraepithelial T cells. EATL occurs in people with coeliac disease, a relatively common autoimmune disorder, with global

Anamarija M Perry MD, Department of Pathology, University of Michigan, North Campus Research Complex Arbor, MI, USA
Email: anaperry@med.umich.edu

prevalence of around 1%, and characterised by intolerance to gluten [3–6]. This is the most common primary intestinal lymphoma in western countries, comprising around 70% of all cases, consistent with higher prevalence of coeliac disease in individuals of non-Hispanic white race. Genetic susceptibility is important for development of coeliac disease and people with HLA-DQ2 and HLA-DQ8 have increased risk. Moreover, risk factors for development of EATL include homozygosity for HLA-DQ2 allele and advanced age. EATL most commonly occurs in sixth and seventh decade but has been reported in adults over a broad age range, with slight male predominance [4,5].

Clinical features

The most common sites of involvement by EATL are jejunum and ileum, however, it can also occur in stomach and colon. Multifocal involvement is frequently seen. Patients with EATL present with symptoms and signs similar to coeliac disease including abdominal pain, diarrhoea, weight loss, nausea and vomiting, as well as B-symptoms. Furthermore, some patients present with intestinal obstruction by tumour mass, signs of acute abdomen due to intestinal perforation, or haemorrhage. Majority of patients who develop EATL have a previous diagnosis of coeliac disease. They can develop symptoms after previous response to gluten-free diet or can be refractory to gluten-free diet and show worsening of symptoms. However, a subset of patients (10–58%) have no previous diagnosis of coeliac disease and get diagnosed concomitant with diagnosis of EATL or later. EATL most commonly spreads to local abdominal lymph nodes (in one-third of cases), and less frequently to the bone marrow, liver, lungs, and skin. Majority of patients have high clinical stage (III/IV) at diagnosis. Prognosis of EATL patients is generally poor with the median survival of <1 year. In some patients, intense chemotherapy followed by autologous stem cell transplantation can improve outcome [3,5].

Gross and microscopic features

Grossly, EATL presents as plaque, mass with ulceration, or stricture. The adjacent mucosa can show loss of mucosal folds.

Morphologically, the entire wall of the intestine is typically diffusely infiltrated by sheets of lymphoma cells, which can show variety of cytological appearances. In most cases, lymphoma cells are medium-sized to large with round to irregular nuclei, vesicular chromatin and prominent nucleoli **(Figure 10.1)**. Frequently, sheets of large cells and anaplastic morphology are present. Angioinvasion and necrosis can be observed. As is frequently the case with T-cell lymphomas, some cases have background (occasionally extensive) inflammatory cells including eosinophils, histiocytes and plasma cells, as well as loosely formed granulomas (i.e. collections of histiocytes). Tumour cells involve the epithelium to variable extent. It is important to carefully examine the intestinal mucosa adjacent to EATL (particularly in jejunum) which usually shows morphologic changes consistent with coeliac disease **(Figure 10.1)**. These include villous atrophy, crypt hyperplasia, increased intraepithelial lymphocytes (IELs), and increase in lymphocytes and plasma cells in the lamina propria [3].

Immunophenotype

Lymphoma cells are positive for CD2, CD3 (cytoplasmic), CD7, and cytotoxic granule-associated proteins (TIA-1, granzyme B and perforin) **(Figure 10.1)**. They are typically negative for CD5, CD56, and double negative for CD4 and CD8. However, positivity for CD8

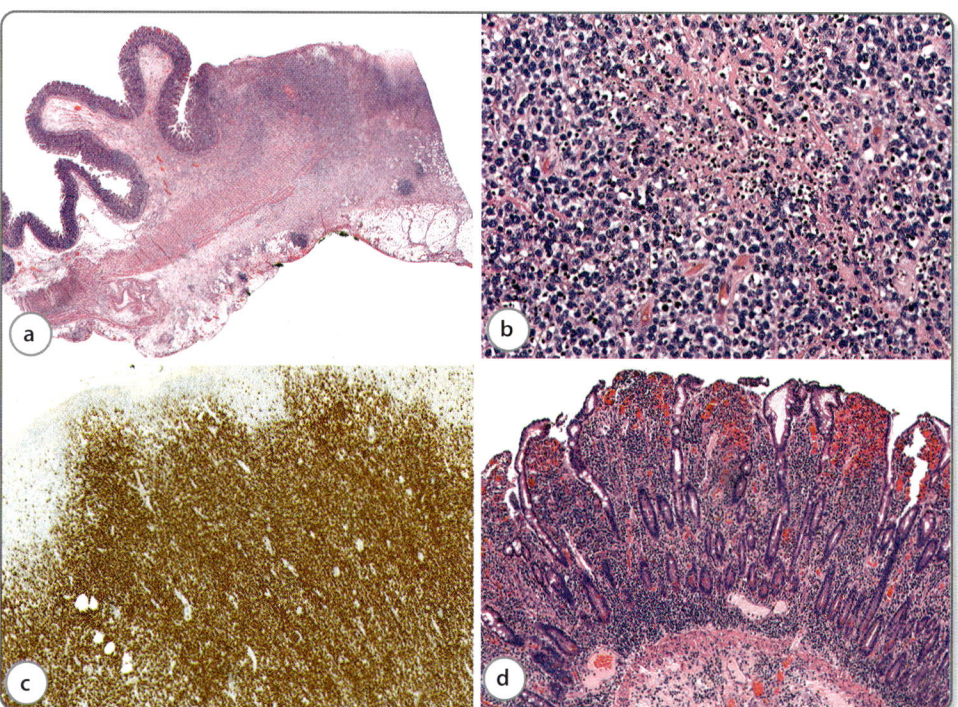

Figure 10.1 Enteropathy associated T-cell lymphoma. (a) Lymphoma diffusely involves the entire wall of the small intestine. Surface ulceration is seen. (b) Lymphoma cells are medium-sized to large. Frequent apoptotic bodies are seen. (c) Lymphoma is diffusely positive for CD3. (d) Adjacent small intestinal mucosa shows changes compatible with coeliac disease.

can be observed in up to 30% of cases, and subset of cases is positive for cytoplasmic T-cell receptor (TCR)-β or TCR-γ. Surface CD3 and TCR are absent. CD30 is variably expressed, more commonly in cases with large and/or anaplastic morphology [3,5].

Genetics

Virtually all cases show clonal T-cell receptor-beta (*TRB*) and/or -gamma (*TRG*) gene rearrangement. Sequencing studies showed recurrent mutations in *JAK-STAT* pathway genes, the most common being *JAK1* (20–50%) and *STAT3* (20–25%). In up to 20% of cases, mutations in *MAPK* pathway genes are seen including *BRAF*, *KRAS*, and *NRAS*. Other recurrently mutated genes include epigenetic modifiers (*TET2, YLPM1*, and *SETD2*), as well as other genes such as *TERT, TP53, BRIP1,* etc. [5,7–10].

Refractory coeliac disease

When discussing EATL, it is important to cover refractory coeliac disease (RCD) which is some cases can precede development of EATL. RCD is defined as persistence or recurrence of gastrointestinal malabsorptive symptoms and abnormal small intestinal histology despite strict adherence to gluten-free diet for ≥12 months. Some patients have primary RCD, while others develop it after a variable period of response to gluten-free diet. The prevalence of RCD varies widely from <1 to 10%. Similar to EATL, the risk factors for RCD include homozygosity for HLA-DQ2 allele and advanced age (i.e. longer exposure to gluten). There are two clinicopathological subtypes of RCD – type I and type II.

Clinical features

Clinical features are similar between the two types of RCD and include signs of malabsorption. However, patients with RCD type II usually show more severe symptoms and more frequently show ulceration and bowel stenosis. The most important clinical difference is much higher 5-year survival for RCD type I (80–96%) compared to type II (45–58%). Moreover, there is a lower risk of progression to EATL in patients with RCD type I (3–14% in 5 years), compared to RCD type II (50% in 5 years) [3,5].

Microscopic features and immunophenotype

Morphologically, both types of RCD, as well as uncomplicated coeliac disease, show similar histologic findings and are difficult to distinguish based on morphology alone. Small IELs are increased in both types and show no significant atypia. RCD type II usually shows more prominent morphologic changes, as well as small aggregates of lymphocytes in the lamina propria in subset of cases. However, IELs have distinct immunophenotypes in two types of RCD. In RCD type I, IELs show normal immunophenotype and are positive for surface and cytoplasmic CD3, CD8, surface TCR, and variably positive for CD5. In contrast, in RCD type II, IELs are positive for cytoplasmic CD3, and negative for surface CD3, surface TCR, CD5, and CD8. To diagnose type II RCD, the aberrant phenotype should be detected on 20% of IELs by flow cytometry or 50% by immunohistochemistry [3,5,11–14].

Genetics

Molecular studies also show differences between the two types of RCD. In type I RCD, *TCR* gene rearrangement studies show polyclonal products in overwhelming majority of cases, with rare cases showing clonal rearrangement. Moreover, genetic and molecular studies showed no alterations. In type II RCD, clonal *TRB* and/or *TRG* gene rearrangement are seen in majority (but not all) cases. Sequencing of RCD type II cases showed deregulated *JAK-STAT* pathway with activating mutations in *JAK1* and *STAT3* genes [11,15].

Monomorphic epitheliotropic intestinal T-cell lymphoma

Monomorphic epitheliotropic intestinal T-cell lymphoma is a primary intestinal lymphoma derived from intraepithelial T cells. This lymphoma used to be called type II EATL, a name that was changed to MEITL in 2017 World Health Organization Classification [3]. MEITL shows no association with coeliac disease and transcriptome sequencing showed distinct expression signatures between EATL and MEITL, warranting definitive separation of these two entities [3,7,16]. MEITL is diagnosed worldwide but is the most common primary intestinal lymphoma in Asia. It is most commonly diagnosed in older individuals with median in seventh decade with a male-to-female ratio of 2:1.

Clinical features

Patients with MEITL commonly present with acute abdomen due to perforation and/ or haemorrhage. Intestinal obstruction by tumour mass is seen in some patients. Small intestine, particularly jejunum is most frequently involved, and multifocal involvement is frequently seen. Most frequently, lymphoma presents as an ulcerated mass in the intestine. As MEITL is not associated with coeliac disease, history of malabsorption is absent. B-symptoms are common. MEITL most commonly spreads locally to lymph nodes, mesentery and pelvic organs, and rarely to other sites such as bone marrow. Advanced clinical stage (III/IV) is reported in 23–73% of cases at diagnosis. MEITL is an aggressive lymphoma with a 5-year survival of 32% [3,5].

Microscopic features

Aptly named, MEITL shows sheets of relatively monotonous (monomorphic), medium-sized lymphoma cells, with round to slightly irregular nuclei, fine chromatin, inconspicuous to small nucleoli, and moderately abundant pale cytoplasm **(Figure 10.2)**. However, subset of cases shows atypical morphology, including significant pleomorphism, larger size, vesicular chromatin, and/or prominent nucleoli. Intestinal villi show distorted architecture with widening and blunting, and lymphoma cells show prominent epitheliotropism **(Figure 10.2)**. Of note, increased IELs can also be seen away from a main tumour mass [3,5,17].

Immunophenotype

Lymphoma cells are positive for CD3, CD8, CD56, and cytotoxic granule-associated proteins (TIA-1 and granzyme B) **(Figure 10.2)**. The cells are negative for CD4, CD5, and CD30.

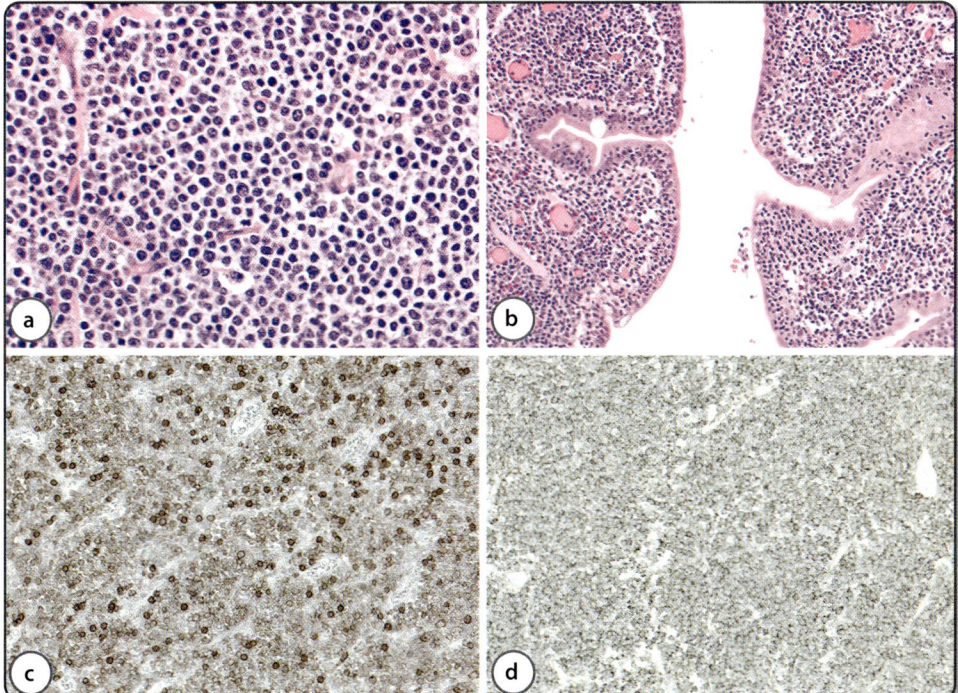

Figure 10.2 Monomorphic epitheliotropic intestinal T-cell lymphoma. (a) Sheets of monotonous medium-sized lymphoma cells with slightly irregular nuclei, inconspicuous nucleoli and moderately abundant pale cytoplasm. (b) Surface mucosa shows prominent epitheliotropism. Lymphoma cells are positive for CD8 (c) and CD56 (d).

Moreover, TCR-γ is often positive (up to 60% of cases), while occasional cases express TCR-β. Aberrant expression of B-cell marker CD20 can be seen in 20% of cases [3,17].

Genetics

Over 90% all cases show clonal *TRB* and/or *TRG* gene rearrangement. Sequencing studies of MEITL showed a mutational profile that overlaps with EATL, with some significant differences. Inactivation of *SETD2* is seen in 76–83% of cases. Mutations in *JAK-STAT* pathway are also common, including *JAK1, JAK3, STAT3, STAT5B*, and *SH2B3*. Other recurrent mutations include *TP53, BCOR, GNAI2*, and *ATM*. Compared to EATL, MEITL shows more common mutations in *MAPK* pathway including mutations in *BRAF, KRAS*, and *NRAS*. Furthermore, whole transcriptome sequencing showed differences between MEITL and EATL with higher expression of *SYK, NCAM1, FASLG*, and *TGBR1* in MEITL. Importantly, expression of SYK is not seen in EATL [7–9,16–18].

Intestinal T-cell lymphoma, not otherwise specified

This category should be used for mature intestinal T-cell lymphomas that do not meet the diagnostic criteria for EATL, MEITL, or other T- or NK-cell lymphomas that can involve GI tract. In some cases where only limited/inadequate biopsy is available (e.g. surface mucosa is not available for evaluation) and subclassification is challenging it might be appropriate to use this diagnosis. This diagnostic category remains in the most recent 2022 International Consensus as well as 2022 World Health Organization Classifications [19,20]. Intestinal T-cell lymphoma, NOS (ITCL, NOS) most commonly occurs in older adults with male predominance. It appears to be more common in Asia.

Clinical features

The most common site of involvement is colon; however, any GI site can be involved. The patients present with different signs and symptoms, depending on the involved site including abdominal pain, diarrhoea, obstruction, perforation or haemorrhage. Approximately half of the patients present in advanced (III/IV) clinical stage. Similar to EATL and MEITL, ITCL, NOS is an aggressive disease with a median survival of 35 months.

Microscopic features and immunophenotype

As expected, these cases show heterogeneous morphology, but cells are usually medium/sized to large. Angiodestruction and necrosis are common.

By immunohistochemistry, most cases are either CD4-positive or CD4/CD8 double negative, and TCR-β positive. Cytotoxic phenotype is frequently seen [3,5].

Genetics

Genetic studies on ITCL, NOS are limited and showed mutations in *JAK1, JAK3, STAT5B, SETD2*, and *TET2*, overlapping with genetic changes seen in EATL and MEITL [21].

Indolent clonal T-cell lymphoproliferative disorder of the gastrointestinal tract

Two types of indolent LPDs occur in the GI tract and are included in the lymphoma classifications – indolent clonal T-cell LPD and indolent NK-cell LPD [19,20].

Indolent T-cell LPD is a clonal T-cell LPD which can involve mucosa in any part of the GI tract, but most commonly involves small intestine and colon. This is a rare condition with around 50 cases reported in the literature so far. However, it is likely unrecognised which results in underdiagnosis or misdiagnosis as benign inflammatory condition (e.g. inflammatory bowel disease or coeliac disease) or more aggressive T-cell lymphoma, such as peripheral T-cell lymphoma, NOS. The disease occurs in adults, most commonly in the fifth and sixth decade, but it was reported over a broad age range (15–77 years). Males are slightly more frequently affected than females [22–28].

Clinical features

Patients present with different symptoms, including abdominal pain, vomiting, diarrhoea, weight loss, and bleeding. In most patients, the disease is localised to the GI tract, but can occasionally involve abdominal lymph nodes, bone marrow, peripheral blood or liver. Clinical course is protracted, with poor response to therapy including conventional chemotherapy protocols used to treat T-cell lymphomas, as well as immunomodulators. Despite that the patients live with persistent disease for a long time. Rare cases of transformation to more aggressive T-cell lymphoma were reported and prognosis in those cases was generally poor. Endoscopically, indolent T-LPD shows different appearances including prominent mucosal folds or nodules, erosions, hyperaemia, or polypoid lesions. Some cases are endoscopically reminiscent of inflammatory bower disease (i.e. ulcerative colitis) [3,5,22,28].

Microscopic features and immunophenotype

Indolent T-cell LPD shows expansion of lamina propria by a non-destructive monotonous lymphoid infiltrate composed of small to occasionally medium-sized lymphoid cells, with minimal to no atypia. Lymphoid cells have round to slightly irregular nuclei, inconspicuous nucleoli and scant cytoplasm (**Figure 10.3**). Some cases show epitheliotropism. Occasionally scattered admixed inflammatory cells, such as eosinophils can be seen. Infiltrate distorts glandular architecture and occasionally involves muscularis mucosae and submucosa, but does not invade deeper into the muscularis propria.

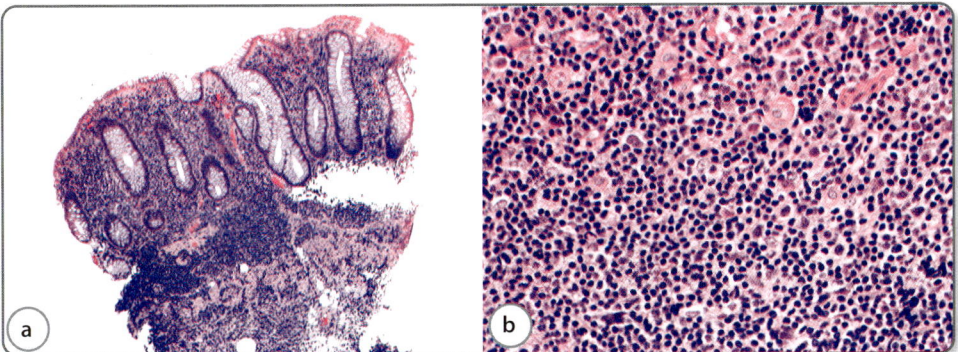

Figure 10.3 Indolent clonal T-cell lymphoproliferative disorder of the gastrointestinal tract. (a) Lymphoid infiltrate in lamina propria distorts but does not destroy colonic glands. (b) Infiltrate is composed of small cells with minimal to no atypia with round nuclei and inconspicuous nucleoli.

By immunohistochemistry, indolent clonal T-LPD is positive for CD3. Cells either express CD4 or CD8 with slightly more CD4-positive cases reported. Occasional CD4/CD8-double positive or double negative cases were reported too. CD5 and CD7 are occasionally aberrantly lost. Furthermore, all reported cases were TCR-β positive and TCR-δ negative. Cases that are CD8 positive express TIA-1 cytotoxic protein. Proliferation index (Ki67) is consistently low (<10%) [3,5,22].

Genetics

By definition, all cases have clonal TCR-β *TRB* and/or -γ *TRG* gene rearrangements. Genetic studies on indolent clonal T-LPD are scarce. Recurrent *STAT3-JAK2* fusions were reported in CD4-positive cases [24,28].

Indolent NK-cell lymphoproliferative disorder of the gastrointestinal tract

Indolent NK-cell LPD is a low-grade neoplasm of NK cells which involves GI tract. This is a rare condition, first described in 2006, with <50 cases reported in the literature. Initial case series described two types of presentation of the same condition, one involving the stomach named "lymphomatoid gastropathy" and the other involving different sites of the GI tract (with frequent multifocal involvement) named "NK-cell enteropathy" [29–32]. Series of patients with lymphomatoid gastropathy was reported from Japan, with median age of patients being 56 years. These individuals were mostly asymptomatic and NK-cell proliferation was discovered incidentally (e.g. during stomach cancer screening) [31]. In contrast, patients with NK-cell enteropathy, reported from the United States and Korea, most frequently presented with abdominal pain, as well as vomiting, diarrhoea, GI bleeding and weight loss. The median age of diagnosis in these series was 46 years [29,32,33]. Endoscopically, lesions in the stomach appear as reddish, are flat or elevated and around 1 cm in size. In other sites of the GI tract, lesions can have different appearances such as nodules, superficial ulcerations and hyperemic foci. Indolent NK-cell LPD is usually localised to the GI tract, with only rare reports of lymph node involvement. The prognosis of indolent NK-cell LPD is favourable and most patients with stomach lesions (i.e. lymphomatoid gastropathy) showed spontaneous regression without therapy, although some relapsed. Subset of reported patients received chemotherapy with limited benefit, similar to indolent clonal T-LPD. However, despite persistence of disease and/or relapse these patients have prolonged survival [29–31].

Microscopic features and immunophenotype

Morphologically, there is an expansion of lamina propria by an infiltrate composed of medium-sized to large cells with round to irregular nuclei, fine chromatin, inconspicuous to small nucleoli, and moderate amount of pale cytoplasm. In early stages, infiltrate displaces the glands, while in advanced stages gland destruction is seen. There is no epitheliotropism. Infiltrate is mostly limited to mucosa with submucosal involvement in occasional cases. Angioinvasion, angiodestruction and necrosis are absent.

Infiltrate is positive for cytoplasmic CD3, CD7, CD56, cytotoxic granule-associated proteins (TIA-1, granzyme B and perforin). Surface CD3, CD4, CD7, and CD8 are negative. EBER in situ hybridisation for Epstein–Barr virus (EBV) is also negative. Proliferative index is variable, but usually low (10–30%) [5,29–31].

Genetics

T-cell receptor gene rearrangement studies showed polyclonal products in all cases. One study reported recurrent *JAK3* mutations in 3/10 cases of indolent NK-cell LPD, supporting the neoplastic nature of this disease [30,34].

OTHER T/NK-CELL LYMPHOMAS INVOLVING THE GASTROINTESTINAL TRACT

Other T- and NK-cell lymphomas, which are not considered primary intestinal lymphomas, can involve the GI tract and should be kept in the differential diagnosis when dealing with these biopsies. One of the extranodal lymphomas that relatively frequently involves the GI tract is extranodal NK-/T-cell lymphoma (ENKTCL), nasal type. This lymphoma will be discussed in more detail. Other T-cell lymphomas, such as anaplastic large cell lymphoma and adult T-cell leukaemia/lymphoma can also occur in the GI tract [3,35–38].

Extranodal NK-/T-cell lymphoma, nasal type

Extranodal NK-/T-cell lymphoma, nasal type, is an uncommon, aggressive extranodal lymphoma of NK- or T-cell lineage that most commonly occurs in the upper aerodigestive tract, but can also occur in other extranodal sites such as GI tract, skin, and soft tissue. GI tract can be involved secondarily in advanced disease or ENKTCL can primarily occur in the GI tract (<10% of cases). ENKTCL is more common in Asia and indigenous populations of Central and South America than in Europe and United States. It most commonly occurs in fifth and sixth decade with male predominance. This lymphoma is strongly associated with EBV and all cases are by definition EBV positive.

Patients with ENKTCL involving the GI tract present with abdominal pain and occasionally signs of perforation. The lymphoma most frequently involves small intestine and colon and presents with mucosal ulcerations, frequently multifocally. Local abdominal lymph nodes are involved in approximately one-third of patients. ENKTCL is an aggressive lymphoma that is treated with intense chemotherapy protocols. Patients with lower clinical stages have better prognosis. According to some studies, involvement of GI tract portends worse prognosis, compared to ENKTCL at other sites.

Morphologically, ENKTCL shows broad cytologic spectrum from small to large and even anaplastic cells. Different cell sizes are frequently admixed. Nuclei are usually irregular and nucleoli are inconspicuous or small (**Figure 10.4**). Angioinvasion and angiodestruction with areas of necrosis are frequently seen. In the GI tract ulceration and destruction of mucosal architecture are commonly seen. By immunohistochemistry, most cases of ENKTCL have an NK-cell phenotype and are positive for CD2, CD56, cytoplasmic CD3, CD7 (variably), TIA-1, granzyme, and perforin. They are negative for CD5, surface CD3, CD4 and CD8. Subset of these cases are of true T-cell lineage (with clonal T-cell gene rearrangement) and these are usually positive for CD5, CD8, and TCR-β or -γ. As mentioned above, EBER in situ hybridisation for EBV is always positive, and this diagnosis should not be made in the absence of EBV (**Figure 10.4**) [39–44].

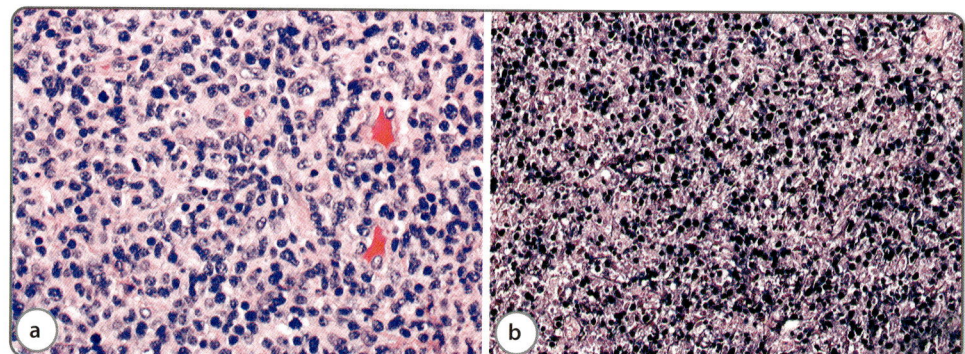

Figure 10.4 Extranodal NK-/T-cell lymphoma, nasal type. (a) Lymphoma cells are medium-sized with markedly irregular nuclei. Frequent mitoses are seen. (b) infiltrate is positive for EBV by EBER in situ hybridisation.

APPROACH TO DIAGNOSING T- AND NK-CELL LYMPHOMAS INVOLVING THE GASTROINTESTINAL TRACT

Most pathologists will agree that the diagnosis of T- and NK-cell lymphomas can be challenging. These lymphomas are relatively uncommon, particularly in western countries, and therefore infrequently encountered by a pathologist. Particularly challenging are small/needle core biopsies with limited tissue, which at times can preclude adequate morphologic assessment and performance of all necessary ancillary studies. Approach to any lymphoma, including lymphomas in the GI tract, should be systematic with consideration of clinical and imaging data (if available). When evaluating a GI biopsy for lymphoma, the following information should be obtained:

- Patient demographics (age and gender)
- Sites involved by lymphoma (i.e. is lymphoma localised to the GI tract and adjacent lymph nodes or it involves multiple sites?); this information is very important when considering whether the lymphoma is primary to the GI tract or the GI tract is secondarily involved by other lymphoma.
- Pertinent clinical history (e.g. previous history of lymphoma or autoimmune disease, history of primary or secondary immunodeficiency, immunosuppressive medications, etc.); when dealing with T-cell lymphoma of the GI tract, key information to obtain is previous history of coeliac disease. However, as mentioned in the EATL section, some patients get diagnosed with coeliac disease concomitant with diagnosis of EATL or even later.

The main diagnostic challenge in T-cell lymphomas of the GI tract is separating different entities. **Table 10.1** summarises clinical, morphologic, immunophenotypic, and genetic characteristics of primary GI T-cell lymphomas. Diagnosis of ITCL, NOS is appropriate for cases that do not meet the morphologic and immunophenotypic criteria for EATL or MEITL. In cases where biopsy material is limited and/or surface epithelium is not available for evaluation, diagnosis of ITCL, NOS can be made and repeat biopsy can be recommended if clinically appropriate. As for NK-cell neoplasms in the GI tract, the main differential diagnosis is between ENKTCL and indolent NK-cell LPD. The easiest way to distinguish between the two is by performing the EBER in situ hybridisation for EBV.

Table 10.1 Comparison of clinical, morphologic, immunophenotypic, and genetic characteristics of primary gastrointestinal T-cell lymphomas				
	EATL	**MEITL**	**ITL, NOS**	**Indolent clonal T-LPD**
Age, gender	Sixth to seventh decade, M>F	Seventh decade, M:F = 2:1	Older adults, M > F	Fifth and Sixth decade, M > F
Most common site(s) of involvement	Jejunum, ileum	Jejunum	Colon	Small intestine and colon
Prognosis	Poor, median survival <1 year	Poor, 5-year survival 32%	Poor, median survival 35 months	Refractory to therapy, but prolonged survival
Gross appearance	Plaque, ulcerated mass, stricture	Ulcerated mass	Mass	Prominent mucosal folds, nodules, erosions, hyperaemia, polypoid lesions
Microscopic appearance	• Infiltrates entire bowel wall • Pleomorphic, medium-sized to large cells, irregular nuclei, prominent nucleoli • Angioinvasion, necrosis • Coeliac disease in adjacent mucosa	• Infiltrates entire bowel wall • Monomorphic appearance, medium-sized cells, round nuclei, fine chromatin, inconspicuous nucleoli • Blunted and widened villi, prominent epitheliotropism	• Infiltrates entire bowel wall • Heterogeneous morphology, pleomorphic • Medium-sized to large cells • Angioinvasion, necrosis	• Mucosa and occasionally submucosa involed • Non-destructive infiltrate of monotonous small to medium-sized lymphoid cells • Round to slightly irregular nuclei, inconspicuous nucleoli, scant cytoplasm
Immunophenotype	• Positive: CD2, cCD3, CD7, TIA-1, granzyme B, perforin; subset cTCR • CD8 posiitve in up to 30% of cases • Negative: sCD3, CD4, CD5, CD56, sTCR	• Positive: CD3, CD8, CD56, TIA-1, granzyme B, TCR γ • Negative: CD4, CD5	• Positive: CD4, TCR β, cytotoxic granules • Some cases CD4/CD8 double negative	• Positive: CD3, either CD4 or CD8, TCR β, TIA-1 • CD5 and CD7 variably lost • Negative: TCR γ
Genetics	• Clonal TRB and/or TRG • Mutations: *JAK1, STAT3, BRAF, KRAS, NRAS*	• Clonal TRB and/or TRG • Mutations: *SETD2* (most common), *JAK1, JAK3, STAT3, STAT5B, SH2B3, GNAI2, BRAF, KRAS, NRAS* • Higher expression of *SYK, NCAM, FASL, TGBR1* compared to EATL	Mutations: *JAK1, JAK3, STAT5B, SETD2, TET2*	• Clonal TRB and/or TRG • *STAT3-JAK2* fusions

EATL, enteropathy-associated T-cell lymphoma; ITL, NOS, intestinal T-cell lymphoma, not otherwise specified; MEITL, monomorphic epitheliotropic intestinal T-cell lymphoma; T-LPD, T-cell lymphoproliferative disorder; TRB, T-cell receptor beta; TRG, T-cell receptor gamma; cCD3, cytoplasmic CD3; sCD3, surface CD3; cTCR, cytoplasmic T-cell receptor; sTCR, surface T-cell receptor.

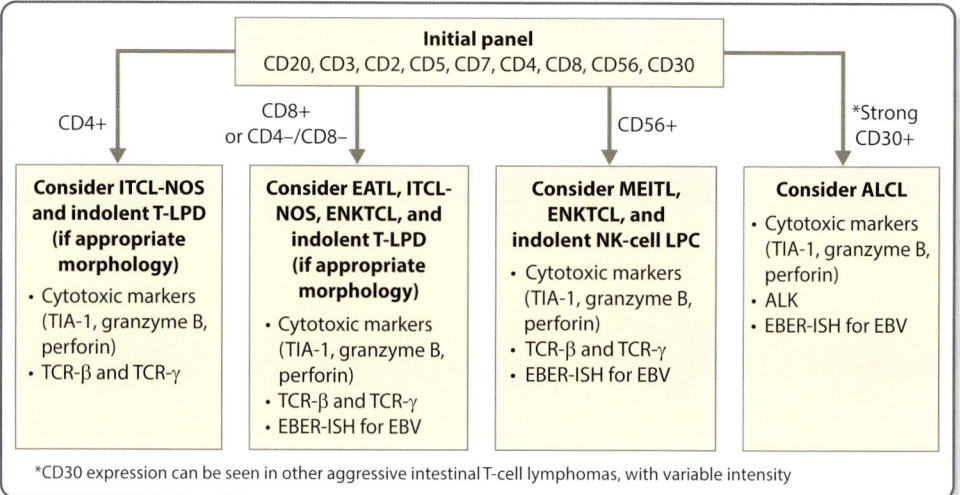

Figure 10.5 Immunohistochemical algorithm for diagnosis of gastrointestinal T- and NK-cell lymphomas.
EATL, enteropathy-associated T-cell lymphoma; ITCL, NOS, intestinal T-cell lymphoma, not otherwise specified; MEITL, monomorphic epitheliotropic intestinal T-cell lymphoma; T-LPD, T-cell lymphoproliferative disorder; TCR, T-cell receptor; EBER-ISH, epstein-barr encoding region

ENKTCL is by definition positive for EBV, while cases of indolent NK-cell LPD should be negative. Furthermore, indolent NK-cell LPD is a superficial lesion, involving usually mucosa and submucosa and not forming a mass, while ENKTCL is an aggressive neoplasm that usually presents as an ulcerated mass.

Immunohistochemical evaluation of T- and NK-cell lymphomas in the GI tract requires a large panel of immunohistochemical stains. Proposed algorithm for diagnosis is shown in **Figure 10.5**. Molecular studies for *TRB* and *TRG* gene rearrangements are typically not needed in cases for EATL, MEITL, and ITCL, NOS, since these lymphomas are morphologically frankly malignant. However, clonality should be performed in suspected cases of RCD, as well as in all cases of indolent T-cell LPD.

Key points for clinical practice

- Gastrointestinal (GI) tract is one of the most common extranodal sites involved by lymphoma.
- Majority if lymphomas in the GI tract are of B-cell lineage, while T- and NK-cell lymphomas comprise around 15% of all GI lymphomas.
- Diagnosis of T- and NK-cell lymphomas of the GI tract can be challenging especially on small endoscopic biopsies.
- Knowledge of clinical history and imaging data is very important for accurate diagnosis and proper classification.
- Enteropathy associated T-cell lymphoma (EATL) in the most common intestinal T-cell lymphoma in the western countries and occurs in people with coeliac disease.

- Intestinal mucosa adjacent to EATL frequently shows histologic features of coeliac disease, a very helpful clue.
- Monomorphic intestinal T-cell lymphoma (MEITL) is the second most common intestinal lymphoma, and is more prevalent in Asia.
- In cases of primary intestinal T-cell lymphomas that do not meet the morphologic and immunophenotypic criteria for EATL, MEITL, or other defined diagnostic entities, or when dealing with a limited biopsy, diagnosis of intestinal T-cell lymphoma, NOS might be appropriate.
- Two indolent LPDs of the GI tract include indolent clonal T-cell LPD and indolent NK-cell LPD.
- Main diagnostic pitfalls in indolent clonal T-LPD include misdiagnosis as benign/inflammatory condition or as more aggressive T-cell lymphoma.
- Indolent NK-cell LPD should be distinguished from extranodal NK/T-cell lymphoma, nasal type which is an aggressive, EBV-positive lymphoma.

REFERENCES

1. van Vliet C, Spagnolo DV. T- and NK-cell lymphoproliferative disorders of the gastrointestinal tract: review and update. Pathology 2020; 52:128–141.
2. Susan SH, Ng SB, Wang S, Tan SY. Diagnostic approach to T- and NK-cell lymphoproliferative disorders in the gastrointestinal tract. Semin Diagn Pathol 2021; 38:21–30.
3. Swerdlow SH CE, Harris NL, Jaffe ES, et al. WHO Classification of Tumours of Haematopoietic and Lymphoid Tissues. Lyon: IARC, 2017.
4. Wang M, Yu M, Kong WJ, Cui M, Gao F. Association between intestinal neoplasms and celiac disease: A review. World J Gastrointest Oncol. 2021; 13:1017–1028.
5. Soderquist CR, Bhagat G. Gastrointestinal T- and NK-cell lymphomas and indolent lymphoproliferative disorders. Semin Diagn Pathol 2020; 37:11–23.
6. Singh P, Arora A, Strand TA, et al. Global Prevalence of Celiac Disease: Systematic Review and Meta-analysis. Clin Gastroenterol Hepatol 2018; 16:823–836, e822.
7. Moffitt AB, Ondrejka SL, McKinney M, et al. Enteropathy-associated T cell lymphoma subtypes are characterized by loss of function of SETD2. J Exp Med 2017; 214:1371–1386.
8. Nicolae A, Xi L, Pham TH, et al. Mutations in the JAK/STAT and RAS signaling pathways are common in intestinal T-cell lymphomas. Leukemia 2016; 30:2245–2247.
9. Roberti A, Dobay MP, Bisig B, et al. Type II enteropathy-associated T-cell lymphoma features a unique genomic profile with highly recurrent SETD2 alterations. Nat Commun 2016; 7:12602.
10. Cording S, Lhermitte L, Malamut G, et al. Oncogenetic landscape of lymphomagenesis in coeliac disease. Gut 2022; 71:497–508.
11. Soderquist CR, Lewis SK, Gru AA, et al. Immunophenotypic Spectrum and Genomic Landscape of Refractory Celiac Disease Type II. Am J Surg Pathol 2021; 45:905–916.
12. Nishimura MF, Nishimura Y, Nishikori A, Yoshino T, Sato Y. Primary Gastrointestinal T-Cell Lymphoma and Indolent Lymphoproliferative Disorders: Practical Diagnostic and Treatment Approaches. Cancers 2021; 13:22.
13. Patey-Mariaud De Serre N, Cellier C, Jabri B, et al. Distinction between coeliac disease and refractory sprue: a simple immunohistochemical method. Histopathology 2000; 37:70–77.
14. van Wanrooij RL, Schreurs MW, Bouma G, et al. Accurate classification of RCD requires flow cytometry. Gut 2010; 59:1732.
15. Ettersperger J, Montcuquet N, Malamut G, et al. Interleukin-15-Dependent T-Cell-like Innate Intraepithelial Lymphocytes Develop in the Intestine and Transform into Lymphomas in Celiac Disease. Immunity 2016; 45:610–625.

16. Mutzbauer G, Maurus K, Buszello C, et al. SYK expression in monomorphic epitheliotropic intestinal T-cell lymphoma. Mod Pathol 2018; 31:505–516.
17. Veloza L, Cavalieri D, Missiaglia E, et al. Monomorphic epitheliotropic intestinal T-cell lymphoma comprises morphologic and genomic heterogeneity impacting outcome. Haematologica 2023; 108:181–195.
18. Nairismagi ML, Tan J, Lim JQ, et al. JAK-STAT and G-protein-coupled receptor signaling pathways are frequently altered in epitheliotropic intestinal T-cell lymphoma. Leukemia 2016; 30:1311–1319.
19. Campo E, Jaffe ES, Cook JR, et al. The International Consensus Classification of Mature Lymphoid Neoplasms: A Report from the Clinical Advisory Committee. Blood 2022; 140:1129–1153
20. Alaggio R, Amador C, Anagnostopoulos I, et al. The 5th edition of the World Health Organization Classification of Haematolymphoid Tumours: Lymphoid Neoplasms. Leukemia. 2022; 36:1720–1748.
21. Lee G, Ryu HJ, Choi JW, et al. Characteristic gene alterations in primary gastrointestinal T- and NK-cell lymphomas. Leukemia 2019; 33:1797–1832.
22. Perry AM, Warnke RA, Hu Q, et al. Indolent T-cell lymphoproliferative disease of the gastrointestinal tract. Blood 2013; 122:3599–3606.
23. Carbonnel F, Lavergne A, Messing B, et al. Extensive small intestinal T-cell lymphoma of low-grade malignancy associated with a new chromosomal translocation. Cancer 1994; 73:1286–1291.
24. Sharma A, Oishi N, Boddicker RL, et al. Recurrent STAT3-JAK2 fusions in indolent T-cell lymphoproliferative disorder of the gastrointestinal tract. Blood 2018; 131:2262–2266.
25. Sena Teixeira Mendes L, Attygalle AD, Cunningham D, et al. CD4-positive small T-cell lymphoma of the intestine presenting with severe bile-acid malabsorption: a supportive symptom control approach. Br J Haematol 2014; 167:265–269.
26. Edison N, Belhanes-Peled H, Eitan Y, et al. Indolent T-cell lymphoproliferative disease of the gastrointestinal tract after treatment with adalimumab in resistant Crohn's colitis. Hum Pathol 2016; 57:45–50.
27. Wang X, Ng CS, Chen C, Yu G, Yin W. An unusual case report of indolent T-cell lymphoproliferative disorder with aberrant CD20 expression involving the gastrointestinal tract and bone marrow. Diagn Pathol 2018; 13:82.
28. Montes-Moreno S, King RL, Oschlies I, et al. Update on lymphoproliferative disorders of the gastrointestinal tract: disease spectrum from indolent lymphoproliferations to aggressive lymphomas. Virchows Arch 2020; 476:667–681.
29. Mansoor A, Pittaluga S, Beck PL, et al. NK-cell enteropathy: a benign NK-cell lymphoproliferative disease mimicking intestinal lymphoma: clinicopathologic features and follow-up in a unique case series. Blood 2011; 117:1447–1452.
30. Matnani R, Ganapathi KA, Lewis SK, et al. Indolent T- and NK-cell lymphoproliferative disorders of the gastrointestinal tract: a review and update. Hematol Oncol 2017; 35:3–16.
31. Takeuchi K, Yokoyama M, Ishizawa S, et al. Lymphomatoid gastropathy: a distinct clinicopathologic entity of self-limited pseudomalignant NK-cell proliferation. Blood 2010; 116:5631–5637.
32. Vega F, Chang CC, Schwartz MR, et al. Atypical NK-cell proliferation of the gastrointestinal tract in a patient with antigliadin antibodies but not celiac disease. Am J Surg Pathol 2006; 30:539–544.
33. Koh J, Go H, Lee WA, Jeon YK. Benign Indolent CD56-Positive NK-Cell Lymphoproliferative Lesion Involving Gastrointestinal Tract in an Adolescent. Korean J Pathol 2014; 48:73–76.
34. Xiao W, Gupta GK, Yao J, et al. Recurrent somatic JAK3 mutations in NK-cell enteropathy. Blood 2019; 134:986–991.
35. Ud Din N, Rahim S, Ansar Z, Ahmed A, Ahmad Z. Anaplastic Large-cell Lymphoma Involving Gastrointestinal Tract: A Clinicopathologic Study of 25 Cases of a Rare Tumor at a Rare Site. Int J Surg Pathol 2022:10668969221137518.
36. Mishra P, Patra S, Srinivasan A, et al. Primary gastrointestinal anaplastic large cell lymphoma: A critical reappraisal with a systematic review of the world literature. J Cancer Res Ther 2021; 17:1307–1313.
37. Miike T, Kawakami H, Kameda T, et al. Clinical characteristics of adult T-cell leukemia/lymphoma infiltration in the gastrointestinal tract. BMC Gastroenterol 2020; 20:298.

38. Sakata H, Fujimoto K, Iwakiri R, et al. Gastric lesions in 76 patients with adult T-cell leukemia/lymphoma. Endoscopic evaluation. Cancer 1996; 78:396–402.

39. Li S, Feng X, Li T, et al. Extranodal NK/T-cell lymphoma, nasal type: a report of 73 cases at MD Anderson Cancer Center. Am J Surg Pathol 2013; 37:14–23.

40. Gualco G, Domeny-Duarte P, Chioato L, et al. Clinicopathologic and molecular features of 122 Brazilian cases of nodal and extranodal NK/T-cell lymphoma, nasal type, with EBV subtyping analysis. Am J Surg Pathol 2011; 35:1195–1203.

41. Tang XF, Yang L, Duan S, Guo H, Guo QN. Intestinal T-cell and NK/T-cell lymphomas: A clinicopathological study of 27 Chinese patients. Ann Diagn Pathol 2018; 37:107–117.

42. Yu BH, Shui RH, Sheng WQ, et al. Primary Intestinal Extranodal Natural Killer/T-Cell Lymphoma, Nasal Type: A Comprehensive Clinicopathological Analysis of 55 Cases. PLoS One 2016; 11:e0161831.

43. Jiang M, Chen X, Yi Z, et al. Prognostic characteristics of gastrointestinal tract NK/T-cell lymphoma: an analysis of 47 patients in China. J Clin Gastroenterol 2013; 47:e74–e79.

44. Au WY, Weisenburger DD, Intragumtornchai T, et al. Clinical differences between nasal and extranasal natural killer/T-cell lymphoma: a study of 136 cases from the International Peripheral T-Cell Lymphoma Project. Blood 2009; 113:3931–3937.

Index

Note: Page numbers in **bold** or *italic* refer to tables or figures respectively.